AF815050

Complementary & Alternative Medicine for Prostate and Urologic Health

Mark A. Moyad

Complementary & Alternative Medicine for Prostate and Urologic Health

Springer

Mark A. Moyad, M.D., M.P.H.
Department of Urology
University of Michigan Medical Center
Ann Arbor, MI, USA

ISBN 978-1-4614-8491-2 ISBN 978-1-4614-8492-9 (eBook)
DOI 10.1007/978-1-4614-8492-9
Springer New York Heidelberg Dordrecht London

Library of Congress Control Number: 2013946656

© Springer Science+Business Media New York 2014
This work is subject to copyright. All rights are reserved by the Publisher, whether the whole or part of the material is concerned, specifically the rights of translation, reprinting, reuse of illustrations, recitation, broadcasting, reproduction on microfilms or in any other physical way, and transmission or information storage and retrieval, electronic adaptation, computer software, or by similar or dissimilar methodology now known or hereafter developed. Exempted from this legal reservation are brief excerpts in connection with reviews or scholarly analysis or material supplied specifically for the purpose of being entered and executed on a computer system, for exclusive use by the purchaser of the work. Duplication of this publication or parts thereof is permitted only under the provisions of the Copyright Law of the Publisher's location, in its current version, and permission for use must always be obtained from Springer. Permissions for use may be obtained through RightsLink at the Copyright Clearance Center. Violations are liable to prosecution under the respective Copyright Law.
The use of general descriptive names, registered names, trademarks, service marks, etc. in this publication does not imply, even in the absence of a specific statement, that such names are exempt from the relevant protective laws and regulations and therefore free for general use.
While the advice and information in this book are believed to be true and accurate at the date of publication, neither the authors nor the editors nor the publisher can accept any legal responsibility for any errors or omissions that may be made. The publisher makes no warranty, express or implied, with respect to the material contained herein.

Printed on acid-free paper

Springer is part of Springer Science+Business Media (www.springer.com)

To Dr. David A. Bloom, the Chair of the University of Michigan Urology Department, where over a 30-year period, he has gone from being my advisor, mentor, friend, therapist, and currently my wonderful boss, and I will always be appreciative of his support, guidance, and ability to see the forest over the tree. This book is also dedicated to my father, Dr. Robert H. Moyad, the best urologist and father I have ever met; to Eva M. Moyad, the selfless spouse of a urologist and best mom; and to my wife, Mia, my best friend and best social worker I have and will ever meet (I know that is a lot of bests—what can I say but I am surrounded by the best).

Preface

Believe it or not, the completion of this book has always been close to the top of my so-called "bucket list" items. This might sound a bit overly profound or histrionic, but it is accurate. When I volunteered in the Urology Department at the University of Michigan at the age of 18 years and then published my first paper in urology and complementary and alternative medicine (CAM) while a student in college (age of 22), I still never envisioned a day where there would be enough material for a CAM book in urology. The dearth of overall attention to CAM and research was disappointing. Fast-forward several decades, initiating and completing some form of CAM research in urology departments around the world goes from rare to ubiquitous! What a pleasure it has been to watch healthcare professionals and patients in urology embrace some CAM options or even lifestyle changes that can profoundly impact their treatment, quality of life, and life expectancy. It has also been a pleasure for me to discourage the use of some CAM options for which no evidence-based merit exists and a potential for real harm is a reality.

It is important for all of us in the area of urology to remember almost every heart-healthy behavior that one can imagine is associated with a potential lower risk of urologic disease. And, most heart-unhealthy behaviors also contribute to a higher risk of diverse urologic diseases. Few medical specialties appear to have such a close correlation with cardiovascular health and risk compared to urology. And, it is this observation that we should never forget, because it allows all of us to visualize the forest as well as the tree, and "first do no harm" becomes a compassionate mantra and not just a cliché. It is an extraordinary and remarkable honor to empower patients with the ability to take control of their health or enhance the effects of their conventional treatment. This book is a symbolic testament and tribute to all those who have helped move CAM forward in my lifetime to the point where it has really become its own unique division or specialty within medicine and urology. Still there is much more work to do, and it is my hope this book inspires the young and the seasoned in urology to never stop appreciating the profound impact you have on your own health and that of others who cross your path for the rest of your life. I hope this book helps you in some tiny way to keep changing the world one starfish at a time.

All my best

Ann Arbor, MI, USA — Mark A. Moyad

Acknowledgments

I want to thank the individuals at Springer, Richard Hruska, and my editor, Diane Lamsback, for putting up with my lack of punctiliousness, but at least we made medical history with this book (first ever comprehensive CAM clinical guide book in urology—yes). Now, it all seems worth it after being married to a computer and thousands of medical references for the last 2 years (sorry, Mia, Nick, Holly, and Chauncey the dog…but at least daddy is home again, so to speak).

Contents

1 The Ideal Eight-Step Urologic Diet and Lifestyle Program: Heart Health = Urologic Health

Introduction

Before recommending the ideal urologic diet and lifestyle program, perhaps health concerns need to be triaged or probability based. Reviewing the most common causes of morbidity and mortality allows for an easier understanding of dietary changes that should be recommended for patients in general. These recommendations need to be simple, logical, and practical for the patient as well as the clinician. Thus, reviewing common causes of mortality is paramount to construing all other recommendations in this chapter.

Cardiovascular disease (CVD) is the number one overall cause of mortality in the USA and in other industrialized countries [1, 2]. Cardiovascular disease is currently the number one cause of death worldwide and is the number one cause of death in virtually every region of the world. Cancer is the second leading cause of death in the USA and in most developed countries and is expected potentially to mirror the number of deaths from CVD in the next several years in various regions of the world. Regardless, CVD has been the number one cause of death in the USA every single year for the last 100 years, with the exception of 1918, which was the year of the influenza pandemic.

If cancer becomes the primary cause of mortality, the majority of what is known concerning lifestyle and dietary change for CVD prevention directly appears to apply to cancer prevention [3]. Heart-healthy changes are tantamount to overall urologic health improvements regardless of the part of the human anatomy that is receiving attention, including the bladder, kidney, penis, or prostate. Heart-healthy changes need to be advocated in urology clinics because this places probability and the research into perspective. Triaging preventive medicine for urologic health is providing probability-based advice via evidence-based medicine.

The largest US and worldwide pharmaceutical-based urologic cancer primary prevention trials exemplify the urgent need for a more proper and balanced perspective. For example, results of the Prostate Cancer Prevention Trial (PCPT) seem to have garnered attention plus controversy regarding the use of finasteride daily versus placebo to reduce the risk of prostate cancer [4–6]. The discussion over the advantages and disadvantages of finasteride will continue, but one observation from this important trial has not received adequate exposure and debate in the medical literature. Over 18,000 men were included in this randomized trial, and 5 men died from prostate cancer in the finasteride and in the placebo arm, but 1,123 men in total died during this primary prevention trial [4]. Thus, prostate cancer was responsible for approximately less than 1 % of the deaths, while the majority of the overall causes of mortality deaths were from CVD and other non-prostate causes. Randomized trials tend to provide an accurate snapshot of day-to-day morbidity and mortality in this regard. This finding places the overall risk of morbidity and mortality in a more proper perspective. Men inquiring about the advantages and disadvantages

M.A. Moyad, *Complementary & Alternative Medicine for Prostate and Urologic Health*,
DOI 10.1007/978-1-4614-8492-9_1, © Springer Science+Business Media New York 2014

of finasteride or dutasteride for prostate cancer prevention need to be reminded that the number one risk to them in general is CVD. The consult about potential prostate cancer risk should occur after this first more relevant point is discussed, emphasized, reiterated, and in some cases even documented in the chart.

The largest urologic health dietary supplement clinical trial to prevent cancer was the selenium and vitamin E supplementation randomized trial (SELECT) [7]. It was terminated approximately 7 years early because of a lack of efficacy and even a potential negative impact with these supplements at these specific dosages. SELECT was the largest randomized primary prevention trial in urologic history, and once again CVD represented the primary cause of mortality overall in this study, with over 500 deaths occurring from this cause compared to the 1 death from prostate cancer in just 5 years follow-up. Heart-healthy programs simply need to receive more emphasis in urology.

The lifestyle recommendations proposed in this chapter essentially serve to impact CVD and urologic health simultaneously. Patients can now be offered lifestyle changes that can potentially impact all-cause morbidity and mortality rather than just disease-specific morbidity and mortality.

General Urologic Recommendation 1

Know and always try to improve on at least four parameters: fasting cholesterol level, blood pressure, glucose, and body mass index (BMI) and/or waist circumference (WC). The gastric bypass surgery data should be referenced in patient discussions to provide motivation for the benefits of weight or waist loss in individuals of all body types.

The lack of general health knowledge exhibited by some patients and even future healthcare professional is concerning. For example, surveys of the general population indicate that a majority of individuals do not know their cholesterol parameters or most risk factors for CVD, and this finding is consistent regardless of age, race, and even gender [8–11]. In my experience when the dual concern of CVD and overall urologic health is emphasized and promoted, patients tend to become familiar with all of their clinical values, numbers, and overall risks. It is of interest that at least in the USA the prevalence of CVD is still high. For example, almost 15 % of men and 10 % of women have CVD between the ages of 20 and 39, and that number increases to approximately 40 % from the ages of 40 to 59 years, over 70 % from 60 to79 years, and over 80 % from 80+ years of age [12]. These prevalence numbers are quite surprising for some patients, but again this places disease risk in perspective.

Patients should also be educated regularly on the normal values of a cholesterol panel because they are regularly updated by expert guideline groups, such as the National Cholesterol Education Program (NCEP) [13, 14]. For example, a man attending a free PSA (prostate-specific antigen) screening would appear to be at risk of ending up with a myopic health and disease perspective unless other screenings, such as blood pressure, cholesterol, weight, and/or glucose, were also proffered. Preliminary empirical evidence of this concern lies in recent data from the Surveillance, Epidemiology and End Results (SEER) tumor registry, which suggests that men diagnosed or treated for prostate cancer need to focus as much on cardiovascular prevention owing to the observed competing causes of mortality [15]. Patients simply need other resources, apart from overburdened primary care practitioners, to emphasize and review basic optimal lipid and general health values [13, 14]. Table 1.1 is a modified quick review for patients and urologic health professionals.

The NCEP suggests a first cholesterol screen at age 20 [13], which is approximately at least 20–30 years before a suggested PSA test or colonoscopy, but few, if any, individuals in my experience have had a lipid test at this early age. Clinicians can assist patients in adhering to this early screening age. For example, when men with a family history of prostate cancer or erectile dysfunction (ED) or an early diagnosis of most diseases inquire about what their children or other family members should do first to prevent this condition from happening to the next generation,

Table 1.1 A partial summary of the urologic health goals for patients in regard to total cholesterol, LDL, HDL, and triglycerides with some modifications that can be utilized in a clinical setting

Blood test parameter	Measurement commentary
Total cholesterol (mg/dL or mmol/L)	*A lower number is better*
<160 or <4.1	Optimal
160–200 or 4.14–5.16	Desirable
200–239 or 5.16–6.19	Borderline high
≥240 or ≥6.22	High
LDL = "bad cholesterol" (mg/dL or mmol/L)	*A lower number is better*
Less than 70 or <1.81	Optimal for some high-risk individuals[a]
Less than 100 or <2.59	Optimal
100–129 or 2.59–3.34	Near optimal
130–159 or 3.37–4.12	Borderline high
160–189 or 4.14–4.90	High
Equal to or greater than 190 or ≥4.92	Very high
HDL= "good cholesterol" (mg/dL or mmol/L)	*A higher number is better*
Less than 40 or <1.04	Low
40–59 or 1.04–1.53	Normal
Equal to or greater 60 or ≥1.55	High (optimal)
Triglyceride (mg/dL or mmol/L)	*A lower number is better*
Less than 150 or <1.70	Normal
150–199 or 1.70–2.25	Borderline high
200–499 or 2.26–5.64	High
Equal to or greater than 500 or ≥5.65	High

[a]Note: High-risk individuals (existing CVD disease or a previous CVD event) may be required to reduce their LDL below 70 mg/dL based on outcomes data provided to the expert panel

a common suggestion that I reiterate for children or adolescents is to just have an initial blood pressure, cholesterol, and glucose screening test and to maintain a healthy weight. In my experience, this tends to surprise and simplify patient concerns because this is an unexpected suggestion. The time is now more appropriate than ever for this approach because of the recent concern about abnormal lipid levels among adolescents screened in the USA, which is approximately 20–43 %, based on a variety of factors, especially weight status (normal, overweight, or obese) [16].

Other novel cardiovascular markers, such as high-sensitivity C-reactive protein (hs-CRP), or traditional ancillary markers, such as hemoglobin A1c, and evidence of subclinical atherosclerotic disease should also be discussed with the patient [3, 12, 17]. Even a referral to a cardiologist may be appropriate for some individuals, because some of these markers may also be related to overall mortality as well as CVD risk and some specific urologic health conditions [18].

Other tangible advantages may occur for the patient and clinician that continue to follow these overall cardiovascular markers. For example, cholesterol levels are an adequate indicator of how well a patient may be adopting lifestyle changes or even medication compliance following a PSA test, ED diagnosis, or after some definitive therapy. If these numbers improve, it may be more likely that the patient is following a urologic health lifestyle program. High-density lipoprotein (HDL) provides a good indicator of the commitment to aerobic exercise and is in a sense the "truth serum" as to how much physical activity has recently occurred. HDL tends to rise, at times substantially, with a greater amount of aerobic physical activity [19], and a higher HDL may be correlated with a lower risk of abnormal prostate conditions [20, 21]. Triglycerides are an indicator of changes in belly (visceral) fat, because this compound is generally stored in this anatomic location with increasing blood levels, and triglycerides have also been associated with some prostate conditions [22].

Blood pressure monitoring should also be emphasized as much as any other value. The Joint National Committee on Prevention, Detection, Evaluation, and Treatment of High Blood Pressure altered the criteria for what defines a healthy blood pressure [23]. Individuals and their partners should be informed that normal blood pressure is less than 120/80 mm Hg, and individuals with a systolic blood pressure of 120–139 mm Hg or diastolic blood pressure of 80–89 mm Hg are actually considered to be "prehypertensive"; lifestyle changes should be advocated in these individuals (Table 1.2) [23].

Blood pressure can be reduced with a healthier lifestyle [24]. This is a good indicator

Table 1.2 A partial summary of the blood pressure guidelines for urologic patients derived from the Joint National Committee on Prevention, Detection, Evaluation, and Treatment of High Blood Pressure

Blood pressure (systolic/diastolic)	What does this mean to patients?
Less than 120/80 mm Hg	Normal = low-risk
120–139/80–89 mm Hg	Prehypertensive (moderately high or pre-high blood pressure) = moderate risk
140/90 mm Hg or greater	Hypertensive (high blood pressure) = high risk

of lifestyle adherence or compliance, and a healthy blood pressure may also lower the risk of ED and benign prostatic hyperplasia (BPH) [25, 26]. Interestingly, one of the more subtle but prevalent etiologies of high blood pressure may be excessive alcohol consumption; this should be discussed with patients as much as sodium restriction [27]. Regardless of patients who adopt healthy lifestyle and behavioral changes should always be given encouragement to continue these changes because of the potentially profound impact these behaviors may have on overall and mental health [28, 29]. Due to the phenomenon of "white coat hypertension" it seems critical to encourage some patients to invest some money in an at-home blood pressure measurement device [30]. These devices have become cost-effective and potentially allow a more accurate assessment of the patient's blood pressure status compared to the one or two values derived annually, for example, from a medical office.

Fasting blood glucose is as important as any other parameter for your patients. Abnormally high blood glucose and diabetes are considered a high-risk cardiovascular correlation, such that these patients are treated as if they already have established cardiovascular disease in terms of lipid control, for example [13]. The association between higher blood glucose levels and urologic disease is also emerging and continues to accumulate data in multiple areas such as BPH and accelerated hypogonadism [31, 32]. The relationship between glucose intolerance and sexual dysfunction is already well established in men and women [33, 34]. Patients appear more motivated to continue healthy lifestyle changes when there is some tangible healthy outcome with the behavioral change, and this becomes more probable when all numbers are utilized in the consult, including cholesterol, blood pressure, and glucose, for example, as opposed to just other single and disease-specific (PSA, etc.) values.

The negative impact of being overweight or obese on overall morbidity and mortality is also well known. Body mass index is moderately reliable as an isolated anthropometric measurement, but at least it is a rapid method to determine who may be overweight or obese [35]. Body mass index is defined as the weight (in kilograms) divided by the square of the height in meters (kilograms per square meter squared). Another method to calculate the BMI is to take weight in pounds and divide it by the height in inches squared and to multiply this number by 704 (pounds/inches^2 × 704). A BMI <25 is considered normal by the World Health Organization (WHO), whereas 25–29 is overweight, ≥30 is defined as obese, and 35 or more is considered morbidly obese. Several of the largest and most recent preventive medicine randomized trials of men or women have demonstrated that most individuals in these studies are indeed overweight at baseline, and this includes trials to prevent specific health abnormalities with prescriptions, supplements, or just dietary change [4, 7, 36, 37]. Thus, it has become so common for participants of clinical trials to be overweight or obese that only a small percentage of individuals in these studies have a BMI in the healthy range.

Waist-to-hip ratio (WHR) may be another rapid measurement to determine obesity [35]. An individual must stand during the entire measurement of WHR. Waist-to-hip ratio more precisely measures abdominal adipose circumference or tissue and fat distribution. The waist is defined as the abdominal circumference midway between the costal margin and the iliac crest. The hip is defined as the largest circumference just below the iliac crest. However, it requires more time and detail, which is why waist circumference alone is perhaps the easiest and fastest method to currently assess obesity, and is my preference together with pant size (waist size). "Belly fat" (visceral adipose tissue) seems to have one of the best predictive values of CVD and potential all-cause mortality risk among all the other weight parameters from some of the largest prospective studies in the world [38–40]. However, the combination of WC with a BMI measurement may have added predictability. Still, WC is also one of the best predictors of heart-unhealthy changes and/or future cardiovascular events, regardless of the age group and ethnic group studied [41, 42].

Waist circumference is also one of the five specific criteria of the metabolic syndrome. Waist circumference has a tangible advantage over BMI, which can be appreciated after an individual commits to resistance exercise. An increase in muscle mass from resistance activities such as weight lifting can actually cause an increase in BMI, which could be frustrating to the patient and clinician [35]. However, this does not generally occur when utilizing the WHR or WC measurement. Informing patients of their official WC and asking pant size allow these parameters to be documented in the chart and allow the patient to identify a goal of maintaining or reducing these numbers by the time of the subsequent clinical visit; therefore, there is a reduced emphasis on just the weight scale or trying to compete with a national standard. A patient with a BMI of 35 and a WC of 40 in. is not as concerning as an individual with similar measurements and a lack of aerobic fitness and some modicum of caloric control, or not being able to reduce their WC value slightly over time is more of an issue. A summary of the basic interpretation of the BMI and WC value is found in Table 1.3 [35].

Kidney stones and renal cell carcinoma (RCC) may have a strong relationship with obesity [43–46]. Obesity is also associated with lower testosterone levels, higher estrogen levels, and a higher risk of CVD, which could partially explain the preliminary finding that obese men have a higher risk of ED [47–49], but recent novel clinical research suggests that an improvement in these parameters occurs rapidly with just a 10 % weight loss from dietary changes alone [50]. I often wonder how many men and healthcare professionals realize that before recommending exogenous testosterone prescriptions or supplements, patients should be made aware of the simple fact that weight loss can result in significant increases in testosterone.

Table 1.3 Body mass index (BMI) and waist circumference (WC) values for men's health discussions

	Classification
BMI number	
Less than 25	Normal weight
25–29	Overweight
30 or more	Obese
WC number	
Less than 35 in. (or 89 cm) in MEN	Normal
35–39 in. (or 89–100 cm) in MEN	Overweight
40 or more in. (101 or more cm) in MEN	Obese
Less than 32.5 in. (or 83 cm) in WOMEN	Normal
32.5–36 in. (or 83–93 cm) in WOMEN	Overweight
37 or more in. (94 or more cm) in WOMEN	Obese

Clinicians should begin to carry and utilize tape measures that can measure WC, and I often argue that this is as critical as the stethoscope. Clinicians should also refer patients on a consistent basis to ancillary diverse services such as nutritionists, therapists, social workers, a variety of professional and even surgical weight-loss programs, if needed, and recent consumer publications on weight loss. Simply becoming familiar with local weight-loss resources is an initial step in the appropriate direction for the patient and clinician. For example, inviting a medical director of a local weight-loss program to give grand rounds on the treatment plans they offer to the community demonstrates, in my opinion, commitment to this cause.

Another method that may provide positive teaching experience is to discuss or at least remind patients about the importance of a healthy weight by mentioning the gastric bypass or surgical weight-loss data. The intent is obviously not to advocate the use of gastric bypass or any type of surgery for every patient but to demonstrate how weight loss clearly and at times quickly impacts health. For example, researchers in the USA and Sweden found in separate studies that obese individuals who had gastric bypass surgery had a 30–40 % lower risk of dying 7–10 years after having the surgery compared to those that did not have the surgery [51–53]. The Swedish study was one of the longest studies ever published at that time of how this procedure impacts long-term health outcomes [52]. Researchers at the Goteborg University compared 4,047 individuals with a BMI of over 34, who received one of three types of surgery (banding, vertical-banded gastroplasty, or gastric bypass) or some dietary advice (control group). Some of the basic characteristics of these patients before the study started were the following:

- About 70 % of the patients were women, and about one-third of the women were postmenopausal.
- The average age was 46–48 years.
- Average weight was 262 pounds.
- Average BMI was 42.
- Average waist-to-hip ratio was about 1.
- Average waist circumference was about 49 in.
- Average cholesterol was 226 mg/dL, and HDL ("good cholesterol") was in the lower 40s.
- Average triglyceride was 197 mg/dL.

After 10.9 years, those that received surgery lost 14–25 % of their original weight compared to 2 % in the other group. Out of the 2,010 surgery patients, 101 died, and there were 129 deaths in the comparison group of 2,037 patients. There was a 29 % significant reduction ($p=0.01$) in the risk of dying from any cause in the surgery group. There were also lower risks of dying from cardiac disease and non-cardiovascular causes such as cancer. However, there was a higher rate of dying from infection (12 vs. 3 patients) and sudden death (20 vs. 14) in the surgery group. The most successful weight loss occurred in the gastric bypass group, where the average reduction in weight was about 30 % loss of their original weight. Interestingly, the risk reduction in disease and death was much larger in the older patients (about 25 %) compared to younger subjects (6 %).

In the US study (funded by a US government grant or branch of the National Institutes of Health), which was retrospective and not prospective, like the first study mentioned, researchers (University of Utah and other centers) looked at 7,925 severely obese individuals who had gastric bypass [51]. These patients were matched to 7,925 control individuals with identical weights and height. About 84 % of the patients were women, the average age was 39 years, and the average BMI was 45–47. After an average follow-up of 7 years, there were 213 deaths in the surgery group versus 321 deaths in the nonsurgical group. A total of 136 lives were saved per 10,000 gastric bypass surgeries after an average of 7.1 years following the actual procedure. The following interesting and significant results were found:

- Deaths from all causes were reduced ($p<0.001$) by 40 %.
- Deaths from diabetes were reduced ($p=0.005$) by 92 %.
- Deaths from cancer were reduced ($p<0.001$) by 60 %.
- Deaths from cardiovascular disease were reduced ($p<0.001$) by 50 %.
- Deaths from heart disease were reduced ($p=0.006$) by 56 %.

However, the surgery group had a 58 % significantly ($p=0.04$) higher risk of dying from accidents, suicides, and other causes not related to the diseases they were studying. None of the nondisease causes of death ("accident unrelated to death, poisoning of undetermined intent, suicide, and other nondisease causes") were significantly different but just higher, but as a combined group there was a significant difference. For example, 63 of the deaths out of 213 in the surgery group were from these causes (15 from suicide) compared to 17 of the 321 deaths in the control group. The researchers did mention that a large number of severely obese individuals have "unrecognized presurgical mood disorder or post-traumatic stress disorder or have been victims of childhood sexual abuse." Some bariatric surgery centers recommend that all patients have a psychological evaluation and if necessary some kind of treatment before surgery and some type of surveillance after surgery, but arguably this should probably be the normal way patients are handled after reading this study. This should be kept in mind when talking to any patient about surgery or another method for weight loss over time.

An examination of more recent surgical series should continue to impress the healthcare professional and patients. In the Swedish Obese Subjects (SOS) study, an ongoing review of outcomes from 25 public surgical departments and 480 primary health centers in Sweden, a total of 2,010 obese patients matched to controls found a 53 % reduction in the number of cardiovascular deaths ($p = 0.002$), and the total of first-time cardiovascular events were reduced by 33 % ($p < 0.001$) [54]. Gastric bypass and other surgical weight-loss randomized controlled data for obese type 2 diabetics from the Cleveland Clinic also continued to demonstrate the profound and immediate changes with weight loss [55]. A significant reduction in the utilization of medications to lower glucose, lipid, and blood pressure occurred within 12 months of their study on 150 patients, which in some cases occurred before the patients were discharged from the hospital! In a similar study from Italy the complete remission rates of type 2 diabetics approached 75–95 % within 2 years [56]. Again, the profound health changes in individuals that lose weight from surgery are an adequate teaching tool for patients to understand the devastating consequences of abnormal weight gain of any type on the human body. Adipose tissue is not inert and secretes a variety of compounds and other inflammatory signals to the rest of the body that essentially cause even innate immune responses to occur against self. In other words, I often tell patients that greater accumulation of adipose tissue is somewhat tantamount to an autoimmune condition.

General Urologic Recommendation 2

Approximately 30–60 min of physical activity a day or more on average should be the goal, which should include lifting weights/resistance exercises several times per week. Equal emphasis should be placed on aerobic and resistance exercise; one is not more important than the other.

Physical activity, defined as at least 180 min of vigorous exercise weekly, was associated with an approximate 70 % lower risk of aggressive prostate cancer, advanced disease, and a potential for improved survival in the Health Professionals Follow-up Study [57]. Over 47,000 men were included in this cohort, with a mean follow-up period of 14 years. Researchers appropriately concluded their publication by recommending at least 30 min a day of physical activity for all individuals due to the overall health benefits of this intervention. Smaller recent investigations have not been able to replicate these profound findings [58, 59], but a recent prospective study that followed men after diagnosis of prostate cancer found a significant reduced progression of their disease in men that were more active even in terms of just walking [60]. Also, a randomized trial demonstrated a significant improvement in continence rates after surgery for men engaged in more than just Kegel exercises but also light activity and a variety of pelvic core strengthening routines [61]. Overall the data are encouraging and strong enough to suggest prostate and renal cell cancer risk reduction with exercise, but the research on bladder and testicular cancer prevention is weak and does not suggest any correlation [62].

Regardless, the morbidity and mortality from CVD is impacted by exercise, but weight lifting also seems to provide additional benefits. For example, data derived from the Health Professionals Follow-up Study, which prospectively followed over 44,000 men for 12 years, found that men jogging for 1 h or more per week had a 42 % reduction ($p < 0.001$ for trend) in the risk of coronary heart disease (CHD) [63]. Men who just walked for 30 min or more per day or who were involved in other physical activities also experienced a risk reduction in CHD versus those who did not engage in these activities. Men performing regular resistance exercise (weight lifting) for just 30 min or more per week experienced a 23 % risk reduction ($p = 0.03$ for trend) in CHD. This was a novel finding because previous prospective studies had not adequately addressed this subject. Weight training can increase fat-free mass and lean body weight, reduce sarcopenia, increase resting metabolic rate, slightly increase testosterone levels, and potentially reduce the risk of abdominal adipose deposition [64, 65]. Weight training or resistance training also appears to improve glucose parameters, including insulin sensitivity, and may slightly improve lipid levels and reduce hypertension [65, 66], which are all potential risk factors for ED and other men's health conditions. Physical activity may also dramatically reduce the impact of sympathetic overload that may be one of the many earliest damaging etiologies of BPH [67]. One of the best past reviews on physical activity and cardiovascular disease found ample evidence for exercise to favorably impact markers of heart disease, including triglycerides, apolipoprotein B reduction, HDL, low-density lipoprotein (LDL) particle size, and a reduction in coronary calcium [68]. Thus, aerobic and resistance activity need to be emphasized equally because of the documented synergism.

The mental health improvements with increased exercise appear to be just as notable as the physical health benefits [69, 70]. For example, one often-referenced trial published over a decade ago included 156 adult volunteers with major depressive disorder (MDD) randomly assigned a 4-month course of aerobic exercise (30 min 3 times/week), sertraline therapy, or a combination of exercise and sertraline [71, 72]. After 4 months patients in all three groups demonstrated significant mental health improvements; however, after 10 months, individuals in the exercise group had significantly lower recurrence rates compared to individuals in the medication group of the study. Exercising during the follow-up period was associated with a 51 % reduction in the risk of a diagnosis of depression at the end of the investigation. Even recent randomized studies of patients with significant comorbidities such as heart failure have significant improvements in physical and mental health with regular exercise [73]. It is important to explain to patients that if the overall results from exercise studies were viewed similar to a specific pharmacologic intervention, then it probably would have already garnered attention worthy of a Nobel Prize in arguably multiple categories of medicine. Also, the ability of exercise to work synergistically with medication is also notable.

Still, despite the plethora of positive research, are healthcare professionals excited about recommending exercise to their patients? The National Health Interview Survey (NHIS) data are recorded throughout the year from the Centers for Disease Control and Prevention (CDC) National Center for Health Statistics (NCHS) by interviewers from the US Census Bureau [74]. It is a household-derived survey, and interviews are usually conducted in the respondent's homes. Questions were asked in 2000, 2005, and 2010, with over 20,000 in each of these years sampled that visited with a physician or other healthcare professional within the past 12 months. In the most recent year of data gathering, which was 2010, about 32 % of adults who had visited with a physician or other healthcare professional had been recommended to begin or continue exercise or some form of physical activity. Between the years of 2000 and 2010, the percentage of adults given exercise advice increased by approximately 10 %, and women were more likely than men to have been advised to exercise, and one-third of patients with cancer were also recommended exercise. Thus, only one in three adults who had seen a physician or healthcare professional in the past 12 months had been told to begin or continue exercise/physical activity. You have the ability to improve these numbers everyday in your practice, and I would encourage you to take advantage of this situation.

General Urologic Recommendation 3

Reduce unhealthy dietary fat intake and increase the consumption of healthy fats, which should simultaneously lower overall caloric intake.

The NCEP recommends that saturated fat be reduced to less than 7 % of total calories to reduce the risk of CVD [13]. In my opinion, this is simply an indirect method to achieve partial caloric reduction [75]. Many foods that contain high levels of saturated fat also contain the highest levels of trans fat ("partially hydrogenated fat"), cholesterol, and, more importantly, total calories. For example, there are almost twice as many calories in 8 oz of whole milk (5 g of saturated fat) compared to skim or soymilk (0 g of saturated fat each), and there are almost four times as many calories in whole milk compared to almond milk. Thus, identifying two similar products, such as milk, meats, dairy, chips, and so forth, and

Table 1.4 Types of dietary fat, some of their primary sources, and the impact on lipid levels and heart health

Type of dietary fat	Commonly found?	Good or bad fat and impacts on lipids versus carbohydrates (sugars)
Monounsaturated fat (includes omega-9)	Health cooking oils (canola, olive, safflower, etc.), nuts, etc.	Good Lowers LDL Increases HDL
Polyunsaturated fat (includes omega-3 fatty acids)	Healthy cooking oils (canola, soybean, etc.), flaxseed, fish, nuts, soybeans, etc.	Good Lowers LDL Increases HDL
Saturated fat (known also as hydrogenated fat)	Non-lean meat, high-fat dairy, some fast food, etc.	Mostly bad (because it is associated with high caloric intake) Increases LDL Increases HDL
Trans fat (also known as partially hydrogenated fat)	Some margarine, fast food, snack foods, deep fried foods, etc.	Bad Increases LDL Lowers HDL

choosing the item lower in saturated fat in general allows for a profound (at times) reduction in total caloric intake, which is critical to helping maintain or reach an appropriate weight or waist size and improving overall heart health.

Yet, simply reducing all saturated fat in an individual's diet is not necessarily a practical and healthy dietary lifestyle change, because some saturated fats in the diet may promote healthy parameters. The current cardiovascular goal of obtaining less than 7 % of calories from saturated fat seems almost ideal from past studies, because getting minimal to no calories from saturated fat not only is too excessive; it actually appears to reduce levels of HDL ("good cholesterol") from past CVD and other health-promoting clinical trials [76, 77]. Aggressively reducing saturated fat consumption also implies that this type of fat, in and of itself, is heart unhealthy, which is not accurate from the largest recent meta-analysis of prospective studies [78]. And, in some countries around the world where overall caloric intake is very low compared to the USA, saturated fat may have some tangible cardiovascular benefits, but this also needs to be placed in perspective [79]. For example, in some regions of the world, such as Japan, a closer look at healthy individuals with the largest intakes of saturated fat would actually lead to their being placed in the lowest category of saturated fat intake in the USA, if they were to immediately migrate to the USA [79]. Regardless, a potential impact of reducing saturated fat, in my opinion, is that it may reduce overall caloric intake and reduce weight and waist gains. Another benefit of reducing saturated fat is that it allows for the opportunity to reduce dietary cholesterol intake and increase the consumption of other monounsaturated and polyunsaturated fats that have shown a greater reduction in CVD from past clinical trials and epidemiologic research [80, 81]. If the patient has normal weight, exercise, and other heart-healthy parameters, then the concern over saturated fat intake should not be as acute, because caloric restriction or caloric control in some form by these individuals is not as beneficial. A summary of the different types of dietary fat, food sources, and impacts on specific lipids is found in Table 1.4 [75].

General Urologic Recommendation 4

Consume a diversity of low-cost fruits and especially vegetables and do not consume high-calorie, high-cost, and high-antioxidant exotic or even traditional fruit juices (unless there is a low-calorie option).

Media attention and research appear to focus on one fruit or vegetable with each passing year. Clinicians need to be able to remain somewhat objective and explain to patients that these media reports do not necessarily represent any major research breakthrough but rather support the ongoing and past research that consuming a diversity of low-cost fruits and especially vegetables is just one practical and logical approach to improving urologic health. Several examples of this controversy exist, including the past attention focused on the compound lycopene in tomatoes in preventing prostate and other cancers based on numerous epidemiologic studies and a notable meta-analysis [82]. However, this meta-analysis concluded by reminding readers that this is just further evidence that a diversity of fruits and vegetables was important for a healthy diet, but this appeared to be misconstrued. Tomatoes were never the only or necessarily the primary source of lycopene. A variety of other healthy products contain this compound, such as apricots, guava, and pink grapefruit [83–86]. Watermelon is also an outstanding source of lycopene and is the largest source per gram compared to any other nutritional source, including tomato products. Regardless, lycopene has minimal overall beneficial data in and of itself to solve various urologic issues, but at least the compound and products that contain this compound are generally safe or even heart healthy [87–89].

The ongoing pomegranate juice and supplement research has experienced a somewhat similar story, but with a slightly different message for clinicians. The first attention-gathering study did not include a placebo group or another group of men that consumed another type of healthy juice product [90], and other studies in urology have questionable methodology and results [91]. Yet, this should not be construed as a lack of efficacy, and some of these companies should be lauded for at least investing in research, but an objective overview of the preliminary research and the caloric contribution of these and other juices is necessary. Many brands of these novel juices contain at least 140 cal per 8-oz serving, which is a caloric contribution similar to commercial regular soft drinks and alcoholic drinks (approximately 100–150 cal) [75]. In partial defense of some of these companies, it is also laudable that some lower-calorie exotic juice options from these same manufacturers are now becoming commercially available. Still, many of these juices are expensive in comparison to cheaper nutritious and lower-calorie products. Additionally, drug and juice interactions are still being researched, which is important because grapefruit juice studies have provided a paradigm of medication interactions [92], but novel juices such as pomegranate may also cause some potential concern with medications metabolized by CYP3A4 [93, 94]. In reality, if a patient believes in pomegranate juice or another product I often recommend a lower-calorie or a no-calorie option and utilize weight and other heart-healthy changes as the primary driving force of whether or not to continue or advocate for or against this patient-driven regimen.

Fruits, and especially vegetables, in general have been associated with a reduced risk of some urologic conditions in past studies [95]. For example, the *Brassica* vegetable group is diverse and includes broccoli, brussels sprouts, cabbage, cauliflower, kale, watercress, and others and may slightly reduce the risk of urologic disease [96]. It is interesting that these products are very low in overall calories. The *Allium* vegetables have also been associated with a reduced risk, and this group includes chives, garlic, leeks, onions, and scallions [97]. Fruits and vegetables have unique and shared anticancer and anti-heart disease compounds that may contribute to improved overall health [95]. The sum of the epidemiologic data continues to support the increased consumption of a diversity of fruits and vegetables to potentially and favorably impact urologic health, but the overall data currently support a slightly greater potential reduction in CVD risk and mortality [98], perhaps through assisting in weight loss or via other heart-healthy compound(s) such as natural salicylates (i.e., aspirin derivatives) or other natural compounds in these products [99]. Clinicians should recommend fruit and vegetable consumption for better overall health, but not for cancer prevention, where the recent large-scale data appear to be less impressive [100, 101]. There are also certain high-risk factors for urologic disease such as bladder cancer and smoking that simply cannot be fully eliminated or erased by improving other aspects of lifestyle, such as increased fruit and vegetable consumption [102]. In other words, triaging lifestyle changes or recommendations from most to least important is critical to a patient's success.

General Urologic Recommendation 5

Consume more (soluble and insoluble) dietary fiber (20–30 g/day or 14 g/1,000 cal consumed), especially from food sources.

General and numerous health benefits derived from consuming dietary fiber have been well documented and include reductions in the following [103–106]:

- Coronary heart disease (CHD) risk
- Stroke
- High blood pressure
- Diabetes
- Obesity

For example, a pooled analysis of past cohort studies of dietary fiber for the reduction of CHD included research from ten international studies and included the USA [107]. Over a period of 6–10 years of follow-up, and after multivariate adjustment, it was revealed that each 10 g/day increase of calorie-adjusted total dietary fiber was correlated with a 14 % reduction in the risk of total coronary events and a 27 % reduction in risk of coronary death. These findings were similar for both genders, and the inverse associations occurred for both soluble ("viscous") and insoluble fiber. Past studies have not observed a consistent benefit with one class of fiber over the other [108, 109]. Recent large US and other international studies have found even more striking overall potential benefits for consuming more dietary fiber. For example, the NIH-AARP US prospective cohort found not only a lower risk of dying from cardiovascular, respiratory, and infectious disease with greater intakes of fiber but a significantly lower risk of dying younger ("total death") in men and women [110]. This study may represent a major shift into the research behind fiber intake because now the potential health impact may be so much larger than first realized, because reductions in the death rates of some of the largest causes of mortality may occur with greater fiber intakes [110, 111].

Even minor additions of fiber can positively impact medication dosages. A total of 15 g of psyllium husk supplementation daily with a 10-mg statin (simvastatin) was demonstrated to be as effective as 20 mg of this statin by itself in reducing cholesterol in a preliminary placebo-controlled study of 68 patients over 12 weeks [112]. Although adding soluble fiber from commercial products appears to be safe and synergistic with cholesterol-lowering medications [113], the first choice for increasing fiber intake should be food sources based on cost-effectiveness and simplicity.

A meta-analysis of 24 randomized placebo-controlled trials of fiber supplementation found a consistent impact on blood pressure reduction [114]. Supplementation with a mean dose of only 11.5 g/day of fiber reduced systolic blood pressure by −1.13 mm Hg and diastolic pressure by −1.26 mm Hg. The reductions were actually greater in older and more hypertensive individuals compared to younger and normotensive participants. Recent international studies continue to support the modest reduction or control in blood pressure with greater intakes of dietary fiber [115].

How much fiber should patients be consuming daily? Daily intakes of total fiber in the USA and many other Western countries is approximately 10–15 g/day, which is approximately only half or even less than half of the total amount consistently recommended by the American Heart Association (AHA) and American Dietetic Association (20–30 g/day) for adequate overall health [105, 106, 116]. Another perspective on recommended fiber intake for children and adults is that for every 1,000 cal of food and beverage consumed, there should be at least 14 g of fiber consumed.

Dietary fiber from food is easily achieved by low-cost sources of soluble and insoluble fiber. For example, I often tell patients to just consume a third of a cup of a bran cereal, which is approximately only the size of one to two liquor shot glasses, with flaxseed and some fruit, and before they leave the door in the morning, approximately 20 g of fiber will have already been ingested toward the 25–30-g goal [75]! Low-cost fiber sources such as flaxseed can provide potentially numerous heart-healthy and urologic-healthy benefits and outcomes [117–122]. Interestingly, the preliminary clinical data for flaxseed and urologic health including symptoms of BPH and prostate cancer molecular changes are arguably as strong as any other nutritional item ever tested in urology, especially when considering the benefit-to-risk ratio. Perhaps the low-cost and non-commercialization of this product on a large scale has led to the lack of adequate education that I have observed on this product. Flaxseed is also one of the highest plant sources of heart-healthy omega-3 fatty acids [118], and chia seed is arguably the largest plant source of fiber and omega-3 [123]. Both of these additions to the male health diet would be ideal.

Yet fiber itself appears to have become overtly commercialized, and in my experience, some patients are turning primarily toward powders and pills to solve their fiber deficit; this is not only costly but also provides primarily small amounts of primarily soluble fiber that make it difficult to reach their total fiber goal utilizing only these sources. For example, I often ask audiences and students how many fiber capsules/pills are needed to be consumed daily to obtain just 20–30 g of fiber, and the answer always seems to provide adequate surprising value (the answer is 30–40 capsules/pills a day or more depending on the commercial source) [75]! A bolus of only soluble fiber without insoluble fiber can also create excessive bloating and other gastrointestinal issues because soluble fiber can be utilized and metabolized extensively by gut flora. Research continues to support the overall and heart-healthy benefits of fiber, especially when it is primarily derived from food sources [105], because these sources also provide a unique and optimal balance of soluble and insoluble fiber.

General Urologic Recommendation 6

Consume moderate (approximately two servings or more) weekly intakes of a variety of healthy fatty fish, but fried and high mercury concentrated fish should be generally discouraged. Other healthy plant-based sources of omega-3 fatty acids (e.g., nuts and healthy plant cooking oils) should also be equally emphasized.

Numerous types of oily fatty fish contain high concentrations of marine-based omega-3 fatty acids (compounds known as "EPA" and "DHA"). Fish are also the best natural food source of vitamin D_3 (cholecalciferol), and they contain high concentrations of high-quality protein and a diversity of minerals [75]. Omega-3 fatty acids from food sources have exhibited numerous benefits in terms of reducing the risk of a variety of prevalent chronic diseases [124, 125], especially some aspects of cardiovascular disease [126–132].

A variety of healthy fatty/oily fish contain high levels of omega-3 fatty acids, vitamin D, and protein, including salmon, tuna, sardines, anchovies, whitefish. Other baked, broiled, raw, but not fried, fish are potentially beneficial [75]. Diversity should be encouraged to increase compliance and exposure to a range of nutrients. The benefit of fish consumption to reduce the risk of certain urologic diseases is preliminary [133, 134], but a fairly recent meta-analysis suggested that the sum of the evidence actually suggests a greater reduction in prostate-cancer mortality compared to morbidity [135]. There is also growing evidence for an ability of omega-3 from fish to reduce the risk of kidney stones [136, 137].

The true clinical impact of mercury from fish on adult individuals remains controversial [138, 139], and it is possible that mercury may reduce some of the benefits of fish consumption [140]. Four types of larger predatory fish have been most concerning (king mackerel, shark, swordfish, and tilefish), because they have the ability to concentrate larger amounts of methylmercury over their longer life spans. However, moderate and recommended consumption (two to three times per week) of most fish should have minimal impact on human mercury serum levels. A large investigation of moderate mercury serum levels in older individuals found little to no negative long-term impacts on neurobehavioral parameters [141]. A randomized trial of mercury exposure from dental amalgam in children also found no significant health issues [142]. The positive impact of consuming fish appears to outweigh the negative impact in the majority of individuals with the exception of women considering pregnancy or who are pregnant. One of the largest US cohorts to recently evaluate this issue found lower cardiovascular disease risk in adult men and women consuming higher amounts of fish regardless of mercury exposure (benefit > risk) [143]. Interestingly, low-cost and low-mercury fish such as anchovies and sardines have some of the highest concentrations of omega-3 oils that are used in omega-3 fatty acid clinical trials utilizing dietary supplements for heart disease and cancer [75]. It should also be kept in mind that the AHA recommends about two servings of fish per week and plant omega-3 consumption [144], which I try to reiterate often to urologic patients. Thus, the healthiest sources of omega-3 compounds in food are coincidentally very low in mercury. Fish-oil supplements for completely healthy individuals or for chronic disease prevention do not have data, and the use of fish oil to prevent heart disease in a primary or secondary prevention setting has mixed results because of potential subgroup benefit or harm [145–148].

Tree nuts share some similar clinical positive impacts of marine omega-3 oils. A consistent reduction in the risk of CHD and/or sudden cardiac death has been associated with an increased consumption of a diversity of nuts in prospective studies, and they can also reduce inflammatory markers that impact a variety of organ systems [149–154]. Nuts contain a variety of potential beneficial compounds, such as ALA (the primary plant-based omega-3 fatty acid), other polyunsaturated fats, monounsaturated fats, vitamin E, magnesium, potassium, fiber, and flavonoids [75]. Nut consumption via an improvement in heart health may also improve urologic health and even erectile health [155]. However, the primary limitation of tree nuts is their high caloric content when going beyond several servings a day. Healthy plant oils utilized for cooking such as soybean, canola, olive oil, safflower, and so forth also contain a high concentration of omega-3 fatty acids, monounsaturated fat, and numerous other vitamins and minerals such as natural vitamin E [75]. Most cooking oils contain 120 cal per tablespoon; therefore, moderation again is the cornerstone to good health and nutrition.

General Urologic Recommendation 7

Educate patients on the first six heart-healthy lifestyle changes, because only 1–2 % of individuals are able to follow these on a regular basis. It is the sum of what is accomplished in moderation that has the highest probability of impacting urologic health compared to just one or several lifestyle changes in extreme (similar to cardiovascular disease prevention). Add other parameters as personally needed and triaged (tobacco cessation, sodium reduction, alcohol in moderation, pill reduction or addition, etc.).

If multiple lifestyle changes or if achieving numerous healthy parameters over time appears to be associated with the largest improvements in health, then this theory should be tested. It has been tested over the years, and the results are profound. For example, data from the National Health and Nutrition Examination Survey (NHANES) was utilized that included 44,959 US adults 20 years of age or older [156]. Mean age was 46–47 years, and approximately half of the participants were women. Median follow-up was 14.5 years. A total of only 1–2 % of the participants met all seven of the health parameters. Amazingly, there was a 51 % reduction in all-cause mortality, 76 % reduction in cardiovascular mortality, and 70 % reduction in ischemic heart disease (IHD) mortality for participants meeting six or more metrics compared to one or fewer. Achieving a higher number of cardiovascular health parameters also appeared to be correlated with a lower risk for all-cancer mortality. The following seven goals/parameters were utilized in this study:

- Avoiding all tobacco products
- Being physically active almost every day of the week
- BMI 25 or less
- Overall diet that is heart healthy (fruits, veggies, fiber, fish, etc.)
- Total cholesterol equal to or less than 200 mg/dL
- Blood pressure equal to or less than 120/80 mm Hg
- Fasting blood glucose less than 100 mg/dL

Another classic example of the benefit of just following one or two of the above healthy lifestyle parameters is derived from the Nurses' Health Study, which reviewed 24 years of follow-up data in 116,564 women who were 30–55 years old in the 1970s and were healthy and not diagnosed with cancer or cardiovascular disease [157].

Table 1.5 US Mediterranean diet study—individuals with scores of 6 or more on the checklist had a lower risk of early mortality compared to those with scores of 4 or less[a]

Beverage or food	Answer yes or no (1 point for each question answered "yes" and 0 points for a "no")
Alcohol: 2 drinks a day or fewer for men and 1 drink or fewer for women	
Fat intake focused on healthy fats, mostly monounsaturated and polyunsaturated (canola, olive, safflower oil, etc.)	
Fish: at least 2 or more servings per week	
Fruit: 4 or more servings a day	
Legumes/beans: 2 or more servings a week	
Meat: 1 or fewer servings a day	
Nuts and seeds: 2 or more servings a week	
Vegetables (other than potatoes): 4 or more servings a day	
Whole grains (e.g., whole/multigrain and whole wheat foods with high amount of fiber and protein): 2 or more servings a day	
Total score	

Just review the checklist, and add up the points
[a]Note: Traditional Mediterranean diets also allow moderate intakes of dairy, such as cheese, milk, and yogurt

During the 24 years of study, a total of 10,282 deaths occurred mostly from cancer (5,223 deaths) and cardiac disease (2,370), but 2,689 deaths occurred from other causes. Regardless of whether the researchers looked at dying from any cause, an interesting trend occurred when multivariate relative risks were utilized. Women who were of normal weight and exercised about 30 min a day had the lowest risk of dying of any cause compared to any other type of woman in this cohort. However, the researchers also found that thin women that hardly exercised had a greater chance of dying of any cause compared to thin women that exercised regularly. Obese women that rarely exercised had the highest chance of dying early, but the researchers also found that obese women (of the same general weight) that exercised about 30 min a day had a lower risk of dying from any cause compared to the obese women that rarely exercised! Thus, the greatest probability of living longer can be found in normal-weight individuals who exercise 30 min daily or more and follow other healthy lifestyle parameters, but even if an individual is overweight or obese and exercises, it still counts as an investment in long-term health. Interestingly, these same data and results can easily be derived from notable male cohort studies [158, 159].

Other past general health comprehensive lifestyle studies have demonstrated that few (less than 5 %) individuals have reported adhering to numerous moderate healthy behaviors at one time [160]. Again, the collective sum of what is accomplished, rather than one or two specific behavioral changes, has the largest impact on cardiovascular markers, CVD, cancer, and all-cause mortality [161]. Thus, I often use checklists derived and modified from the Mediterranean diet US study [162], the INTERHEART study, and other lifestyle studies to ensure verve and compliance in patients [75, 163–167]. These studies essentially found that regardless of race, age, genetics, and geographic location, the ability to essentially maintain numerous consistent features of lifestyle and/or diet was associated with an 85–95 % reduced risk of a cardiovascular event, and similar behaviors and changes in other recent studies demonstrated an improved ability to live far beyond average life expectancy with minimal mental or physical morbidity. The critical primary characteristics in these individuals included behavioral changes, with no benefit or detriment derived from a dietary supplement.

Table 1.5 is a modified, often utilized handout or checklist that I created and provide to individuals seeking to increase their odds or probability of living longer and better through dietary changes adapted from a Mediterranean diet [75]. How many patients or even colleagues have all of these features or need to work on these changes? How many urologic health conditions could be prevented or improved with these heart-healthy changes?

Applying comprehensive heart-healthy lifestyle data to determine its true objective efficacy in urologic health may not appear to be simple, but in reality it is not difficult. When discussed with patients, the observations from this research are quite profound throughout urology. For example, a unique 2-year randomized trial from Italy of vigorous aerobic exercise and diet to improve ED should have received more clinical attention [168, 169]. It still should change the way healthcare professionals treat men with ED. A total of 110 obese men (BMI of 36–37 = morbidly obese) with ED, WHR of 1.01–1.02, age 43 years, ED score of 13–14 out of 25 (IIEF), and without diabetes, high cholesterol, or hypertension were included in this trial. A total of 55 men were included in an aggressive intervention group that involved caloric restriction and increased physical activity via personalized dietary counseling (Mediterranean-style diet) and regular appointments with a personal trainer. Another group of 55 men were in the control group and were given general educational information about exercise and healthy food choices. After 2 years, the BMI significantly decreased on average from 36.9 to 31.2 in the intervention group, and serum levels of interleukin-6 and C-reactive protein (higher levels are potential indicators of more vascular inflammation) also decreased significantly. The average physical activity level increased significantly from 48 min per week to 195 min per week in the intervention group, and the mean erectile function score increased significantly from 13.9 to 17. A total of 17 men in the intervention group actually reported an erectile function score of 22 or higher (normal function). Several changes were independently and significantly associated with a higher rate of improved erections, including a lower BMI or BMI reduction, increased physical activity, and a lower C-reactive protein levels. Approximately 33 % of the men in this study with ED regained normal erectile function after 2 years of following healthy behaviors, primarily from exercise, weight reduction, caloric control, and healthy dietary changes. A major limitation of this trial was the lack of analysis of psychological factors and social intervention. However, because these lifestyle changes could have improved mood and self-esteem and reduced depression, this could have also been a reason for improved erectile function. Still, the combined healthy changes in the intervention group that occurred after 2 years were notable and diverse and included the following:

- Total caloric reduction of −390 cal/day (2,340–1,950).
- Complex carbohydrate increase and simple sugar reduction.
- Fiber consumption increased by 10 g/day (15–25).
- Protein consumption increase.
- No change in the overall percentage of fat in the diet (30 % of calories), but a reduction in saturated fat (14–9 %) and an increased intake in monounsaturated fat (9–14 %).
- Ratios of omega-6 to omega-3 fatty acids were reduced by half (12–6).
- Cholesterol was reduced from dietary sources by 84 mg/day (360–276).
- Exercise time (mainly walking) increased from about 7 min/day to almost 30 min/day.
- Average weight loss was 33 pounds (226.6–193.6).
- Average BMI decreased by almost 6 points (36.9–31.2).
- WHR decreased by 0.09 (1.02–0.93).
- Erectile function scores increased by 3 points (13.9–17 points).
- Systolic (127–124 mm Hg) and diastolic (86–82 mm Hg) blood pressure decreased by 3–4 points.
- Total cholesterol decreased by 11 mg/dL (213–202), but HDL (good cholesterol) increased by 9 points (39–48 mg/dL).
- Triglycerides decreased by 19 mg/dL (169–150).
- Glucose decreased by 8 mg/dL (103–95), and insulin level also decreased by 7 points (21–14 μU/ml).
- C-reactive protein (CRP) was reduced by 1.4 mg/L (3.3–1.9).
- Interleukin 6 was reduced by 1.4 pg/mL (4.5–3.1).
- Interleukin-8 (IL-8, another inflammatory marker) was reduced by 1.2 pg/mL (5.3–4.1).

Of course, other lifestyle modifications, including tobacco cessation, should be considered to reduce all-cause mortality, including cancer [170, 171], and potentially to reduce the risk of specific urologic health conditions [172–174]. Urologic healthcare professionals have an opportunity to improve tobacco cessation rates, especially when dealing with a newly diagnosed urologic cancer patient [175]. Many urologic health professionals find themselves at critical moments in a patient's care that could determine the future adherence to life-changing lifestyle changes.

Moderate alcohol consumption, regardless of the source, also seems to reduce cardiovascular events [175, 176]. However, alcohol follows a U-shaped curve, which is why when consumed in excess, the detriments of alcohol outweigh the benefits. Sodium intake also follows a U-shaped curve. However, arguably one of the best clinical trials that could have an educational role in urology concerning sodium consumption was from the Dietary Approaches to Stop Hypertension (DASH) diet study [177–180]. Basically, the DASH study was organized and financed by the National Heart, Lung, and Blood Institute (NHLBI) to look at the effects of overall dietary changes on blood pressure and then sodium restriction in addition to these dietary changes. The DASH study involved 459 adults age 22 years or older with a systolic blood pressure lower than 160 mm Hg and a diastolic blood pressure 80–95 mm Hg, which is considered prehypertension or stage 1 hypertension. None of these individuals were taking blood pressure medications. Approximately 50 % of the individuals were women, and 60 % were African Americans, and the participants were assigned to one of three groups over an 8-week period:

1. A control or moderate diet similar to a normal American diet, but lower in calcium, magnesium, and potassium intake.
2. Similar to the control diet but more fruits and vegetables.
3. A DASH diet, which included fruits and vegetables, low-fat dairy, whole grains, chicken, fish, and nuts and was low in fats, low in red meat, low in sweets, and low in beverages that are high in sugar.

Thus, the DASH diet is high in calcium, magnesium, potassium, and fiber, but low in saturated fat, low in trans fat, and low in cholesterol. All three diets contained the same amount of sodium or salt at 3,000 mg per day, but participants were allowed 500 mg of extra sodium daily if they wanted. Alcohol consumption was limited to two drinks or fewer per day, and weight was not supposed to be decreased or increased during the study. It is interesting that the 3,000 mg of salt per day is actually still about 20 % below the US average, but it is still above the recommended average consumption of 2,400 mg of day. After the original DASH study was concluded, researchers conducted a similar study of a control diet compared to the DASH diet. In each diet group (control or DASH), participants ingested three different rotating levels of sodium intake in random order for 30 days each, including 3,000 mg of salt per day, 2,400 mg of salt per day, or 1,500 mg of salt per day. Therefore, each individual ingested all three sodium daily amounts on his or her assigned diet, which was either DASH or control diet. Researchers found that reducing salt intake lowered systolic and diastolic blood pressure significantly in both the control and DASH dietary groups. The impressive findings in this part of the study were as follows:

- The DASH diet itself lowered blood pressure at all the levels of sodium ingestion.
- Reducing salt intake to 1,500 mg per day reduced the blood pressure by two times as much as the higher sodium intakes.
- The impact of lowering salt intake AND following the DASH diet on blood pressure was much greater when it was combined; so overall dietary changes and salt reduction is a far more powerful combination then either change by itself.
- Overall, the combined impact of the DASH diet and reducing sodium to 1,500 mg a day was a decrease of –8.9 mm Hg systolic and –4.5 mm Hg diastolic.
- Overall, the combined impact of the DASH diet and reducing sodium to 1,500 mg a day in normal blood pressure patients was a decrease of –7.1 mm Hg systolic and –3.7 mm Hg diastolic.

- Overall, the combined impact of the DASH diet and reducing sodium to 1,500 mg a day in high blood pressure patients was a decrease of −11.5 mm Hg systolic and −5.7 mm Hg diastolic.

These findings are groundbreaking in terms of lifestyle changes to reduce blood pressure! Patients should be first given the choice of eating an overall healthy diet and lowering salt intake before necessarily being offered medication, or regardless of medication status they should be offered this diet and salt reduction to reduce blood pressure. Also, another groundbreaking conclusion, even patients with normal blood pressure can significantly reduce their blood pressure with dietary change and a lowering intake of salt. Whether a person has high blood pressure or not and whether or not they are on a blood pressure medication, the message is very clear. Moderately changing diet to reduce blood pressure includes the following changes derived from the DASH diet:

- More grains (7–8 daily servings)
- More vegetables (4–5 servings a day)
- More fruits (4–5 servings a day)
- Low-fat or no-fat dairy products (2–3 servings a day)
- Low to moderate meat, poultry, or fish (2 or less servings a day)
- More nuts, seeds, and dry beans (4–5 servings a week)
- Low fats and oils (2–3 servings a day; the DASH diet had 27 % of total calories as fat, which is moderate)
- Low in sweets (5 servings a week, also low in fat)
- 1,500 mg or less of sodium per day or 2,400 mg a day, depending on the individual situation, and keep in mind that most sodium reduction comes from eating healthier and reducing intake of processed foods—not from the salt shaker

Again, the findings from the government-funded DASH study are profound and should be reviewed by urologic healthcare professionals and patients. The impact of the DASH protocol is now beginning to show potentially dramatic results in urology. For example, in the Health Care Professionals Follow-up Study of 45,821 men with 18 years of follow-up and the Nurses' Health Study I and II of approximately 195,000 women with 14–18 years of follow-up, researchers constructed a DASH diet score and evaluated kidney stone risk [181]. A total of 5,645 kidney stones were documented during this time period. The group with higher DASH scores (greater intakes of potassium, magnesium, oxalate, calcium, and vitamin C and lower sodium intake) experienced a 40–45 % reduction in the risk of a kidney stone. Again, this suggests that the sum of personal lifestyle behaviors and parameters has a far more powerful impact on heart and urologic disease compared to one or just a few changes. I find it compelling that a comprehensive heart-healthy lifestyle program appears to have the greatest risk reduction on urologic conditions such as stone disease.

General Urologic Recommendation 8

Less is more when it comes to the consumption of pills for preventive health.

Unless a patient qualifies for a pill, there is no convincing evidence that high doses of concentrated antioxidants prevent urologic conditions in healthy individuals. Heart-healthy dietary supplements or prescription medications when needed will arguably demonstrate the largest impact in urologic disease prevention or adjuvant treatment.

What is missing from the first seven ideal urologic recommendations for your patients? Absent is the utilization of pills (supplements or prescriptions) to prevent cardiovascular or urologic disease, especially in otherwise healthy individuals, because the benefit has not been found or the participants in the aforementioned studies were not regularly consumers of pills and medications. Is this a surprise?

For example, despite minimal scientific evidence, multivitamins are the largest selling and utilized supplements in the USA by men and women, with over 40 % of the population using them [182, 183]. They are also the primary supplement utilized by participants in notable prostate cancer screening studies [184], male health prevention trials [185], male physicians [186], and notable women's studies [187]. Why such overall and diverse endorsement without data? Perhaps it is the perception of the evidence compared to the reality, but in reality the vast majority of the observational data has been unimpressive thus far [188]. Thus, until higher quality evidence finds some realistic benefit with these supplements, the potential even for some harm when taking them in excess seems concerning, especially in terms of urologic health [189, 190]. For example, an increased risk of advanced and fatal prostate cancer was found in one of the largest prospective epidemiologic studies of multivitamins for those taking more than one per day, and the greater use of other supplements was also associated with an even greater risk [190]. Men with a family history of prostate cancer experienced the largest and most significant elevated risks of this condition. Other large male observational studies have found somewhat similar results [191, 192]. It is interesting that some recent studies in breast cancer have somewhat mirrored these negative findings [193, 194]. Overall, the data are not impressive thus far in a positive or negative direction, and it is plausible that a good deal of confounding occurs.

Multivitamins are replete in my experience with higher doses of B vitamins, which have also recently been found to potentially have no impact on health or increase the risk of prostate cancer from one of the largest and most recent meta-analysis of clinical trials [195, 196]. Since there is no consistent suggestion of benefit with a greater intake of multivitamins and since there is a suggestion of either no impact or serious harm, it would be prudent to wait for more clarity [197, 198] or, in my opinion, begin to tell most men and patients to reduce their dosage of adult multivitamins (review the Physicians Health Study 2 in the prostate cancer chapter).

A partial level of insight may have been provided in the Supplementation en Vitamines et Mineraux Antioxydants (SUVIMAX) randomized, placebo-controlled trial, which included several vitamins and minerals at very moderate or low dosages that are not usually utilized in clinical trials [199] and are commonly found in current children's or older adult formulations, from my experience. SUVIMAX was a randomized, double-blind, placebo-controlled primary prevention trial (participants were healthy at the start of the trial) of healthy individuals. A total of 13,017 French adults (7,876 women aged 35–60 years and 5,141 men aged 45–60 years) were included in this study. All of the individuals took either a placebo or a daily capsule that consisted of the following:

- 120 mg of vitamin C
- 30 mg of vitamin E
- 6 mg of beta-carotene
- 100 mcg of selenium
- 20 mg of zinc

These individuals were then followed for 7.5 years. Nothing notable occurred in the group as a whole, but men experienced a nonsignificant ($p=0.54$) 18 % reduction in ischemic cardiovascular risk, a significant ($p=0.008$) 31 % reduction in risk of being diagnosed with cancer, and a significant ($p=0.02$) 37 % reduction in the risk of dying from any cause. It appeared that taking a low-dose multivitamin minimally based formula could provide a potential benefit for some men. The researchers from this study suggested that men benefited only because they had lower levels of these vitamins and minerals in their blood from less than optimal dietary patterns at the beginning of the study, compared to the women who consumed a more healthy diet on average. A follow-up secondary observation to this study (8.8–9 years) found that this low-dose multivitamin reduced the risk of prostate cancer by 48 % in men with a low PSA (less than 3), but in men with a higher PSA, a multivitamin may have been associated with a higher risk of being diagnosed with prostate cancer [200]. In other words, if a man has an elevated PSA, he should be careful about taking dietary supplements to reduce risk. This multivitamin did not impact PSA or IGF levels, suggesting that risk was impacted by other methods. It was also interesting in this study that older age (average age of men, 51 years), higher BMI, and men with higher PSA levels had significantly increased risks for prostate cancer. Side effects from the low-dose multivitamin were similar to placebo. One limitation in this study was that no information was collected on family history of prostate cancer. Yet, this clinical trial is arguably one of the best pieces of evidence to date for men's and women's health and the consumption of a mixed dietary supplement product. Thus, I will repeat an often-cited mantra of mine that it would be wise not to take anything larger than a children's multivitamin per day until someone can demonstrate that "more is better," which, as mentioned earlier, is not the case.

Regardless, how much more evidence do healthcare professionals and patients need in urology, especially when the recent results of the SELECT trial, the largest chemoprevention trial of supplements in urologic history, showed a significant increased risk of prostate cancer when utilizing 400 IU daily of vitamin E [201]? Also, there was a nonsignificant increased risk of aggressive prostate cancer in all the dietary supplement groups compared to placebo [201] and an increased risk of hemorrhagic stroke in another similar randomized trial [202].

The results of the first randomized US trial of adult men only (Physicians Health Study II) utilizing a daily multivitamin are available now and are providing more clarity (see the prostate cancer chapter for the latest results) that one (not more) very low-dose multivitamin pill is more than adequate for adults [203]. Also, other dietary supplements do not have adequate chemoprevention data in healthy individuals in urology; for example, there are studies of vitamin D supplements that suggest harm can be caused by excessive intakes [204]. Still, I do believe that dietary supplements have a clear role in urology for men at high risk for certain conditions or those who have been diagnosed with specific conditions or for dealing with some side effects of treatment. When clinicians and patients are better educated on these studies, there will be a realization that just like prescription medications, some dietary supplements have a role in medicine and urology. For example, monitoring vitamin D blood levels in completely healthy individuals is questionable [205], but in higher-risk osteoporosis patients, such as men on LHRH medications for prostate cancer, it appears to be clinically appropriate [206]. Vitamin D, like most dietary supplements in my opinion, tends to mimic or follow hormone-like functions and rules, which means they generally follow a U-shaped risk curve (similar to alcohol and other hormones) for urologic health [201, 202, 207, 208]. In other words, deficiency or excessive doses of many nutrients found in supplements tend to be a problem (similar to prescription medications). This is another reason to promote healthier lifestyles and reserve dietary supplementation for those that truly qualify.

Interestingly, the additional issue is that until a supplement or drug is found to be safe and heart healthy, I am not an advocate for recommending it to patients. Dietary supplements should be advocated for urologic condition–specific situations. It is interesting that in the field of prostate cancer prevention, or even urologic-specific partial amelioration of disease, for example, perhaps the most intriguing medications for prevention in my opinion may be heart-healthy prescriptions or over-the-counter medicines that have been tested for long periods of time outside of urology. In other words, these pills now all have generic options. For example, aspirin, metformin, and statins are garnering some impressive indirect data [209–223]. Yet, these medications all have the ability to cause more harm than good in the wrong patient [221]. I believe effective chemoprevention of a urologic cancer or condition with a supplement will be accomplished when a particular supplement, for example, is able to mimic some of the mechanisms of heart-healthy effects observed with aspirin, metformin, and/or statins [209–223]. In the worst-case scenario, if the pill does not work but reduces the risk of the number one cause of death in men (cardiovascular disease), then I believe it is a step forward in medicine and urology and not a lateral or backward move, which appears to be the norm lately [4, 7, 201, 202].

Conclusion

Other simplistic lifestyle changes could have been proposed in this manuscript, but why belabor the minutiae over the profound? Let me remind the reader of the seven researched heart-healthy (reduce or reanalyze pill counts is my eighth goal) goals/parameters that could have such a profound impact on overall health and longevity:

- Avoiding all tobacco products
- Being physically active almost every day of the week
- BMI of 25 or less
- Overall diet that is heart healthy (fruits, veggies, fiber, fish, etc.)
- Total cholesterol equal to or less than 200 mg/dL
- Blood pressure equal to or less than 120/80 mm Hg
- Fasting blood glucose less than 100 mg/dL

Again, only 1–2 % of patients can achieve these parameters? Is it possible that as we spend hundreds of millions of taxpayer dollars trying to identify the ideal dietary supplement or pharmacologic agent for urologic health the ideal lifestyle program has already been staring right into our eyes?! Clinicians now have access to a wealth of data that suggests that an ideal urologic diet and lifestyle program does exist to reduce the primary causes of morbidity and mortality in women and men and a plethora of these recommendations were outlined in this chapter. A quick overall review of this eight-step heart and urologic health program can be found in Table 1.6.

Healthcare professionals, especially in urology, should embrace lifestyle and dietary changes for everything from cancer to kidney stones, and several ways to demonstrate your commitment to lifestyle changes in your medical practice, from my experience, are outlined in Table 1.7. One of the most common questions I am asked by healthcare practitioners around the world is how to encourage healthy lifestyle changes in such a short time that is allotted with each patient. Some of the most successful tips that have worked in my experience are briefly reviewed for the healthcare professional in Table 1.7.

A commitment to these changes in all aspects of our behavior is not an easy task. It is difficult today when attending global urologic meetings to find an ample amount of time dedicated to diet and lifestyle. In fact, a recent or past glance at the official condition-specific or general treatment guidelines in urology is an example of the dearth of ideas or suggestions on lifestyle recommendations [224, 225]. Our inability to make lifestyle guidelines a part of all aspects of urology from BPH/LUTS to erectile dysfunction is not an issue of data or evidence-based studies or even a lack of randomized trials but instead an educational and awareness issue. When the field of urology begins to place as much emphasis on lifestyle as we do on pills and procedures, I believe a dramatic shift in patient behavior will also begin to occur. I believe urology has done as well as any other field of medicine in trying to emphasize lifestyle research and teaching, but what does that tell you about how the rest of medicine is doing? Currently, there is a global obesity epidemic that has already had profound negative impacts on all aspects of urology, and perhaps if the glass of life is really half-full in your urologic practice, this may be the best opportunity in the history of urology to impact the overall quality and quantity of the lives of the individuals who put their complete trust in your care. If the enthusiasm displayed by

Table 1.6 A review of Dr. Moyad's ideal urologic lifestyle program and checklist

8-Step ideal urologic lifestyle program review (reviewed and discussed by patient and healthcare professional)	Your score (1 point if ideal or "normal" and 0 points if "abnormal" or needs more work)
Cholesterol?	
Blood pressure?	
Glucose?	
BMI and/or waist circumference?	
Overall diet healthy (healthy fats, fruits and veggies, fiber, fish, omega-3 from plants, sodium intake, alcohol in moderation, etc.)	
Aerobic exercise daily	
Resistance exercise several times a week	
What pills do I really need, and which ones can be reduced or eliminated as I adhere to more healthy lifestyle changes?	
Additional personalized recommendations for your patients:	

Table 1.7 Dr. Moyad's ten suggestions on how to immediately improve patient adherence/compliance in your medical practice with healthy urologic lifestyle changes

Improving adherence/compliance to the ideal urologic lifestyle and diet program	Example and/or commentary
1. Simplify recommendations for patients (less than one sentence is enough in many cases)	1. Heart health = urologic health or heart health = penile or sexual health or heart healthy = prostate healthy, heart healthy = bladder/kidney healthy, etc.
2. Practice and also appear to be exactly what you preach (perception should match the reality)	2. Clinicians should not only appear to be fit but follow the specific lifestyle recommendations they advocate
3. Motivate patients to practice what you preach by teaming up at least once a year	3. Pick a charity event annually, such as a fun run, biking event, and walk, that you and your patients can participate in yearly
4. Get to know ancillary behavioral assistance in your community and provide specific examples to your patients, which will provide credibility	4. Familiarize yourself with local nutritionists, trainers, health clubs, weight-loss programs, health classes, etc. and precisely what these services have to offer the patient
5. Do not solve the world's problems in one visit. Pick a single goal for your patients or triage their preventive health and then write a quick lifestyle prescription to the patient or letter for the patient's employer	5. Better to know and recommend a variety of smoking cessation programs when talking to tobacco-utilizing patients compared to spending additional time on environmental toxins or specific dietary changes. Also, better to be able to discuss the specifics of weight-loss programs compared to specific dietary supplements for obese patients. Write an exercise prescription on a pad just like a drug prescription and occasionally write employer of your patient asking for some exercise time to help reduce employer and employee insurance costs
6. Office pictures are worth a thousand words. Show patients the moment they walk into and through your office that lifestyle changes are paramount to your practice setting	6. Handouts in the waiting room, BMI or waist circumference posters in the exam rooms, advertisements for exercise and cooking classes, a variety of health magazines, etc.
7. Office staff are just as important as you in sending the message	7. All members of the office staff should be as excited about lifestyle changes, including providing information to patients on goals, local classes, fitness events, and health coupons
8. Encourage the patient's spouse or another family member to attend the office visit	8. Ask the scheduling staff to remind the patient that you like to have at least one other family member in the room to improve quality of the patient visit
9. Encourage patients to give back to the community in your practice ("spiritual health screening"), which will develop cohesiveness and charity within and outside the practice setting	9. Ask patients to volunteer, donate blood, and exercise for charity or another identified community need
10. Personalize your practice to the patients whenever the opportunity arises	10. Dr_______ top 10 lifestyle tips after prostate cancer treatment. Feel free to give one-page handouts on your specific lifestyle recommendations before or after a particular procedure. Provide personal health book or DVD recommendations, etc.

practitioners of all ages that I come in contact with lately from around the world is an indication of the verve for these lifestyle changes to be implemented in clinical practice, then I am more optimistic than ever that the field of urology will provide the leadership needed to assist in reversing numerous unhealthy parameters.

References

1. Lloyd-Jones D, Adams RJ, Brown TM, Carnethon M, Dai S, D Simone G, American Heart Association Statistics Committee and Stroke Statistics Subcommittee, et al. Heart disease and stroke statistics-2010 update: a report from the American Heart Association. Circulation. 2010;121:e46–215.

2. World Heart Federation web site. Available at: http://www.world-heart-federation.org. Accessed 20 March 2010.
3. Eyre H, Kahn R, Robertson RM, Clark NG, Doyle C, Hong Y, American Cancer Society; American Diabetes Association, and the American Heart Association, et al. Preventing cancer, cardiovascular disease, and diabetes: a common agenda for the American Cancer Society, the American Diabetes Association, and the American Heart Association. Circulation. 2004;109:3244–55.
4. Thompson IM, Goodman PJ, Tangen CM, Lucia MS, Miller GS, Ford LG, et al. The influence of finasteride on the development of prostate cancer. N Engl J Med. 2003;349:215–24.
5. Scardino PT. The prevention of prostate cancer-The dilemma continues. N Engl J Med. 2003;349:297–9.
6. Kaplan SA, Roehrborn CG, Meehan AG, Liu KS, Carides AD, Binkowitz BS, et al. PCPT: Evidence that finasteride reduces risk of most frequently detected intermediate- and high-grade (Gleason score 6 and 7) cancer. Urology. 2009;73:935–9.
7. Lippman SM, Klein EA, Goodman PJ, Lucia MA, Thompson IM, Ford LG, et al. Effect of selenium and vitamin E on risk of prostate cancer and other cancers: the Selenium and Vitamin E Cancer Prevention Trial (SELECT). JAMA. 2009;301:39–51.
8. Nash IS, Mosca L, Blumenthal RS, Davidson MH, Smith SC, Paternak RC. Contemporary awareness and understanding of cholesterol as a risk factor: Results of an American Heart Association National Survey. Arch Intern Med. 2003;163:1597–600.
9. Hickey A, O'Hanlon A, McGee H, Donnellan C, Shelley E, Horgan F, et al. Stroke awareness in the general population: knowledge of stroke risk factors and warning signs in older adults. BMC Geriatr. 2009;9:35.
10. Jones SP, Jenkinson AJ, Leathley MJ, Watkins CL. Stroke knowledge and awareness: an integrative review of the evidence. Age Ageing. 2010;39:11–22.
11. Reiner Z, Sonicki Z, Tedeschi-Reiner E. The perception and knowledge of cardiovascular risk factors among medical students. Croat Med J. 2012;53: 278–84.
12. Rogers VL, Go AS, Lloyd-Jones DM, Benjamin EJ, Berry JD, Borden WB, et al. Heart disease and stroke statistics—2012 update: a report from the American Heart Association. Circulation. 2012;125:e2–220.
13. Expert Panel on Detection, Evaluation, and Treatment of High Blood Cholesterol in Adults. Executive summary of the Third Report of the National Cholesterol Education Program (NCEP) Expert panel on Detection, Evaluation, and Treatment of High Blood Cholesterol in Adults (Adult Treatment Panel III). JAMA. 2001;285:2486–98.
14. Grundy SM, Cleeman JI, Merz CN, Brewer Jr HB, Clark LT, Hunninghake DB, et al. Implications of recent clinical trials for the National Cholesterol Education Program Adult Treatment Panel III Guidelines. Circulation. 2004;110:227–39.
15. Ketchandji M, Kuo YF, Shahinian VB, Goodwin JS. Cause of death in older men after the diagnosis of prostate cancer. J Am Geriatr Soc. 2009;57:24–30.
16. Centers for Disease Control and Prevention. Prevalence of abnormal lipid levels among youths-United States 1999–2006. MMWR Morb Mortal Wkly Rep. 2010;59:29–33.
17. Ridker PM. Clinical application of C-reactive protein for cardiovascular disease detection and prevention. Circulation. 2003;107:363–9.
18. Chang ST, Chu CM, Hsu JT, Hsiao JF, Chung CM, Ho C, et al. Independent determinants of coronary artery disease in erectile dysfunction patients. J Sex Med. 2010;7(4 Pt 1):1478–87.
19. Kraus WE, Houmard JA, Duscha BD, Knetzger KJ, Wharton MB, McCartney JS, et al. Effects of the amount and intensity of exercise on plasma lipoproteins. N Engl J Med. 2002;347:1483–92.
20. Hammarsten J, Hogstedt B. Hyperinsulinaemia as a risk factor for developing benign prostatic hyperplasia. Eur Urol. 2001;39:151–8.
21. Mondul AM, Weinstein SJ, Virtamo J, Albanes D. Serum total and HDL cholesterol and risk of prostate cancer. Cancer Causes Control. 2011;22:1545–52.
22. Van Hemelrijck M, Garmo H, Holmberg L, Walldius G, Jungner I, Hammar N, et al. Prostate cancer risk in the Swedish AMORIS study: the interplay among triglycerides, total cholesterol, and glucose. Cancer. 2011;117:2086–95.
23. Chobanian AV, Bakris GL, Black HR, Cushman WC, Green LA, Izzo Jr JL, Joint National Committee on Prevention, Detection, Evaluation, and Treatment of High Blood Pressure; National Heart, Lung, and Blood Institute; National High Blood Pressure Education Program Coordinating Committee, et al. Hypertension. 2003;42:1206–52.
24. Whelton SP, Chin A, Xin X, He J. Effect of aerobic exercise on blood pressure: a meta-analysis of randomized, controlled trials. Ann Intern Med. 2002;136:493–503.
25. Ponholzer A, Temmi C, Mock K, Marszalek M, Obermayr R, Madersbacher S. Prevalence and risk factors for erectile dysfunction in 2869 men using a validated questionnaire. Eur Urol. 2005;47:80–5.
26. Chong C, Fong L, Lai R, Lau WK, Hartmann M, Chia SE. The prevalence of lower urinary tract symptoms and treatment-seeking behaviour in males over 40 years in Singapore: a community-based study. Prostate Cancer Prostatic Dis. 2012;15: 273–7.
27. Hillborn M, Saloheimo P, Juvela S. Alcohol consumption, blood pressure, and the risk of stroke. Curr Hypertens Rep. 2011;13:208–13.
28. Strijk JE, Proper KI, Klaver L, van der Beek AJ, van Mechelen W. Associations between VO_{2max} and vitality in older workers: a cross-sectional study. BMC Public Health. 2010;10:684.
29. Blair SN, Morris JN. Healthy hearts- and the universal benefits of being physically active: physical activity and health. Ann Epidemiol. 2009;19:253–6.

30. Baguet JP. Out-of-office blood pressure: from measurement to control. Integr Blood Press Control. 2012;5:27–34.
31. Kim WT, Yun SJ, Choi YD, Kim GY, Moon SK, Choi YH, et al. Prostate size correlates with fasting blood glucose in non-diabetic benign prostatic hyperplasia patients with normal testosterone levels. J Korean Med Sci. 2011;26:1214–8.
32. Corona G, Monami M, Rastrelli G, Aversa A, Sforza A, Lenzi A, et al. Type 2 diabetes mellitus and testosterone: a meta-analysis study. Int J Androl. 2011;34(6 Pt 1):528–40.
33. Isidro ML. Sexual dysfunction in men with type 2 diabetes. Postgrad Med J. 2012;88:152–9.
34. Copeland KL, Brown JS, Creasman JM, Van Den Eeden SK, Subak LL, Thom DH, et al. Diabetes mellitus and sexual function in middle-aged and older women. Obstet Gynecol. 2012;120(2 Pt 1):331–40.
35. Moyad MA. Current methods used for defining, measuring, and treating obesity. Semin Urol Oncol. 2001;19:247–56.
36. Writing Group for the Women's Health Initiative Investigators. Risks and benefits of estrogen plus progestin in healthy postmenopausal women: principal results from the Women's Health Initiative randomized controlled trial. JAMA. 2002;288:321–33.
37. Shike M, Latkany L, Riedel E, Fleisher M, Schatzkin A, Lanza E, et al. Lack of effect of a low-fat, high-fruit, -vegetable, and -fiber diet on serum prostate-specific antigen of men without prostate cancer: results from a randomized trial. J Clin Oncol. 2002;20:3592–8.
38. Pischon T, Boeing H, Hoffmann K, Bergmann M, Schulze MB, Overvad K, et al. General and abdominal adiposity and risk of death in Europe. N Engl J Med. 2008;359:2105–20.
39. Jacobs EJ, Newton CC, Wang Y, Patel AV, McCullough ML, Campbell PT, et al. Waist circumference and all-cause mortality in a large US cohort. Arch Intern Med. 2010;170:1293–301.
40. Seidell JC. Waist circumference and waist/hip ratio in relation to all-cause mortality, cancer and sleep apnea. Eur J Clin Nutr. 2010;64:35–41.
41. Zhu S, Heymsfield SB, Toyoshima H, Wang Z, Pietrobelli A, Heshka S. Race-ethnicity-specific waist circumference cutoffs for identifying cardiovascular disease risk factors. Am J Clin Nutr. 2005;81:409–15.
42. Chandramohan G, Kalantar-Zadeh K, Kermah D, Marie Go SC, Vaziri ND, Norris KC. Relationship between obesity and pulse pressure in children: results of the National Health and Nutrition Survey (NHANES) 1988–1994. J Am Soc Hypertens. 2012;6:277–83.
43. Taylor EN, Stampfer MJ, Curhan GC. Obesity, weight gain, and the risk of kidney stones. JAMA. 2005;293:455–62.
44. Scales Jr CD, Smith AC, Hanley JM, Saigal CS, Urologic Diseases in America Project. Prevalence of kidney stones in the United States. Eur Urol. 2012;62:160–5.
45. Moyad MA. Obesity, interrelated mechanisms, and exposures and kidney cancer. Semin Urol Oncol. 2001;19:270–9.
46. Mathew A, George PS, Ildaphonse G. Obesity and kidney cancer risk in women: a meta-analysis (1992–2008). Asian Pac J Cancer Prev. 2009;10: 471–8.
47. Riedner CE, Rhoden EL, Ribeiro EP, Fuchs SC. Central obesity is an independent predictor of erectile dysfunction in older men. J Urol. 2006;176: 1519–23.
48. Bacon CG, Mittleman MA, Kawachi I, Giovannucci E, Glasser DB, Rimm EB. Sexual function in men older than 50 years of age: results from the Health Professionals Follow-up Study. Ann Intern Med. 2003;139:161–8.
49. Walczak MK, Lokhandwala N, Hodge MB, Guay AT. Prevalence of cardiovascular risk factors in erectile dysfunction. J Gend Specif Med. 2002;5:19–24.
50. Khoo J, Piantadosi C, Worthley S, Wittert GA. Effects of low-energy diet on sexual function and lower urinary tract symptoms in obese men. Int J Obes. 2010;34:1396–403.
51. Adams TD, Gress RE, Smith SC, Halverson RC, Simper SC, Rosamond WD, et al. Long-term mortality after gastric bypass surgery. N Engl J Med. 2007;357:753–61.
52. Sjostrom L, Narbro K, Sjostrom CD, Karason K, Larsson B, Wedel H, Swedish Obese Subjects Study, et al. N Engl J Med. 2007;357:741–52.
53. Bray GA. The missing link-lose weight, live longer. N Engl J Med. 2007;357(8):818–9.
54. Sjostrom L, Peltonen M, Jacobson P, et al. Bariatric surgery and long-term cardiovascular events. JAMA. 2012;307:56–65.
55. Schauer PR, Kashyap SR, Wolski K, Brethauer SA, Kirwan JP, Pothier CE, et al. Bariatric surgery versus intensive medical therapy in obese patients with diabetes. N Engl J Med. 2012;366:1567–76.
56. Mingrone G, Panunzi S, De Gaetano A, Guidone C, Iaconelli A, Leccesi L, et al. Bariatric surgery versus conventional medical therapy for type 2 diabetes. N Engl J Med. 2012;366:1577–85.
57. Giovannucci EL, Liu Y, Leitzmann MF, Stampfer MJ, Willett WC. A prospective study of physical activity and incident and fatal prostate cancer. Arch Intern Med. 2005;165:1005–10.
58. Crespo CJ, Garcia-Palmieri MR, Smit E, Lee IM, McGee D, Muti P, et al. Physical activity and prostate cancer mortality in Puerto Rican men. J Phys Act Health. 2008;5:918–29.
59. Moore SC, Peters TM, Ahn J, Park Y, Schatzkin A, Albanes D, et al. Physical activity in relation to total, advanced, and fatal prostate cancer. Cancer Epidemiol Biomarkers Prev. 2008;17:2458–66.
60. Richman EL, Kenfield SA, Stampfer MJ, Paciorek A, Carroll PR, Chan JM. Physical activity after diagnosis and risk of prostate cancer progression: data from the cancer of the prostate strategic urologic research endeavor. Cancer Res. 2011;71:3889–95.

61. Park SW, Kim TN, Nam JK, Ha HK, Shin DG, Lee W, et al. Recovery of overall exercise ability, quality of life, and continence after 12-week combined exercise intervention in elderly patients who underwent radical prostatectomy: a randomized controlled study. Urology. 2012;80:299–305.
62. Leitzmann MF. Physical activity and genitourinary cancer prevention. Recent Results Cancer Res. 2011;186:43–71.
63. Tanasescu M, Leitzmann MF, Rimm EB, Willett WC, Stampfer MJ, Hu FB. Exercise type and intensity in relation to coronary heart disease in men. JAMA. 2002;288:1994–2000.
64. Poehlman ET, Melby C. Resistance training and energy balance. Int J Sport Nutr. 1998;8:143–59.
65. Braith RW, Stewart KJ. Resistance exercise training: its role in the prevention of cardiovascular disease. Circulation. 2006;113:2642–50.
66. Hurley BF, Roth SM. Strength training in the elderly. Sports Med. 2000;30:249–68.
67. Platz EA, Kawachi I, Rimm EB, Colditz GA, Stampfer MJ, Willett WC, et al. Physical activity and benign prostatic hyperplasia. Arch Intern Med. 1998;158:2349–56.
68. Ahmed HM, Blaha MJ, Nasir K, Rivera JJ, Blumenthal RS. Effects of physical activity on cardiovascular disease. Am J Cardiol. 2012;109:288–95.
69. Blake H, Mo P, Malik S, Thomas S. How effective are physical activity interventions for alleviating depressive symptoms in older people? A systematic review. Clin Rehabil. 2009;23:873–87.
70. Deslandes A, Moraes H, Ferreira C, Veiga H, Silveira H, Mouta R, et al. Exercise and mental health: many reasons to move. Neuropsychobiology. 2009;59:191–8.
71. Blumenthal JA, Babyak MA, Moore KA, Craighead WE, Herman S, Khatri P, et al. Effects of exercise training on older patients with major depression. Arch Intern Med. 1999;159:2349–56.
72. Babyak M, Blumenthal JA, Herman S, Khatri P, Doraiswamy M, Moore K, et al. Exercise treatment for major depression: maintenance of therapeutic benefit at 10 months. Psychosom Med. 2000;62:633–8.
73. Blumenthal JA, Babyak MA, O'Connor C, Keteyian S, Landzberg J, Howlett J, et al. Effects of exercise training on depressive symptoms in patients with chronic heart failure: the HF-ACTION randomized trial. JAMA. 2012;308:465–74.
74. Barnes PM, Schoenborn CA. Trends in adults receiving a recommendation for exercise or other physical activity from a physician or other health professional. NCHS Data Brief. 2012;86:1–8.
75. Moyad MA. Dr Moyad's no Bogus science health advice. Ann Arbor, MI: Ann Arbor Media Group; 2009.
76. Yu JN, Cunningham JA, Rosenberg Thouin S, Gurvich T, Liu D. Hyperlipidemia. Prim Care. 2000;27:541–87.
77. Ornish D, Weidner G, Fair WR, Marlin R, Pettengill EB, Raisin CJ, et al. Intensive lifestyle changes may affect the progression of prostate cancer. J Urol. 2005;174:1065–9.
78. Siri-Tarino PW, Sun Q, Hu FB, Krauss RM. Meta-analysis of prospective cohort studies evaluating the association of saturated fat with cardiovascular disease. Am J Clin Nutr. 2010;91:535–46.
79. Yamagishi K, Iso H, Yatsuya H, Tanabe N, Date C, Kikuchi S, JACC Study Group, et al. Dietary intake of saturated fatty acids and mortality from cardiovascular disease in Japanese: the Japan Collaborative Cohort Study for Evaluation of Cancer Risk (JACC) Study. Am J Clin Nutr. 2010;92:759–65.
80. Mozaffarian D, Micha R, Wallace S. Effects of coronary heart disease of increasing polyunsaturated fat in place of saturated fat: a systematic review and meta-analysis of randomized controlled trials. PLoS Med. 2010;7:e1000252.
81. Chiuve SE, Rimm EB, Sandhu RK, Bernstein AM, Rexrode KM, Manson JE, et al. Dietary fat quality and risk of sudden cardiac death in women. Am J Clin Nutr. 2012;96:498–507.
82. Giovannucci E. Tomatoes, tomato-based products, lycopene, and cancer: review of the epidemiologic literature. J Natl Cancer Inst. 1999;91:317–31.
83. Moyad MA. The ABCs of nutrition and supplements for prostate cancer. Ann Arbor, MI: JW Edwards; 2000.
84. http://www.usda.gov. Accessed 25 Oct 2010.
85. Clinton SK. Lycopene: chemistry, biology, and implications for human health and disease. Nutr Rev. 1998;56:35–51.
86. Mourvaki E, Gizzi S, Rossi R, Rufini S. Passionflower fruit-a "new" source of lycopene? J Med Food. 2005;8:104–6.
87. Ilic D, Forbes KM, Hassed C. Lycopene for the prevention of prostate cancer. Cochrane Database Syst Rev. 2011;11, CD008007.
88. Ilic D, Misso M. Lycopene for the prevention and treatment of benign prostatic hyperplasia and prostate cancer: a systematic review. Maturitas. 2012;72:269–76.
89. Ried K, Fakler P. Protective effect of lycopene on serum cholesterol and blood pressure: meta-analyses of intervention trials. Maturitas. 2011;68:299–310.
90. Pantuck AJ, Leppert JT, Zomorodian N, Aronson W, Hong J, Barnard RJ, et al. Phase II study of pomegranate juice for men with rising prostate-specific antigen following surgery or radiation for prostate cancer. Clin Cancer Res. 2006;12(13):4018–26.
91. Forest CP, Padma-Nathan H, Liker HR. Efficacy and safety of pomegranate juice on improvement of erectile dysfunction in male patients with mild to moderate erectile dysfunction: a randomized, placebo-controlled, double-blind, cross-over study. Int J Impot Res. 2007;19:564–7.
92. Uno T, Yasui-Furukori N. Effect of grapefruit juice in relation to human pharmacokinetic study. Curr Clin Pharmacol. 2006;1:157–61.
93. Komperda KE. Potential interaction between pomegranate juice and warfarin. Pharmacotherapy. 2009;29:1002–6.
94. Jarvis S, Li C, Bogle RG. Possible interaction between pomegranate juice and warfarin. Emerg Med J. 2010;27:74–5.

95. Cohen JH, Kristal AR, Stanford JL. Fruit and vegetable intakes and prostate cancer risk. J Natl Cancer Inst. 2000;92:61–8.
96. Kristal AR, Lampe JW. Brassica vegetables and prostate cancer risk: a review of the epidemiological evidence. Nutr Cancer. 2002;42:1–9.
97. Hsing AW, Chokkalingam AP, Gao Y-T, Madigan MP, Deng J, Gridley G, et al. Allium vegetables and risk of prostate cancer: a population-based study. J Natl Cancer Inst. 2002;94:1648–51.
98. Walker C, Reamy BV. Diets for cardiovascular disease prevention: what is the evidence? Am Fam Physician. 2009;79:571–8.
99. Duthie GG, Wood AD. Natural salicylates: foods, functions and disease prevention. Food Funct. 2011;2:515–20.
100. Boffetta P, Couto E, Wichmann J, Ferrari P, Trichopoulos D, Bueno-de-Mesquita HB, et al. Fruit and vegetable intake and overall cancer risk in the European Prospective Investigation into Cancer and Nutrition (EPIC). J Natl Cancer Inst. 2010;102: 529–37.
101. Buchner FL, Bueno-de-Mesquita HB, Ros MM, Kampman E, Egevad L, Overvad K, et al. Variety in vegetable and fruit consumption and risk of bladder cancer in the European Prospective Investigation into Cancer and Nutrition. Int J Cancer. 2011;128:2971–9.
102. Grant EJ, Ozasa K, Preston DL, Suyama A, Shimizu Y, Sakata R, et al. Effects of radiation and lifestyle factors on risks of urothelial carcinoma in the life span study of atomic bomb survivors. Radiat Res. 2012;178:86–98.
103. Van Horn L. Fiber, lipids, and coronary heart disease. Nutrition Committee Advisory. Circulation. 1997;95:2701–4.
104. Brown L, Rosner B, Willett WW, Sacks FM. Cholesterol-lowering effects of dietary fiber: a meta-analysis. Am J Clin Nutr. 1999;69:30–42.
105. Anderson JW, Baird P, Davis Jr RH, Ferreri S, Knudtson M, Koraym A, et al. Health benefits of dietary fiber. Nutr Rev. 2009;67:188–205.
106. Slavin JL. Position of the American Dietetic Association: health implications of dietary fiber. J Am Diet Assoc. 2008;108:1716–31.
107. Pereira MA, O'Reilly E, Augustsson K, Fraser GE, Goldbourt U, Heitmann BL, et al. Dietary fiber and risk of coronary heart disease: a pooled analysis of cohort studies. Arch Intern Med. 2004;164:370–6.
108. Pietinen P, Rimm EB, Korhonen P, Hartman AM, Willett WC, Albanes D, et al. Intake of dietary fiber and risk of coronary heart disease in a cohort of Finnish men: the Alpha-Tocopherol, Beta-Carotene Cancer Prevention Study. Circulation. 1996;94:2720–7.
109. Rimm EB, Ascherio A, Giovannucci E, Spiegelman D, Stampfer MJ, Willett WC. Vegetable, fruit, and cereal fiber intake and risk of coronary heart disease among men. JAMA. 1996;275:447–51.
110. Park Y, Subar AF, Hollenbeck A, Schatzkin A. Dietary fiber intake and mortality in the NIH-AARP diet and health study. Arch Intern Med. 2011;171: 1061–8.
111. Eshak ES, Iso H, Date C, Kikuchi S, Watanabe Y, Wada Y, et al. Dietary fiber intake is associated with reduced risk of mortality from cardiovascular disease among Japanese men and women. J Nutr. 2010;140:1445–53.
112. Moreyra AE, Wilson AC, Koraym A. Effect of combining psyllium fiber with simvastatin in lowering cholesterol. Arch Intern Med. 2005;165:1161–6.
113. Agrawal AR, Tandon M, Sharma PL. Effect of combining viscous fibre with lovastatin on serum lipids in normal human subjects. Int J Clin Pract. 2007;61:1812–8.
114. Streppel MT, Arends LR, van't Veer P, Grobbee DE, Geleijnse JM. Dietary fiber and blood pressure: a meta-analysis of randomized placebo-controlled trials. Arch Intern Med. 2005;165:150–6.
115. Vernay M, Aidara M, Salanave B, Deschamps V, Malon A, Oleko A, et al. Diet and blood pressure in 18–74 year old adults: the French Nutrition and Health Survey (ENNS, 2006–2007). J Hypertens. 2012;30:1920–7.
116. Marlett JA, McBurney MI, Slavin JL, American Dietetic Association. Position of the American Dietetic Association: health implications of dietary fiber. J Am Diet Assoc. 2002;102:993–1000.
117. Pan A, Yu D, Demark-Wahnefried W, Franco OH, Lin X. Meta-analysis of the effects of flaxseed interventions on blood lipids. Am J Clin Nutr. 2009;90:288–97.
118. Rodriguez-Leyva D, Dupasquier CM, McCullough R, Pierce GN. The cardiovascular effects of flaxseed and its omega-3 fatty acid, alpha-linolenic acid. Can J Cardiol. 2010;26:489–96.
119. Demark-Wahnefried W, Price DT, Polascik TJ, Robertson CN, Anderson EE, Paulson DF, et al. Pilot study of dietary fat restriction and flaxseed supplementation in men with prostate cancer before surgery: exploring the effects on hormonal levels, prostate-specific antigen, and histopathologic features. Urology. 2001;58:47–52.
120. Demark-Wahnefried W, Robertson CN, Walther PJ, Polascik TJ, Paulson DF, Vollmer RT. Pilot study to explore effects of low-fat, flaxseed-supplemented diet on proliferation of benign prostatic epithelium and prostate-specific antigen. Urology. 2004;63:900–4.
121. Demark-Wahnefried W, Polascik TJ, George SL, Switzer BR, Madden JF, Ruffin 4th MT, et al. Flaxseed supplementation (not dietary fat restriction) reduces prostate cancer proliferation rates in men presurgery. Cancer Epidemiol Biomarkers Prev. 2008;17:3577–87.
122. Zhang W, Wang X, Liu Y, Tian H, Flickinger B, Empie MW, et al. Effects of dietary flaxseed lignan extract on symptoms of benign prostatic hyperplasia. J Med Food. 2008;11:207–14.
123. Jin F, Nieman DC, Sha W, Xie G, Qiu Y, Jia W. Supplementation of milled chia seeds increases plasma ALA and EPA in postmenopausal women. Plant Foods Hum Nutr. 2012;67:105–10.
124. Morris MC, Evans DA, Bienias JL, Tangney CC, Bennett DA, Wilson RS, et al. Consumption of fish

and n-3 fatty acids and risk of incident Alzheimer disease. Arch Neurol. 2003;60:940–6.
125. Morris MC. The role of nutrition in Alzheimer's disease: epidemiological evidence. Eur J Neurol. 2009;16 Suppl 1:1–7.
126. Moyad MA. An introduction to dietary/supplemental omega-3 fatty acids for general health and prevention: Part I. Urol Oncol. 2005;23:28–35.
127. Moyad MA. An introduction to dietary/supplemental omega-3 fatty acids for general health and prevention: Part II. Urol Oncol. 2005;23:36–48.
128. Bucher HC, Hengstler P, Schindler C, Meier G. N-3 polyunsaturated fatty acids in coronary heart disease: a meta-analysis of randomized controlled trials. Am J Med. 2002;112:298–304.
129. Kris-Etherton PM, Harris WS, Appel LJ, Nutrition Committee. Fish consumption, fish oil, omega-3 fatty acids, and cardiovascular disease. Circulation. 2002;106:2747–57.
130. Harris WS. N-3 fatty acids and serum lipoproteins: human studies. Am J Clin Nutr. 1997;65(5 Suppl): 1645S–54.
131. Cabo J, Alonso R, Mata P. Omega-3 fatty acids and blood pressure. Br J Nutr. 2012;107 Suppl 2:S195–200.
132. Albert CM, Campos H, Stampfer MJ, Ridker PM, Manson JE, Willett WC, et al. Blood levels of long-chain n-3 fatty acids and the risk of sudden death. N Engl J Med. 2002;346:1113–8.
133. Augustsson K, Michaud DS, Rimm EB, Leitzmann MF, Stampfer MJ, Willett WC, et al. A prospective study of intake of fish and marine fatty acids and prostate cancer. Cancer Epidemiol Biomark Prev. 2003;12:64–7.
134. Yang YJ, Lee SH, Hong SJ, Chung BC. Comparison of fatty acid profiles in the serum of patients with prostate cancer and benign prostatic hyperplasia. Clin Biochem. 1999;32:405–9.
135. Szymanski KM, Wheeler DC, Mucci LA. Fish consumption and prostate cancer risk: a review and meta-analysis. Am J Clin Nutr. 2010;92:1223–33.
136. Siener R, Jansen B, Watzer B, Hesse A. Effect of n-3 fatty acid supplementation on urinary risk factors for calcium oxalate stone formation. J Urol. 2011;185: 719–24.
137. Yasui T, Suzuki S, Itoh Y, Tozawa K, Tokudome S, Kohri K. Eicosapentaenoic acid has a preventive effect on the recurrence of nephrolithiasis. Urol Int. 2008;81:135–8.
138. Guallar E, Sanz-Gallardo MI, van't Veer P, Bode P, Aro A, Gomez-Aracena J, et al. Mercury, fish oils, and the risk of myocardial infarction. N Engl J Med. 2002;347:1747–54.
139. Yoshizawa K, Rimm EB, Morris JS, Spate VL, Hsieh CC, Spiegelman D, et al. Mercury and the risk of coronary heart disease in men. N Engl J Med. 2002;347:1755–60.
140. Virtanen JK, Laukkanen JA, Mursu J, Voutilainen S, Tuomainen TP. Serum long-chain n-3 polyunsaturated fatty acids, mercury, and risk of sudden cardiac death in men: a prospective population-based study. PLoS One. 2012;7:e41046.
141. Weil M, Bressler J, Parsons P, Bolla K, Glass T, Schwartz B. Blood mercury levels and neurobehavioral function. JAMA. 2005;293:1875–82.
142. DeRouen TA, Martin MD, Leroux BG, Townes BD, Woods JS, Leitao J, et al. Neurobehavioral effects of dental amalgam in children: a randomized clinical trial. JAMA. 2006;295:1784–92.
143. Mozaffarian D, Shi P, Morris JS, Spiegelman D, Grandjean P, Siscovick DS, et al. Mercury exposure and risk of cardiovascular disease in two U.S. cohorts. N Engl J Med. 2011;364:1116–25.
144. Kris-Etherton PM, Harris WS, Appel LJ, AHA Nutrition Committee, American Heart Association. Omega-3 fatty acids and cardiovascular disease: new recommendations from the American Heart Association. Arterioscler Thromb Vasc Biol. 2003;23:151–2.
145. GISSI-Prevenzione Investigators. Dietary supplementation with n-3 polyunsaturated fatty acids and vitamin E after myocardial infarction: results from the GISSI-Prevenzione trial. Lancet. 1999;354:447–55.
146. Marchioli R, Barzi F, Bomba E, Chieffo C, Di Gregorio D, Di Mascio R, et al. Early protection against sudden cardiac death by n-3 polyunsaturated fatty acids after myocardial infarction: time-course analysis of the results of the Gruppo Italiano per lo Studio della Sopravvivenza nell'Infarto Miocardico (GISSI)-Prevenzione. Circulation. 2002;105:1897–903.
147. Yokoyama M, Origasa H, Matsuzaki M, Matsuzawa Y, Saito Y, Ishikawa Y, et al. Effects of eicosapentaenoic acid on major coronary events in hypercholesterolaemic patients (JELIS): a randomized open-label, blinded endpoint analysis. Lancet. 2007;369:1090–8.
148. Kwak SM, Myung SK, Lee YJ, Seo HG, Korean Meta-Analysis Study Group, et al. Efficacy of omega-3 fatty acid supplements (eicosapentaenoic acid and docosahexaenoic acid) in the secondary prevention of cardiovascular disease: a meta-analysis of randomized, double-blind, placebo-controlled trials. Arch Intern Med. 2012;172:686–94.
149. O'Neil CE, Keast DR, Nicklas TA, Fulgoni 3rd VL. Nut consumption is associated with decreased health risk factors for cardiovascular disease and metabolic syndrome in U.S. adults: NHANES 1999–2004. J Am Coll Nutr. 2011;30:502–10.
150. Albert CM, Gaziano JM, Willett WC, Manson JE. Nut consumption and decreased risk of sudden cardiac death in the physicians' health study. Arch Intern Med. 2002;162:1382–7.
151. Ellsworth JL, Kushi LH, Folsom AR. Frequent nut intake and risk of death from coronary heart disease and all causes in postmenopausal women: the Iowa Women's Health Study. Nutr Metab Cardiovasc Dis. 2001;11:372–7.
152. Fraser GE, Shavlik DJ. Risk factors for all-cause and coronary heart disease mortality in the oldest-old: the Adventist Health Study. Arch Intern Med. 1997;157:2249–58.

153. Sabate J, Wien M. Nuts, blood lipids and cardiovascular disease. Asia Pac J Clin Nutr. 2010;19:131–6.
154. Casas-Agustench P, Bullo M, Salas-Salvado J. Nuts, inflammation and insulin resistance. Asia Pac J Clin Nutr. 2010;19:124–30.
155. Aldemir M, Okulu E, Neselioglu S, Erel KO. Pistachio diet improves erectile function parameters and serum lipid profiles in patients with erectile dysfunction. Int J Impot Res. 2011;23:32–8.
156. Yang Q, Cogswell ME, Flanders WD, Hong Y, Zhang Z, Loustalot F, et al. Trends in cardiovascular health metrics and associations with all-cause and CVD mortality among US adults. JAMA. 2012;307:1273–83.
157. Hu FB, Willett WC, Tricia L, Stampfer MJ, Colditz GA, Manson JE. Adiposity as compared with physical activity in predicting mortality among women. N Engl J Med. 2004;351(26):2694–703.
158. Ajani UA, Lotufo PA, Gaziano JM, Lee IM, Spelsberg A, Buring JE, et al. Body mass index and mortality among US male physicians. Ann Epidemiol. 2004;14:731–9.
159. Baik I, Ascherio A, Rimm EB, Giovannucci E, Spiegelman D, Stampfer MJ, et al. Adiposity and mortality in men. Am J Epidemiol. 2000;152:264–71.
160. Platz EA, Willet WC, Colditz GA, Rimm EB, Spiegelman D, Giovannucci E. Proportion of colon cancer risk that might be preventable in a cohort of middle-aged US men. Cancer Causes Control. 2000;11:579–88.
161. Trichopoulou A, Costacou T, Bamia C, Trichopoulos D. Adherence to a mediterranean diet and survival in a Greek population. N Engl J Med. 2003;348:2599–608.
162. Mitrou PN, Kipnis V, Thiebaut AC, Reedy J, Subar AF, Wirfalt E, et al. Mediterranean dietary pattern and prediction of all-cause mortality in a U.S. population: results from the NIH-AARP Diet and Health Study. Arch Int Med. 2007;167:2461–8.
163. Yusuf S, Hawken S, Ounpuu S, Dans T, Avezum A, Lanas F, on behalf of the INTERHEART Study Investigators, et al. Effect of potentially modifiable risk factors associated with myocardial infarction in 52 countries (the INTERHEART study): case-control study. Lancet. 2004;364:937–52.
164. Joshi P, Islam S, Pais P, Reddy S, Dorairaj P, Kazmi K, et al. Risk factors for early myocardial infarction in South Asians compared with individuals in other countries. JAMA. 2007;297:286–94.
165. Wilcox BJ, He Q, Chen R, Yano K, Masaki KH, Grove JS, et al. Midlife risk factors and healthy survival in men. JAMA. 2006;296:2343–50.
166. Yates LB, Djousse L, Kurth T, Buring JE, Gaziano JM. Exceptional longevity in men: modifiable factors associated with survival and function to age 90 years. Arch Int Med. 2008;168:284–90.
167. Terry DF, Pencina MJ, Vasan RS, Murabito JM, Wolf PA, Hayes MK, et al. Cardiovascular risk factors predictive for survival and morbidity-free survival in the oldest-old Framingham Heart Study participants. J Am Geriatr Soc. 2005;53:1944–50.
168. Esposito K, Giugliano F, Di Palo C, Giugliano G, Marfella R, D'Andrea F, et al. Effect of lifestyle changes on erectile dysfunction in obese men. JAMA. 2004;291(24):2978–84.
169. Giugliano D, Giugliano F, Esposito K. Sexual dysfunction and the Mediterranean diet. Public Health Nutr. 2006;9:1118–20.
170. Critchley JA, Capewell S. Mortality risk reduction associated with smoking cessation in patients with coronary heart disease: a systematic review. JAMA. 2003;290:86–97.
171. Ehdale B, Furberg H, Zabor EC, Ostroff JS, Shariat SF, Bochner BH, et al. Impact of smoking status at diagnosis on disease recurrence and death in upper tract urothelial carcinoma. BJU Int. 2012;111:589–95.
172. Plaskon LA, Penson DF, Vaughan TL, Stanford JL. Cigarette smoking and risk of prostate cancer in middle-aged men. Cancer Epidemiol Biomarkers Prev. 2003;12:604–9.
173. Roberts WW, Platz EA, Walsh PC. Association of cigarette smoking with extraprostatic prostate cancer in young men. J Urol. 2003;169:512–6.
174. Rodriguez C, Tatham LM, Thun MJ, Calle EE, Heath Jr CW. Smoking and fatal prostate cancer in a large cohort of adult men. Am J Epidemiol. 1997;145:466–75.
175. Bassett JC, Gore JL, Chi AC, Kwan L, McCarthy W, Chamie K, et al. Impact of bladder cancer diagnosis on smoking behavior. J Clin Oncol. 2012;30:1871–8.
176. Mukamal KJ, Conigrave KM, Mittleman MA, Camargo Jr CA, Stampfer MJ, Willett WC, et al. Roles of drinking pattern and type of alcohol consumed in coronary heart disease in men. N Engl J Med. 2003;348:109–18.
177. Pai JK, Mukamal KJ, Rimm EB. Long-term alcohol consumption in relation to all-cause and cardiovascular mortality among survivors of myocardial infarction: the Health Professionals Follow-up Study. Eur Heart J. 2012;33:1598–605.
178. Appel LJ, Moore TJ, Obarzanek E, Vollmer WM, Svetkey LP, Sacks FM, et al. A clinical trial of the effects of dietary patterns on blood pressure. DASH Collaborative Research Group. N Engl J Med. 1997;336:1117–24.
179. Sacks FM, Svetkey LP, Vollmer WM, Appel LJ, Bray GA, Harsha D, et al. Effects on blood pressure of reduced dietary sodium and the Dietary Approaches to Stop Hypertension (DASH) diet. DASH-Sodium Collaborative Research Group. N Engl J Med. 2001;344:3–10.
180. Karanja N, Erlinger TP, Pao-Hwa L, Miller ER, Bray GA. The DASH diet for high blood pressure: from clinical trial to dinner table. Cleve Clin J Med. 2004;71(9):745–53.
181. Taylor EN, Fung TT, Curhan GC. DASH-Style diet associates with reduced risk for kidney stones. J Am Soc Nephrol. 2009;20:2253–9.
182. Rock CL. Multivitamin–multimineral supplements: who uses them? Am J Clin Nutr. 2007;85(suppl):277S–9.

183. Gahche J, Bailey R, Burt V, Hughes J, Yetley E, Dwyer J, et al. Dietary supplement use among U.S. adults has increased since NHANES III (1988–1994). NCHS Data Brief 2011;(61):1–8.
184. Barqawi A, Gamito E, O'Donnell C, Crawford ED. Herbal and vitamin supplement use in a prostate cancer screening population. Urology. 2004;63:288–92.
185. Kristal AR, Arnold KB, Schenk JM, Neuhouser ML, Goodman P, Penson DF, et al. Dietary patterns, supplement use, and the risk of symptomatic benign prostatic hyperplasia: results from the prostate cancer prevention trial. Am J Epidemiol. 2008;167:925–34.
186. Muntwyler J, Hennekens CH, Manson JE, Buring JE, Gaziano M. Vitamin supplement use in a low-risk population of US male physicians and subsequent cardiovascular mortality. Arch Intern Med. 2002;162:1472–6.
187. Shikany JM, Patterson RE, Agurs-Collins T, Anderson G. Antioxidant supplement use in Women's Health Initiative participants. Prev Med. 2003;36:379–87.
188. Neuhouser ML, Wassertheil-Smoller S, Thomson C, Aragaki A, Anderson GL, Manson JE, et al. Multivitamin use and risk of cancer and cardiovascular disease in the Women's Health Initiative cohorts. Arch Intern Med. 2009;169:294–304.
189. Giovannucci E, Chan AT. Role of vitamin and mineral supplementation and aspirin use in cancer survivors. J Clin Oncol. 2010;28:4081–5.
190. Lawson KA, Wright ME, Subar A, Mouw T, Hollenbeck A, Schatzkin A, et al. Multivitamin use and risk of prostate cancer in the National Institutes of Health-AARP Diet and Health Study. J Natl Cancer Inst. 2007;99:754–64.
191. Stevens VL, McCullough ML, Diver WR, Rodriguez C, Jacobs EJ, Thun MJ, et al. Use of multivitamins and prostate cancer mortality in a large cohort of US men. Cancer Causes Control. 2005;16:643–50.
192. Neuhouser ML, Barnett MJ, Kristal AR, Ambrosone CB, King IB, Thornquist M, et al. Dietary supplement use and prostate cancer risk in the Carotene and Retinol Efficacy Trial. Cancer Epidemiol Biomarkers Prev. 2009;18:2202–6.
193. Larsson SC, Akesson A, Bergkvist L, Wolk A. Multivitamin use and breast cancer incidence in a prospective cohort of Swedish women. Am J Clin Nutr. 2010;91:1268–72.
194. Berube S, Diorio C, Brisson J. Multivitamin-multimineral supplement use and mammographic breast density. Am J Clin Nutr. 2008;87:1400–4.
195. Clarke R, Halsey J, Lewington S, Lonn E, Armitage J, Manson JE, et al. Effects of lowering homocysteine levels with B vitamins on cardiovascular disease, cancer, and cause-specific mortality. Arch Intern Med. 2010;170:1622–31.
196. Collin SM, Metcalfe C, Refsum H, Lewis SJ, Zuccolo L, Smith GD, et al. Circulating folate, vitamin B12, homocysteine, vitamin B12 transport proteins, and risk of prostate cancer: a case–control study, systematic review, and meta-analysis. Cancer Epidemiol Biomarkers Prev. 2010;19:1632–42.
197. Ng K, Meyerhardt JA, Chan JA, Niedzwiecki D, Hollis DR, Saltz LB, et al. Multivitamin use is not associated with cancer recurrence or survival in patients with stage III colon cancer: findings from CALGB 89803. J Clin Oncol. 2010;28:4354–63.
198. Li Q, Chuang SC, Eluf-Neto J, Menezes A, Matos E, Koifman S, et al. Vitamin or mineral supplement intake and the risk of head and neck cancer: pooled analysis in the INHANCE consortium. Int J Cancer. 2012;131:1686–99.
199. Hercberg S, Galan P, Preziosi P, Bertrais S, Mennen L, Malvy D, et al. The SU.VI.MAX study: a randomized, placebo-controlled trial of the health effects of antioxidant vitamins and minerals. Arch Intern Med. 2004;164:2335–42.
200. Meyer F, Galan P, Douville P, Bairati I, Kegle P, Bertrais S, et al. Antioxidant vitamin and mineral supplementation and prostate cancer prevention in the SU.VI.MAX trial. Int J Cancer. 2005;116:182–6.
201. Klein EA, Thompson Jr IM, Tangen CM, Crowley JJ, Lucia MS, Goodman PJ, et al. Vitamin E and the risk of prostate cancer: the Selenium and Vitamin E cancer prevention trial (SELECT). JAMA. 2011;306:1549–56.
202. Sesso HD, Buring JE, Christen WG, Kurth T, Belanger C, MacFadyen J, et al. Vitamins E and C in the prevention of cardiovascular disease in men: the Physicians' Health Study II randomized controlled trial. JAMA. 2008;300:2123–33.
203. Christen WG, Gaziano JM, Hennekens CH. Design of Physicians' Health Study II-a randomized trial of beta-carotene, vitamins E and C, and multivitamins, in prevention of cancer, cardiovascular disease, and eye disease, and review of results of completed trials. Ann Epidemiol. 2000;10:125–34.
204. Barnett CM, Beer TM. Prostate cancer and vitamin D: what does the evidence really suggest? Urol Clin North Am. 2011;38:333–42.
205. Isenor JE, Ensom MH. Is there a role for therapeutic drug monitoring of vitamin D level as a surrogate marker for fracture risk. Pharmacotherapy. 2010;30:254–64.
206. Smith MR, Egerdie B, HernandezToriz N, Feldman R, Tammela TL, Saad F, Denosumab HALT Prostate Cancer Study Group, et al. N Engl J Med. 2009;361:745–55.
207. Michaelsson K, Baron JA, Snellman G, Gedeborg R, Byberg L, Sundstrom J, et al. Plasma vitamin D and mortality in older men: a community-based prospective cohort study. Am J Clin Nutr. 2010;92:841–8.
208. Sanders KM, Stuart AL, Williamson EJ, Simpson JA, Kotowicz MA, Young D, et al. Annual high-dose oral vitamin D and falls and fractures in older women. JAMA. 2010;303:1815–22.
209. Rothwell PM, Fowkes FG, Belch JK, Ogawa H, Warlow CP, Meade TW. Effect of daily aspirin on long-term risk of death due to cancer: analysis of individual patient data from randomized trials. Lancet. 2011;377:31–41.
210. Jalving M, Gietema JA, Lefrandt JD, de Jong S, Reyners AK, Gans RO, et al. Metformin: taking

away the candy for cancer? Eur J Cancer. 2010;46: 2369–80.

211. Diabetes Prevention Program Research Group. 10-year follow-up of diabetes incidence and weight loss in the Diabetes Prevention Program Outcomes Study. Lancet. 2009;374:1677–86.
212. Platz EA, Till C, Goodman PJ, Parnes HL, Figg WD, Albanes D, et al. Men with low serum cholesterol have a lower risk of high-grade prostate cancer in the placebo arm of the Prostate Cancer Prevention Trial. Cancer Epidemiol Biomarkers Prev. 2009;18: 2807–13.
213. Murtola TJ, Visakorpi T, Lahtela J, Syvala H, Tammela TL. Statins and prostate cancer prevention: where we are now and future directions. Nat Clin Pract Urol. 2008;5:376–87.
214. St Sauver JL, Jacobsen SJ, Jacobson DJ, McGree ME, Girman CJ, Nehra A. Statin use and decreased risk of benign prostatic enlargement and lower urinary tract symptoms. BJU Int. 2011;107:443–50.
215. Dadkhah F, Safarinejad MR, Asgari MA, Hosseini SY, Lashay A, Amini E. Atorvastatin improves the response to sildenafil in hypercholesterolemic men with erectile dysfunction and not initially responsive to sildenafil. Int J Impot Res. 2010;22:51–60.
216. Solomon KR, Freeman MR. The complex interplay between cholesterol and prostate malignancy. Urol Clin N Am. 2011;38:243–59.
217. Moyad MA. Why a statin and/or another proven heart healthy agent should be utilized in the next major cancer chemoprevention trial: part I. Urol Oncol. 2004;22:466–71.
218. Moyad MA. Why a statin and/or another proven heart healthy agent should be utilized in the next major cancer chemoprevention trial: part II. Urol Oncol. 2004;22:472–7.
219. Moyad MA. Heart healthy equals prostate healthy equals statins: the next cancer chemoprevention trial. Part I. Curr Opin Urol. 2005;15:1–6.
220. Moyad MA. Heart healthy equals prostate healthy equals statins: the next cancer chemoprevention trial. Part II. Curr Opin Urol. 2005;15:7–12.
221. De Berardis G, Lucisano G, D'Ettorre A, Pellegrini F, Lepore V, Tognoni G, et al. Association of aspirin use with major bleeding in patients with and without diabetes. JAMA. 2012;307:2286–94.
222. Dell'Aglio DM, Perino LJ, Kazzi Z, Abramson J, Schwartz MD, Morgan BW. Acute metformin overdose: examining pH, lactate level, and metformin concentrations in survivors versus nonsurvivors: a systematic review of the literature. Ann Emerg Med. 2009;54:818–23.
223. Zaharan NL, Williams D, Bennett K. Statins and risk of treated incident diabetes in a primary care population. Br J Clin Pharmacol. 2013;75:1118–24.
224. American Urological Association. Guidelines at a glance: a quick reference for Urologists-2012. Linthicum, MD: American Urological Association; 2012.
225. Montague DK, Jarow JP, Broderick GA, Dmochowski RR, Heaton JP, Lue TF, Erectile Dysfunction Guideline Update Panel, et al. Chapter 1: The management of erectile dysfunction: an AUA update. J Urol. 2005;174:230–9.

2 BPH/LUTS: Heart Healthy = Prostate Healthy

Introduction

There is little question currently that BPH prevention and perhaps partial treatment may occur via heart-healthy processes [1, 2]. Almost all documented heart-healthy interventions or lifestyle changes can prevent some aspect of BPH/LUTS. It is also interesting that some of the older and emerging cardiovascular risk markers may also be predictive of LUTS severity. For example, the Boston Area Community Health survey looked at a random sample of 5,502 adults aged 30–79 years [3]. LUTS was defined as an American Urological Association Symptom Index (AUASI) of 8 or higher. Significant correlation was found among men and women for LUTS and higher CRP, which suggested that LUTS is also an inflammatory process. Of course, there are also some processes of BPH that are clearly out of the realm of complete lifestyle control; for example, it is also well recognized that aging and/or genetics plays a role in the etiology of BPH for many men [4–7]. It is interesting that some of these past studies suggest a very strong genetic and familial component with BPH. Regardless, the focus of this chapter is on lifestyle changes or parameters that may or may not impact BPH.

Alcohol

Regular alcohol intake appears to lower the risk of BPH, and the form of alcohol and perhaps quantity does not appear to make a difference. It is interesting that an experimental technique that involves an intraprostatic injection of approximately 6–12 mL of absolute ethanol at 5–10 sites in the prostate ("transurethral ethanol ablation") has had moderate success thus far in treating BPH. Significant positive changes have been observed in International Prostate Symptom Score (IPSS), maximum flow rate (Q_{max}), mean residual volume (PVR), and prostate volume within several months. This technique causes a coagulative necrosis of the tissues via dehydration and nerve ending alpha-receptor destruction [8–10]. Obviously intraprostatic injection of alcohol is different from consumption of alcohol, but perhaps not radically different.

Earlier and even recent prospective or other epidemiologic studies, such as the Health Professionals Follow-up Study and others, continue to suggest that moderate and even larger alcohol intakes could be associated with a lower risk of BPH [11–15], which could be more efficacious in those with a lower body mass index (BMI). Additionally, the derivation of the alcohol

M.A. Moyad, *Complementary & Alternative Medicine for Prostate and Urologic Health*,
DOI 10.1007/978-1-4614-8492-9_2, © Springer Science+Business Media New York 2014

(beer, hard liquor, or wine) did not matter. Regardless, arguably the most convincing evidence that alcohol might lower BPH risk was a meta-analysis of 19 studies that included 120,091 men; 16 studies were candidates for pooled analysis, and 12 of these considered BPH to be the primary outcome [16]. Alcohol intakes across most levels of consumption were associated with a significant reduction in BPH. For example, even an alcohol intake of 36 g/day or more was correlated with a 35 % reduction in risk ($p < 0.001$). Interestingly, the inverse relationships appeared to be more robust with increased intake, but all dosage intakes provided protection. Yet the protection afforded with alcohol was not observed with LUTS. The authors point to the potential beneficial effects of alcohol as further evidence that "systemic metabolic disturbances may drive BPH pathogenesism" so that a multitude of heart-healthy protective mechanisms could protect against BPH. It is also plausible that lower androgen levels in heavy drinkers [13], a reduced sympathetic tone, and even HDL increases could be other mechanisms whereby BPH is prevented or progression rates are reduced [17].

Blood Pressure/Hypertension

Prescription alpha-blockers for BPH were first developed and utilized for hypertension [18]. Thus, it should not be a surprise that high blood pressure mitigation or the prevention of hypertension may reduce BPH. The metabolic syndrome, which includes obesity, dyslipidemia, hypertension, and glucose abnormality, appears to be correlated with BPH risk [19]. Thus, again, it is not a surprise that hypertension can increase the risk of or exacerbate BPH [20].

Caffeine/Coffee

Few studies have been conducted on caffeine sources, especially coffee and BPH. The scarce data demonstrate either no impact of coffee on BPH [21–23] or a slightly increased risk [12]. In reality, many of these past studies are from Europe (Italy), where coffee drinking itself is associated with other behaviors, which would make it difficult to truly isolate the impact of this kind of consumption. Regardless, in my opinion patients should be encouraged to consume coffee or caffeine in moderation, not only for their quality of life but because more recent overall general health data have reported multiple potential positive outcomes from reduced rates of liver, brain, and other neurologic diseases [24].

Caloric Intake

Preliminary evidence is beginning to accumulate that some form of caloric restriction might delay the onset of numerous diseases and theoretically improves survival from a variety of diseases [25]. Interestingly, at least in laboratory and animal studies, there have been consistent reductions in the following parameters with some form of caloric restriction:

- Fat mass
- Inflammatory markers
- Insulin
- Insulin insensitivity
- IGF-1
- Oxidative stress
- Sympathetic activity
- Thyroid axis
- Visceral fat

Thus, it is not surprising that caloric control has some evidence in animals that it may inhibit prostate cell proliferation rates [26, 27]. Some of the researchers from the randomized, placebo-controlled trial known as the Prostate Cancer Prevention Trial (PCPT) decided to try to answer a critical dietary question [28]. A total of 3,341 men from the placebo arm of the PCPT were evaluated during 6 years of the trial. The original trial included 5 mg of daily finasteride versus placebo to prevent prostate cancer, but this study analyzed observational data from the placebo arm of this trial. Low caloric intake was independently associated with a significantly lower PSA velocity ($p = 0.05$). Thus, it is probable that a lower caloric intake could be associated with a healthier profile and reduces prostate cell proliferation rates.

It is interesting that a recent clinical trial of 31 abdominally obese type 2 diabetic men actually tested whether a severe caloric restriction diet (−1,000 cal/day) or a high-protein reduced-calorie diet (−600 cal/day) could impact urologic markers [29]. Remarkably, within 8 weeks there were significant improvements with both diets with glucose, LDL, IIEF-5, sexual desire inventory (SDI), and IPSS. After 8 weeks, all of the participants were then maintained on the −600 calorie, high-protein diet for 44 weeks; after 1 year the results were maintained, including reductions in inflammatory markers and further improvements in IIEF-5, SDI, and IPSS scores. Thus, just 5–10 % body weight reduction in a short or over a longer period has immediate and sustainable impacts on a variety of urologic parameters, including BPH/LUTS.

It should also be noted that as interesting as it is that some form of caloric restriction has an impact on health parameters, it is not an easy task to follow on a regular basis. Although weight-loss goals can be achieved for some individuals without any exercise at all, it should also be reiterated that exercise provides a mental health boost and reduction of the more unhealthy visceral fat that caloric restriction is not able to achieve in human clinical trials [30]. In addition, I am often asked if caloric restriction of some form matters in the minority of individuals who excessively exercise. In other words, if an individual is able to maintain heart-healthy parameters, including weight, but consumes an excessive amount of calories and eliminates them through exercise (like some Olympic athletes), is that permissible and healthy? Research has not adequately addressed this issue, but it appears that caloric excess in the setting of excessive exercise and the maintenance of heart-healthy parameters is also a healthy scenario, but this again is based on opinion, because there is a lack of clinical data addressing this interesting issue.

Cardiovascular Disease Markers (LDL, HDL Triglycerides, Etc.) and Inflammation

Despite being mentioned earlier, it is important to reiterate and slightly expand on the concept that increases in cardiovascular and inflammatory markers appear to be associated with an increase in BPH or the progression of this condition [1–3]. There is some preliminary data to suggest that one or more abnormal lipid markers may increase the risk of BPH in some individuals [31], but this should not be a surprise, because the prostate itself produces and stores large amounts of cholesterol [32]. Thus, any abnormalities in cholesterol metabolism might cause detrimental effects on prostate tissue. Reductions in LDL and triglycerides and improvements in HDL could prevent or delay the progression of BPH.

For example, CRP tends to be a marker of systemic inflammation but may also be a marker of intraprostatic inflammatory changes [33], and prostatitis and infections of the prostate also appear to be related to BPH and/or clinical outcomes of some BPH patients [34, 35]. It should also be of interest that a preliminary cohort study found a lower risk of BPH and the progression of this condition with regular use of nonsteroidal anti-inflammatory drugs (NSAIDs) [36] and a randomized trial of celecoxib (100 mg at 9 PM) versus placebo for refractory nocturia from BPH found a significant improvement in this parameter [37]. This evidence suggests that at least reducing inflammation might favorably impact this disease. Interventions that positively impact lipid and inflammatory markers may improve BPH prognosis when utilized early and in the right patient [38, 39], but whether or not they will improve outcomes any better than existing BPH treatments is highly questionable [40].

Diabetes/Glucose Intolerance/Metabolic Syndrome

There is a strong association in the medical literature of glucose intolerance and BPH incidence and progression. Higher glucose and insulin levels may act as a mitogen on prostate tissue and appear to accelerate BPH, and this has been known for quite some time [41–46]. Insulin resistance is a key component of the metabolic syndrome, and these synergistic negative parameters may provide a multifactorial etiology for this condition. For example, excessive insulin may stimulate the liver to produce more insulin-like growth factor (IGF-1), and multiple areas along the IGF pathway, including in and around the prostate, may be impacted [47–49]. Additionally, secretion of other growth factors, such as fibroblast growth factor (FGF), can also occur in diabetic prostate tissue [50].

Fiber/Flaxseed/Omega-3/Soy or Soy Protein

Food products that contain fiber may reduce all-cause mortality [51], are generally heart healthy, and provide protection against a vast array of aging conditions [52–58]. An ability to lower blood pressure, cholesterol, glucose, inflammation, and weight simply suggests it may be an ideal BPH preventive agent, but there is minimal research for fiber in this area of medicine. Preliminary clinical evidence suggests that fiber may lower PSA and slow the growth of proliferative benign prostate tissue [59, 60].

Perhaps the potential positive clinical data for fiber can be found in the low-cost food product flaxseed, which has generated preliminary positive data. Flaxseed is high in fiber and plant estrogens (lignans), is one of the largest sources of plant omega-3 fatty acids (alpha-linolenic acid), and has a history of favorably impacting lipid levels [61–63]. A preliminary clinical trial that examined tissue from BPH patients before and after three rounded tablespoons of ground flaxseed (30 g total per day for 6 months) daily along with a low-fat diet found significant reductions in PSA, cholesterol, and proliferation rates [64]. A subsequent randomized trial from this same group found that proliferation rates were impacted more by flaxseed alone compared to a low-fat diet in men with prostate cancer [65]. It is also of interest that a recent flaxseed-derived supplement made of purified lignan extract (secoisolariciresinol diglucoside, or SDG) at 300 or 600 mg/day showed favorable and significant results compared to a placebo in a clinical trial of 87 participants over a 4-month period [66]. IPSS were reduced by approximately 7 points in the intervention arms compared to 3.5 points in the placebo group with additional improvements in quality of life. Similar SDG derivatives of a variety of doses have also now been found to preliminarily and significantly reduce cholesterol and glucose values [67, 68]. Whether or not ingesting low-cost flaxseed as well as an SDG supplement will reduce BPH symptoms has not been studied, but it is worth an attempt for some patients.

It should be of some interest that dietary soy products have a somewhat similar characteristic to flaxseed because they contain fiber and omega-3 from plants and are one of the largest food concentration sources of phytoestrogens (isoflavones) [69]. Older laboratory studies have found that genistein, one of soy's principal isoflavones, could reduce the growth of BPH and prostate cancer tissue in histoculture [70]. Otherwise, the overall medical literature in the area of BPH and soy is minimal, based on a lack of research with some scant positive data from case–control studies [71]. A 40-mg soy isoflavone supplement given for 1 year ($n = 1{,}670$) did not perform much better than placebo, but the groups (control and intervention) in this trial experienced significant within-group positive effects on BPH parameters [72]. In the meantime because of the heart-healthy properties of dietary soy, it should be encouraged for BPH patients, which is why I recommend it. It is an outstanding source of high-quality protein that can help improve lipid values and cardiovascular outcomes and be utilized with pharmacologic agents. Only 15–30 g/day of soy protein is needed for some tangible numerical results [73]. The American Heart Association provided an earlier recommendation of 25–50 g of soy protein per day for cholesterol reduction [74]. Perhaps the addition of a high-quality protein powder to a patient's diet as a substitute for calories or unhealthy food sources may be just as effective [75]. Regardless, if fiber or flaxseed or even soy protein is recommended to your patients with or without BPH, the good news is that past studies have not found any clinically relevant or profound negative changes in androgen levels in men with these healthy foods [64, 65, 76], but, in some rare cases, a potential slight reduction in testosterone level [77].

Fruits and Vegetables

There are only a minimal number of studies examining the relationship between fruit and vegetable consumption and the risk of BPH [14, 71, 78, 79]. The totality of the evidence thus far demonstrates a consistent pattern of BPH reduction with increasing vegetable intake only [14]. One of the largest prospective epidemiologic studies in the world to evaluate the impact of fruit, vegetable, and nutrient consumption with the risk of BPH is the Health Professionals Follow-Up Study (HPFS) [78]. The average age of the men was 52–54 years, and every 2 years the health status of the participants was determined by questionnaires and medical records for a period of over 14 years. BPH cases were men that reported having surgery or who had an AUASI of 15–35, which included 6,092 men compared to 7,800 men without BPH with an AUA score of 7 or less (n=18,373). Men with an AUASI of 8–14 were not included in this study (n=7,800). Vegetable consumption is significantly (p trend=0.03) and inversely correlated with BPH, with the highest consumption being associated with 11 % reduction in risk. However, fruit intake was not associated with the risk of BPH. The most significant reduction in the risk of BPH was found for increasing vitamin C intake from food (p for trend=0.009). Vitamin E intake from foods was not associated with the risk of BPH. Thus, a diet high in vegetable intake may lower the risk of BPH. Still, the highest intake of fruits and vegetables was almost ten servings a day in this study! However, I find it most interesting that men with the highest intake of healthy foods also were less likely to smoke, more likely to drink in moderation, more physically active, and had the highest intake of dietary fiber per day. In other words, this study sends a very important message, which is the sum of what one does in moderation provides a bigger benefit than one or two healthy behavioral changes in extreme.

A case–control study from Milan, Italy, of 1,369 patients compared to 1,451 controls utilizing trained interviewers found a 59 % reduction in BPH in the highest category of intake of Allium vegetables, specifically onion and garlic intake, even after controlling for confounding factors and utilizing a multivariate odds ratio [79]. An earlier study from this same research group supported the findings that vegetables may reduce the risk of BPH [21]. Again, the epidemiologic research dating back over a period of over 30 years continues to suggest that vegetable consumption reduces the risk of BPH [80, 81].

Physical Activity/Exercise

Perhaps one of the greatest lifestyle changes that has been consistently documented to prevent BPH/LUTS or the progression of this condition is regular physical activity. A meta-analysis of 11 studies involving over 43,000 men found that moderate to vigorous physical activity reduced the risk of BPH or LUTS by approximately 25 % compared to sedentary lifestyle [82]. Men would have to engage in at least 30 min of light to moderate physical activity per day, approximately 6–7 days a week, to potentially maximize their benefits in this area.

A past study of obesity and BPH in the HPFS found that physical activity was correlated with a lower risk of BPH possibly by maintaining a healthy weight and through other heart-healthy mechanisms [83]. A follow-up retrospective study to the HPFS identified 1,890 men who had BPH surgery or 1,853 men who scored 15 or more points out of 35 on the seven questions from the American Urological Association Symptom Score (AUASS) [84]. A total of 21,745 men were considered controls because they scored 7 points or less on the same symptom score. Researchers controlled for age, race, alcohol intake, and smoking status. Greater physical activity was significantly and inversely related to total BPH (25 % reduction), surgery for BPH (24 % reduction), and symptomatic BPH (25 % reduction). Interestingly, walking was the most prevalent physical activity, and men who walked 2–3 h a week had a 25 % reduction in risk for total BPH. Men that were more physically active were also less likely to smoke, were leaner, less likely to have diabetes, and more likely to consume alcohol and more calories. In the Physicians' Health Study, men who exercised had a reduced risk of BPH surgery compared to sedentary men [85]. However, men who exercised experienced an increased risk with increasing amount of exercise that may have resulted because of the small number of men ($n = 320$) studied or because men in this cohort who exercise regularly are more likely to be treated for BPH compared to men who do not exercise as much. The Massachusetts Male Aging Study included 1,709 men followed for 9 years, and increasing levels of physical activity was associated with a reduced risk of BPH [86]. Men in the highest level of physical activity had an odds ratio of 0.5 (50 % reduction) compared to men in the lowest levels of physical activity.

Perhaps the first of its kind randomized trial of an exercise regimen demonstrated a benefit for men with BPH [87]. This study from Korea investigated the impact of regular tai chi exercise on LUTS, quality of life, and sex hormone levels in men with BPH. A total of 56 participants (mean age of approximately 70 years) were randomized into the tai chi or control group. The tai chi intervention consisted of 11 basic and 9 combination movements for a total of 20 overall movements. The first 15 min consisted of warm-up stretching exercises, the next 40 min involved the 20 primary movements, and there was a 5-min cool-down stretching exercise. Men in the tai chi group attended classes three times per week for a total of 12 weeks. Participants were also asked to practice their exercises two times per day at home (morning and evening). The control group members were contacted twice by phone over 12 weeks to confirm their inactivity levels. No significant baseline differences were found between the tai chi and control group in terms of marriage status, education, employment, income, perceived health status, surgical prostate history, medication use for prostate issues, or exercise status. IPPS decreased significantly in the tai chi group compared to control (−4.14 vs. +0.71) after 12 weeks, and quality of life also significantly improved with this exercise intervention, including specific reductions in urination discomfort, worry and concern (significant difference), and interference with daily activities. There was no impact of tai chi on insulin or glucose, but a significant increase in testosterone in the exercise group. Two serious limitations of this novel clinical trial were the 50 % dropout rate that occurred in both the intervention and the control group, which the researchers attributed to the older age of the participants and compliance enforcement issues and a lack of monitoring other heart-healthy parameters to provide other potential mechanisms of action, such as blood pressure responses, in the intervention compared to the control group. It should not be surprising that tai chi or other forms of exercise or even meditation and stress reduction techniques could improve BPH symptoms via a variety of diverse heart-healthy mechanisms. For example, a systematic review of 26 past tai chi studies that included nine randomized trials found that in 22 past studies there were blood pressure reductions with tai chi of 3- to 32-mm Hg systolic and 2- to 18-mm Hg diastolic [88]. A recent randomized trial of 96 elderly participants without BPH and a mean age of 69 years found a significant improvement in sleep quality, cognitive performance, and balance compared to the control group after 6 months of twice-a-week 60-min tai chi sessions [89]. However, the dropout rate was 19 %, which again demonstrates that a commitment to exercise is not a simple task. Hence, multiple healthy beneficial changes could translate into tangible changes for BPH patients that can be used with or without other conventional options.

Thus, when considering the totality of the data, there is a striking reduction in the risk of BPH and outcomes with regular physical activity, which is attributed to a variety of mechanisms from lower sympathetic tone, reduction in weight gain, glucose normalization, favorable lipid profile, and so forth [90].

Smoking/Tobacco

There are no strong positive or negative associations with tobacco utilization and BPH, with some studies reporting reductions [15, 91, 92] and others an increased risk in heavy smokers, for example, 35 or more cigarettes/day [11], which could be due to sympathetic overload with excessive tobacco utilization [93]. Overall there is no strong association with tobacco and risk of BPH [93], but the impact of tobacco on morbidity and mortality is enough of a reason to promote immediate smoking cessation [94, 95].

Weight/Waist Circumference/BMI

Prostate volume and an increase in the severity of obstructive urinary symptoms appear to be correlated with an increase in adipose tissue [44, 45, 96]. Estimates of up to 1.0 mL/year growth in prostate tissue have emerged from past studies of obese patients that harbor multiple other heart-unhealthy parameters [44, 45]. Data from the Baltimore Study of Longitudinal Aging (prospective community cohort) found prostate volume increases with each single point increase in BMI and a striking 3.5 times higher risk of prostate enlargement in obese compared to non-obese participants [42]. Another study of 409 consecutive men in the United States analyzed for waist circumference (WC) differences and outcomes found that WC was correlated significantly with a greater prostate volume, PSA, and IPSS and a greater likelihood of other metabolic syndrome issues [97]. It is of interest that 10 % body weight loss in just 8 weeks led to a significant mean reduction in IPSS scores of over 6 points in non-diabetic obese men and just over 2 points in diabetic men [98], which should encourage clinicians to promote weight loss as early as possible to potentially improve urinary function with or without conventional medicine.

Conclusion

BPH/LUTS has a multifactorial etiology, but patients need simplistic advice apart from just medical intervention on how to prevent and slow the progression of this disease, which can have such profound effects on quality of life. The plethora of evidence continues to point toward heart disease risk factors as initiating and promoting BPH [1, 2, 99], and clinicians need to embrace the concept that heart health is tantamount to prostate health.

Table 2.1 is a summary of the major findings of this review on lifestyle factors and BPH that can be easily explained to patients. Trying to explain how to combat this condition in any other fashion is much too time-consuming and confusing, in my opinion. There is no question that certain non-lifestyle factors beyond the clinician's control, such as socioeconomic status and genetics, also play some role in promoting BPH [100], but the vast majority of the evidence points toward positive heart-healthy lifestyle changes as a potential method to combat this condition right now!

Table 2.1 A review of lifestyle factors that may or may not prevent BPH/LUTS and/or the progression of this condition

Lifestyle factors that could affect the risk and progression of BPH	Does it impact BPH/LUTS? Commentary
Alcohol	Yes Associated with a reduced risk with regular consumption, and source and quantity of alcohol do not appear to matter (moderation is the rule). HDL increase, reduced androgen levels, and reduced sympathetic tone may be part of the reason. Keep in mind that excessive alcohol consumption can increase sympathetic tone/blood pressure
Aging, genetics, and family history	Yes Consistent data suggest that BPH is profoundly increased with genetic/family history of BPH. Obviously these are not lifestyle factors, but patients need to be aware of these non-lifestyle influences
Blood pressure	Yes Hypertension appears to increase the risk of BPH via sympathetic overdrive and other factors

(continued)

Table 2.1 (continued)

Lifestyle factors that could affect the risk and progression of BPH	Does it impact BPH/LUTS? Commentary
Caffeine/coffee	No Caffeine from a favorite beverage in moderation should still be encouraged because of overall healthy benefits
Caloric intake (fat, protein, etc.)	Yes Larger caloric intakes that cause heart-unhealthy changes appear to increase risk of BPH via weight gain and other metabolic disturbances. Greater caloric intakes without weight gain or without heart-unhealthy parameter changes may not increase BPH (so-called Olympic athlete effect)
Cardiovascular disease	Yes Lower cardiovascular disease risk is associated with lower risk of BPH via multiple heart-healthy parameters
Cholesterol/lipid levels/ inflammatory markers	Yes Lower HDL, higher triglycerides, and high LDL and CRP increase the risk of BPH, and the prostate itself is highly sensitive to cholesterol disturbances
Diabetes/glucose intolerance/ metabolic syndrome	Yes Higher insulin and glucose levels appear to act as a mitogen or growth factors for prostate tissue. Every abnormal metabolic syndrome parameter (dyslipidemia, waist size, glucose, blood pressure) can increase the risk of BPH
Fiber/flaxseed/soy/ omega-3 intake	Yes All of these dietary factors now have ample evidence that they are heart healthy and may reduce the risk of BPH
Fruit and vegetable consumption	Yes for vegetables and no for fruit Increasing vegetable intake appears protective against BPH, but fruit consumption does not. Most of the evidence suggests any type of vegetable consumption may be protective, and the caloric content of most vegetables tends to be low, but the fiber and healthy nutritional content is excellent for many vegetables
Glucose (fasting)	Yes Higher insulin and glucose levels appear to act as a mitogen or growth factors for prostate tissue
Physical activity/exercise/ stress reduction/tai chi or other stress-reducing exercises (yoga, pilates, meditation, etc.)	Definitely Multiple mechanisms from improving HDL and cholesterol, blood pressure and glucose normalization, sympathetic signal reduction, androgen stability, and a reduction in adipose tissue
Smoking/tobacco	No Not a consistent positive or negative impact, but the profound data on early morbidity and mortality rates from smoking-related diseases (bladder, kidney, lung, etc.) should be sufficient impetus to begin some form of smoking cessation immediately
Weight/waist size/BMI	Yes Increased aromatase activity, higher blood pressure, glucose, lipid, and inflammatory markers also may stimulate prostate tissue growth. A 5–10 % reduction in weight may improve a variety of urologic parameters, including urinary and quality-of-life symptom scores

References

1. Moyad MA. Lifestyle changes to prevent BPH: heart-healthy=prostate healthy. Urol Nurs. 2003;23:439–41.
2. Moyad MA, Lowe FC. Educating patients about lifestyle modifications for prostate health. Am J Med. 2008;121(8 Suppl 2):S34–42.
3. Kupelian V, McVary KT, Barry MJ, Link CL, Rosen RC, Aiyer LP, et al. Association of C-reactive protein and lower urinary tract symptoms in men and women: results from Boston Area Community Health Survey. Urology. 2009;73:950–7.
4. Partin AW, Page WF, Lee BR, Sanda MG, Miller RN, Walsh PC. Concordance rates for benign prostatic disease among twins suggest hereditary influence. Urology. 1994;44:646–50.

5. Sanda MG, Beaty TH, Stutzman RE, Childs B, Walsh PC. Genetic susceptibility of benign prostatic hyperplasia. J Urol. 1994;152:115–9.
6. Sanda MG, Doehring CB, Binkowitz B, Beaty TH, Partin AW, Hale E, et al. Clinical and biological characteristics of familial benign prostatic hyperplasia. J Urol. 1997;157:876–9.
7. Rohrmann S, Fallin MD, Page WF, Reed T, Partin AW, Walsh PC, et al. Concordance rates and modifiable risk factors for lower urinary tract symptoms in twins. Epidemiology. 2006;17:419–27.
8. Faruque MS, Alam MK, Ullah MA, Rahman MH, Kibria MG, Haque MM, et al. Evaluation of transurethral ethanol ablation of prostate for symptomatic benign prostatic hyperplasia. Mymensingh Med J. 2012;21:265–9.
9. Goya N, Ishikawa N, Ito F, Ryoji O, Tokumoto T, Toma H, Yamaguchi Y. Ethanol injection therapy of the prostate for benign prostatic hyperplasia: preliminary report on application of a new technique. J Urol. 1999;162:383–6.
10. Savoca G, De Stefani S, Gattuccio I, Paolinelli D, Stacul F, Belgrano E. Percutaneous ethanol injection of the prostate as minimally invasive treatment for benign prostatic hyperplasia: preliminary report. Eur Urol. 2001;40:504–8.
11. Platz EA, Rimm EB, Kawachi I, Colditz GA, Stampfer MJ, Willett WC, et al. Alcohol consumption, cigarette smoking, and risk of benign prostatic hyperplasia. Am J Epidemiol. 1999;149:106–15.
12. Gass R. Benign prostatic hyperplasia: the opposite effects of alcohol and coffee intake. BJU Int. 2002;90:649–54.
13. Crispo A, Talamini R, Gallus S, Negri E, Gallo A, Bosetti C, et al. Alcohol and the risk of prostate cancer and benign prostatic hyperplasia. Urology. 2004;64:717–22.
14. Kristal AR, Arnold KB, Schenk JM, Neuhouser ML, Goodman P, Penson DF, et al. Dietary patterns, supplement use, and the risk of symptomatic benign prostatic hyperplasia: results from the prostate cancer prevention trial. Am J Epidemiol. 2008;167:925–34.
15. Lee YJ, Jeong SJ, Byun SS, Lee JJ, Han JW, Kim KW. Prevalence and correlates of nocturia in community-dwelling older men: results from the Korean Longitudinal Study on Health and Aging. Korean J Urol. 2012;53:263–7.
16. Parsons JK, Im R. Alcohol consumption is associated with a decreased risk of benign prostatic hyperplasia. J Urol. 2009;182:1463–8.
17. Shen W, Yao HQ, Deng ZX, Zhang XM, Zhang LC, Hu WL. Arteriosclerotic risk factors and benign prostatic hyperplasia. Zhonghua Nan Ke Xue. 2010;16:29–33.
18. de Mey C. Cardiovascular effects of alpha-blockers used for the treatment of symptomatic BPH: impact on safety and well-being. Eur Urol. 1998;34 Suppl 2:18–28.
19. Abdollah F, Briganti A, Suardi N, Castiglione F, Gallina A, Capitanio U, et al. Metabolic syndrome and benign prostatic hyperplasia: evidence of a potential relationship, hypothesized etiology, and prevention. Korean J Urol. 2011;52:507–16.
20. Zhang X, Zhang J, Chen J, Zhang C, Li Q, Xu T, et al. Prevalence and risk factors of nocturia and nocturia-related quality of life in the Chinese population. Urol Int. 2011;86:173–8.
21. Bravi F, Bosetti C, Dal Maso L, Talamini R, Montella M, Negri E, et al. Food groups and risk of benign prostatic hyperplasia. Urology. 2006;67:73–9.
22. Prezioso D, Catuogno C, Galassi P, D'Andrea G, Castello G, Pirritano D. Life-style in patients with LUTS suggestive of BPH. Eur Urol. 2001;40 Suppl 1:9–12.
23. Signorello LB, Tzonou A, Lagiou P, Sarnoli E, Zavitsanos X, Trichopoulos D. The epidemiology of benign prostatic hyperplasia: a study in Greece. BJU Int. 1999;84:286–91.
24. Patil H, Lavie CJ, O'Keefe JH. Cuppa joe: friend or foe? Effects of chronic coffee consumption on cardiovascular and brain health. Mo Med. 2011;108:431–8.
25. Heilbronn LK, Ravussin E. Calorie restriction and aging: review of the literature and implications for studies in humans. Am J Clin Nutr. 2003;78:361–9.
26. Varady KA, Roohk DJ, Hellerstein MK. Dose effects of modified alternate-day fasting regimens on in vivo proliferation and plasma insulin-like growth factor-1 in mice. J Appl Physiol. 2007;103:547–51.
27. Blando J, Moore T, Hursting S, Jiang G, Saha G, Beltran L, et al. Dietary energy balance modulates prostate cancer progression in Hi-Myc mice. Cancer Prev Res (Phila). 2011;4:2002–14.
28. Kristal AR, Chi C, Tangen CM, Goodman PJ, Etzioni R, Thompson IM. Associations of demographic and lifestyle characteristics with prostate-specific antigen (PSA) concentration and rate of PSA increase. Cancer. 2006;106:320–8.
29. Khoo J, Piantadosi C, Duncan R, Worthley SG, Jenkins A, Noakes M, et al. Comparing effects of a low-energy diet and a high-protein low-fat diet on sexual and endothelial function, urinary tract symptoms, and inflammation in obese diabetic men. J Sex Med. 2011;8:2868–75.
30. Coker RH, Williams RH, Yeo SE, Kortebein PM, Bodenner DL, Kern PA, et al. The impact of exercise training compared to caloric restriction on hepatic and peripheral insulin resistance in obesity. J Clin Endocrinol Metab. 2009;94:4258–66.
31. Parsons JK, Bergstrom J, Barrett-Connor E. Lipids, lipoproteins and the risk of benign prostatic hyperplasia in community-dwelling men. BJU Int. 2008;101:313–8.
32. Freeman MR, Solomon KR. Cholesterol and benign prostate disease. Differentiation. 2011;82:244–52.
33. Rohrmann S, De Marzo AM, Smit E, Giovannucci E, Platz EA. Serum C-reactive protein concentration and lower urinary tract symptoms in older men in the Third National Health and Nutrition Examination Survey (NHANES III). Prostate. 2005;62:27–33.
34. Sutcliffe S, Giovannucci E, De Marzo AM, Willett WC, Platz EA. Sexually transmitted infections,

prostatitis, ejaculation frequency and the odds of lower urinary tract symptoms. Am J Epidemiol. 2005;162:898–906.
35. Sutcliffe S, Rohrmann S, Giovannucci E, Nelson KE, De Marzo AM, Issacs WB, et al. Viral infections and lower urinary tract symptoms in the Third National Health and Nutrition Examination Survey. J Urol. 2007;178:2181–5.
36. St Sauver JL, Jacobson DJ, McGree ME, Lieber MM, Jacobsen SJ. Protective association between nonsteroidal anti-inflammatory drug use and measures of benign prostatic hyperplasia. Am J Epidemiol. 2006;164:760–8.
37. Falahatkar S, Mokhtari G, Pourreza F, Asgari SA, Kamran AN. Celecoxib for treatment of nocturia caused by benign prostatic hyperplasia: a prospective, randomized, double-blind, placebo-controlled study. Urology. 2008;72:813–6.
38. Padayatty SJ, Marcelli M, Shao TC, Cunningham GR. Lovastatin-induced apoptosis in prostate stromal cells. J Clin Endocrinol Metab. 1997;82:1434–9.
39. Marino G, Pugno E, Cevoli R, Griffa D, Pastorini S, Cocimano V. Phamracologic treatment of benign prostatic hypertrophy (BPH): a combination of mepartricin and simvastatin. Analysis and results. Minerva Urol Nefrol. 1991;43:279–82.
40. Stamatiou KN, Zaglavira P, Skolarikos A, Sofras F. The effects of lovastatin on conventional medical treatment of lower urinary tract symptoms with finasteride. Int Braz J Urol. 2008;34:555–61.
41. Kim WT, Yun SJ, Choi YD, Kim GY, Moon SK, Choi YH, et al. Prostate size correlates with fasting blood glucose in non-diabetic benign prostatic hyperplasia patients with normal testosterone levels. J Korean Med Sci. 2011;26:1214–8.
42. Parsons JK, Carter HB, Partin AW, Windham BG, Metter EJ, Ferrucci L, et al. Metabolic factors associated with benign prostatic hyperplasia. J Clin Endocrinol Metab. 2006;91:2562–8.
43. Parson JK. Modifiable risk factors for benign prostatic hyperplasia and lower urinary tract symptoms: new approaches to old problems. J Urol. 2007;178:395–401.
44. Hammarsten J, Hogstedt B. Clinical, anthropometric, metabolic and insulin profile of men with fast annual growth rates of benign prostatic hyperplasia. Blood Press. 1999;8:29–36.
45. Hammarsten J, Hogstedt B. Calculated fast-growing benign prostatic hyperplasia—a risk factor for developing clinical prostate cancer. Scand J Urol Nephrol. 2002;36:330–8.
46. Sarma AV, St Sauver JL, Hollingsworth JM, Jacobson DJ, McGree ME, Dunn RL, et al. Diabetes treatment and progression of benign prostatic hyperplasia in community-dwelling black and white men. Urology. 2012;79:102–8.
47. Wang Z, Olumi AF. Diabetes, growth hormone-insulin-like growth factor pathways and association to benign prostatic hyperplasia. Differentiation. 2011;82:261–71.
48. Cohen P, Peehl DM, Baker B, Liu F, Hintz RL, Rosenfeld RG. Insulin-like growth factor axis abnormalities in prostate stromal cells from patients with benign prostatic hyperplasia. J Clin Endocrinol Metab. 1994;79:1410–5.
49. Boudon C, Rodier G, Lechevallier E, Mottet N, Barenton B, Sultan C. Secretion of insulin-like growth factors and their binding proteins by human normal and hyperplastic prostatic cells in primary culture. J Clin Endocrinol Metab. 1996;81:612–7.
50. Wang Z, Ikeda K, Wada Y, Foster HE, Weiss RM, Latifpour J. Expression and localization of basic fibroblast growth factor in diabetic rat prostate. BJU Int. 2000;85:945–52.
51. Park Y, Subar AF, Hollenbeck A, Schatzkin A. Dietary fiber intake and mortality in the NIH-AARP diet and health study. Arch Intern Med. 2011;171:1061–8.
52. Eshak ES, Iso H, Date C, Kikuchi S, Watanabe Y, Wada Y, et al. Dietary fiber intake is associated with reduced risk of mortality from cardiovascular disease among Japanese men and women. J Nutr. 2010;140:1445–53.
53. Moreyra AE, Wilson AC, Koraym A. Effect of combining psyllium fiber with simvastatin in lowering cholesterol. Arch Intern Med. 2005;165:1161–6.
54. Agrawal AR, Tandon M, Sharma PL. Effect of combining viscous fibre with lovastatin on serum lipids in normal human subjects. Int J Clin Pract. 2007;61:1812–8.
55. Streppel MT, Arends LR, van't Veer P, Grobbee DE, Geleijnse JM. Dietary fiber and blood pressure: a meta-analysis of randomized placebo-controlled trials. Arch Intern Med. 2005;165:150–6.
56. Vernay M, Aidara M, Salanave B, Deschamps V, Malon A, Oleko A, et al. Diet and blood pressure in 18–74 year old adults: the French Nutrition and Health Survey (ENNS, 2006–2007). J Hypertens. 2012;30(10):1920–7.
57. Marlett JA, McBurney MI, Slavin JL, for the American Dietetic Association. Position of the American Dietetic Association: health implications of dietary fiber. J Am Diet Assoc. 2002;102:993–1000.
58. Kaczmarczyk MM, Miller MJ, Freund GG. The health benefits of dietary fiber: beyond the usual suspects of type 2 diabetes mellitus, cardiovascular disease and colon cancer. Metabolism. 2012;61:1058–66.
59. Barnard RJ, Kobayashi N, Aronson WJ. Effect of diet and exercise intervention on the growth of prostate epithelial cells. Prostate Cancer Prostatic Dis. 2008;11:362–6.
60. Tariq N, Jenkins DJA, Vidgen E, et al. Effect of soluble fiber diets on serum prostate specific antigen in men. J Urol. 2000;163:114–8.
61. Pan A, Yu D, Demark-Wahnefried W, Franco OH, Lin X. Meta-analysis of the effects of flaxseed interventions on blood lipids. Am J Clin Nutr. 2009;90:288–97.

62. Rodriguez-Leyva D, Dupasquier CM, McCullough R, Pierce GN. The cardiovascular effects of flaxseed and its omega-3 fatty acid, alpha-linolenic acid. Can J Cardiol. 2010;26:489–96.
63. Bravi F, Bosetti C, Dal Maso L, Talmini R, Montella M, Negri E, et al. Macronutrients, fatty acids, cholesterol, and risk of benign prostatic hyperplasia. Urology. 2006;67:1205–11.
64. Denmark-Wahnefried W, Robertson CN, Walther PJ, Polascik TJ, Paulson DF, Vollmer RT. Pilot study to explore effects of low-fat, flaxseed-supplemented diet on proliferation on benign prostatic epithelium and prostate-specific antigen. Urology. 2004;63:900–4.
65. Demark-Wahnefried W, Polascik TJ, George SL, Switzer BR, Madden JF, Ruffin IV MT, et al. Flaxseed supplementation (not dietary fat restriction) reduces prostate cancer proliferation rates in men presurgery. Cancer Epidemiol Biomarkers Prev. 2008;17:3577–87.
66. Zhang W, Wang X, Liu Y, Tian H, Flickinger B, Empie MW, et al. Effects of dietary flaxseed lignan extract on symptoms of benign prostatic hyperplasia. J Med Food. 2008;11:207–14.
67. Zhang W, Wang X, Liu Y, Tian H, Flickinger B, Empie MW, Sun SZ. Dietary flaxseed lignan extract lowers plasma cholesterol and glucose concentrations in hypercholesterolaemic subjects. Br J Nutr. 2008;99:1301–19.
68. Fukumitsu S, Aida K, Shimizu H, Toyoda K. Flaxseed lignan lowers blood cholesterol and decreases liver disease risk factors in moderately hypercholesterolemic men. Nutr Res. 2010;30:441–6.
69. Moyad MA. No bogus science health advice. Ann Arbor, MI: Spry; 2010.
70. Geller J, Sionit L, Partido C, Li L, Tan X, Youngkin T, et al. Genistein inhibits the growth of human-patient BPH and prostate cancer in histoculture. Prostate. 1998;34:75–9.
71. Ambrosini GL, de Klerk NH, Mackerras D, Leavy J, Fritschi L. Dietary patterns and surgically treated benign prostatic hyperplasia: a case control study in Western Australia. BJU Int. 2008;101:853–60.
72. Wong WC, Wong EL, Li H, You JH, Ho S, Woo J, et al. Isoflavones in treating watchful waiting benign prostate hyperplasia: a double-blinded, randomized controlled trial. J Altern Complement Med. 2012;18:54–60.
73. Anderson JW, Bush HM. Soy protein effects on serum lipoproteins: a quality assessment and meta-analysis of randomized, controlled studies. J Am Coll Nutr. 2011;30:79–91.
74. Erdman Jr JW. Soy protein and cardiovascular disease: a statement for healthcare professionals from the nutrition committee of the AHA. Circulation. 2000;102:2555–9.
75. Sacks FM, Lichtenstein A, Van Horn L, Harris W, Kris-Etherton P, Winston M, et al. Soy protein, isoflavones, and cardiovascular health: an American Heart Association Science Advisory for professionals from the Nutrition Committee. Circulation. 2006;113:1034–44.
76. Hamilton-Reeves JM, Vazquez G, Duval SJ, Phipps WR, Kurzer MS, Messina MJ. Clinical studies show no effects of soy protein or isoflavones on reproductive hormones in men: results of a meta-analysis. Fertil Steril. 2010;94:997–1007.
77. Demark-Wahnefried W, Price DT, Polascik TJ, Robertson CN, Anderson EE, Paulson DF, et al. Pilot study of dietary fat restriction and flaxseed supplementation in men with prostate cancer before surgery: exploring the effects of hormonal levels, prostate-specific antigen, and histopathologic features. Urology. 2001;58:47–52.
78. Rohrmann S, Giovannucci E, Willett WC, Platz EA. Fruit and vegetable consumption, intake of nutrients, and benign prostatic hyperplasia in US men. Am J Clin Nutr. 2007;85:523–9.
79. Galeone C, Pelucchi C, Talamini R, Negri E, Dal Maso L, Montella M, et al. Onion and garlic intake and the odds of benign prostatic hyperplasia. Urology. 2007;70:672–6.
80. Araki H, Watanabe H, Mishina T, Nakao M. High-risk group for benign prostatic hypertrophy. Prostate. 1983;4:253–64.
81. Gu F. Changes in the prevalence of benign prostatic hyperplasia in China. Chin Med J (Engl). 1997;110:163–6.
82. Parsons JK, Kashefi C. Physical activity, benign prostatic hyperplasia, and lower urinary tract symptoms. Eur Urol. 2008;53:1228–35.
83. Giovannucci E, Rimm EB, Chute CG, Kawachi I, Colditz GA, Stampfer MJ, et al. Obesity and benign prostatic hyperplasia. Am J Epidemiol. 1994;140: 989–1002.
84. Platz EA, Kawachi I, Rimm EB, Colditz GA, Stampfer MJ, Willett WC, et al. Physical activity and benign prostatic hyperplasia. Arch Intern Med. 1998;158:2349–56.
85. Gann PH, Hennekens CH, Longcope C, Verhoek-Ottedahl W, Grodstein F, Stampfer MJ. A prospective study of plasma hormone levels, nonhormonal factors, and development of benign prostatic hyperplasia. Prostate. 1995;26:40–9.
86. Meigs JB, Mohr B, Barry MJ, Collins MM, McKinlay JB. Risk factors for clinical benign prostatic hyperplasia in a community-based population of healthy aging men. J Clin Epidemiol. 2001;54:935–44.
87. Jung S, Lee EN, Lee SR, Kim MS, Lee MS. Tai chi for lower urinary tract symptoms and quality of life in elderly patients with benign prostate hypertrophy: a randomized controlled trial. Evid Based Complement Alternat Med. 2012;2012: 624692.
88. Yeh GY, Wang C, Wayne PM, Phillips RS. The effect of tai chi exercise on blood pressure: a systematic review. Prev Cardiol. 2008;11:82–9.
89. Nguyen MH, Kruse A. A randomized controlled trial of Tai chi for balance, sleep quality and cognitive performance in elderly Vietnamese. Clin Interv Aging. 2012;7:185–90.

90. Sea J, Poon KS, McVary KT. Review of exercise and the risk of benign prostatic hyperplasia. Phys Sportsmed. 2009;37:75–83.
91. Kang D, Andriole GL, Van De Vooren RC, Crawford D, Chia D, Urban DA, et al. Risk behaviours and benign prostatic hyperplasia. BJU Int. 2004;93:1241–5.
92. Sarma AV, Jacobson DJ, St Sauver JL, Lieber MM, Girman CJ, Nehra A, et al. Smoking and acute urinary retention: the Olmsted County study of urinary symptoms and health status among men. Prostate. 2009;69:699–705.
93. Yun AJ, Doux JD. Opening the floodgates: benign prostatic hyperplasia may represent another disease in the compendium of ailments caused by global sympathetic bias that emerges with aging. Med Hypotheses. 2006;67:392–4.
94. Fagerstrom K. The epidemiology of smoking: health consequences and benefits of cessation. Drugs. 2002;62 Suppl 2:1–9.
95. Park HY, Sin D. Smoking kills, quitting heals: the importance of smoking cessation in COPD. Clin Respir J. 2011;5:185–6.
96. Parsons JK, Sarma AV, McVary K, Wei JT. Obesity and benign prostatic hyperplasia: clinical connections, emerging etiological paradigms and future directions. J Urol. 2009;182(6 Suppl):S27–31.
97. Lee RK, Chung D, Chughtai B, Te AE, Kaplan SA. Central obesity as measured by waist circumference is predictive of severity of lower urinary tract symptoms. BJU Int. 2012;110:540–5.
98. Khoo J, Piantadosi C, Worthley S, Wittert GA. Effects of a low-energy diet on sexual function and lower urinary tract symptoms in obese men. Int J Obes (Lond). 2010;34:1396–403.
99. Berger AP, Bartsch G, Deibl M, Alber H, Pachinger O, Fritsche G, et al. BJU Int. 2006;98:1038–42.
100. Fowke JH, Munro H, Signorello LB, Blot WJ, Penson DF, Urologic Diseases of America Project. Association between socioeconomic status (SES) and lower urinary tract symptom (LUTS) severity among black and white men. J Gen Intern Med. 2011;26:1305–10.

3 Complementary and Alternative Medicine Interventions for BPH/LUTS

Introduction

A plethora of CAM interventions, primarily dietary supplements, have been utilized in some preliminary clinical trials that have demonstrated an ability to reduce the symptoms of benign prostatic hyperplasia /lower urinary tract symptoms (BPH/LUTS) [1, 2]. It is my opinion that regardless of ample preliminary positive data, there are few clinicians and researchers (including myself) that believe a dietary supplement or CAM works faster or better compared to a pharmaceutical agent or out-patient conventional procedure. However, clinicians must keep in mind that for some patients the benefit-versus-risk scenario arguably favors a safe and cost-effective dietary supplement, in my opinion, that can be used initially for men with mild to moderate BPH along with lifestyle changes (heart healthy = prostate healthy), before or in addition to a conventional agent or procedure. In this chapter, a brief clinical review is offered for each CAM intervention that contains some data in the medical literature.

Acupuncture

Acupuncture has a potential role in multiple areas of urology—for example, hot flash reduction from androgen-deprivation treatment (ADT) [3], overactive bladder [4], monosymptomatic nocturnal enuresis [5], stress, and other forms of incontinence [6]—so it should not be surprising that acupuncture may have some role in alleviating BPH/LUTS [7]. Acupuncture can be delivered traditionally with needle insertion in a specific anatomical area or be primarily auricular or given as electroacupuncture. However, there are not enough data to recommend acupuncture for BPH/LUTS, and some small past studies suggest no clinical efficacy with this procedure [8]. Yet, theoretically by reducing blood pressure in some patients temporarily and other forms of sympathetic activity or insomnia in some clinical trials [9–11], it appears that some men could benefit by using acupuncture for adjuvant treatment of BPH/LUTS. Again this is based on theoretical benefits and no overt positive data. Patients should be careful about the out-of-pocket costs of any alternative medicine such as acupuncture, and in most clinical trials treatments are given just once or twice every 1–2 weeks and not daily.

Beta-Sitosterol (A Plant Sterol) Dietary Supplements

Phytosterols are found in a variety of plants and plant oils [12]. Phytosterols are similar in structure to cholesterol, except for minor structural differences. They are not synthesized in humans and minimally absorbed, excreted more rapidly from the liver compared to cholesterol, and not found in high concentrations in human tissues. The main phytosterols found in diet are sitosterol, stigmasterol, and campesterol. Beta-sitosterol is arguably the phytosterol found in

M.A. Moyad, *Complementary & Alternative Medicine for Prostate and Urologic Health*,
DOI 10.1007/978-1-4614-8492-9_3, © Springer Science+Business Media New York 2014

largest quantity in the diet. Phytosterols block the uptake of exogenous cholesterol from dietary and bile sources in the intestinal tract. LDL cholesterol is reduced by phytosterols, and HDL and triglycerides are not impacted. The blockage of cholesterol absorption may produce a relative cholesterol pool reduction that is followed by upregulation of cholesterol synthesis and LDL receptors, which can increase LDL removal. This is somewhat similar to how some healthy dietary fats found in many healthy foods, such as almonds or pistachios, may also reduce LDL and improve some specific urologic outcomes [13, 14].

An ample quantity of (over 40) clinical trials utilizing phytosterols themselves have been conducted that have ranged from 1 to 12 months in duration [12, 15, 16]. Plant sterols added to foods such as yogurt, margarine, orange juice, mayonnaise, olive oil, and milk have been shown to reduce LDL by approximately 10–15 % (mean of 10–11 %) when approximately 2,000 mg or more per day is ingested. And, 1,600–3,000 mg of plant sterol supplemental or tablet consumption can also reduce LDL by approximately 4–15 %. Plant sterols may also reduce the absorption of some fat-soluble vitamins, so there has been some debate as to whether multivitamin consumption should occur with the use of these products, and I agree that this should also be encouraged.

It is interesting that the primary mechanism of action of these sterols via cholesterol uptake reduction and a minor anti-inflammatory mechanism suggests, in my opinion, that they are weaker or less potent mimics of the drug ezetimibe (Zetia, Merck & Co., West Trenton, NJ), which can reduce LDL by approximately 20 % with a 10-mg dose [17, 18]. Laboratory research suggests ezetimibe favorably impacts prostate tissue and reduces BPH [19]. Ezetimibe is also commonly added to statin therapy or other lipid-lowering agents to achieve synergistic impacts and more favorably reduce LDL [17, 18]. Thus, it should not be surprising that beta-sitosterol by itself or with other lipid-lowering medications could reduce BPH progression and LUTS. For example, despite some data to suggest no impact of statins on established BPH over a short period of time [20, 21], other epidemiologic and past laboratory studies suggest potentially favorable impacts on BPH prevention and progression with cholesterol-lowering prescribed medications [22–25].

There are two critical and similar reviews that were published in 1999 that have allowed beta-sitosterol supplements to become a potential option for BPH [26, 27]. It is interesting that since this time period no other definitive clinical trials (positive or negative) have been published.

The first systematic review by Wilt et al. appeared in BJU International and identified studies from 1966 to 1998 [26]. A total of four clinical trials that included 519 men met the inclusion criteria [28–31]. All four were randomized, double-blind, placebo-controlled trials that included men with mild to moderate symptomatic BPH, and the intervention was given from 4 to 26 weeks. Beta-sitosterol significantly improved symptom scores and flow measures compared to placebo. For the two studies using IPSS scores, there was a −4.9 point difference (35 % urinary symptom score improvement), a 31 % improvement in quality-of-life score (one study), and the weighted mean difference for peak urinary flow rate and residual volume was 3.91 mL/s (45 % improvement) and −28.62 ml (24 % improvement) when all four studies were included. Beta-sitosterol had no impact on prostate size. It is interesting that a past animal study found that purified beta-sitosterol can inhibit 5-alpha reductase [32], but the inhibitory activity was dramatically lower compared to what has been observed with the drug finasteride, for example, in laboratory studies.

One of the four studies utilized in the meta-analyses utilized a unique form of beta-sitosterol known as "B-sitosterol-B-D-glucoside" (WA184), but this form did not improve urinary flow measures [28] compared to the positive benefits observed with higher doses (20 or 65 mg TID or 60–195 total per day) of beta-sitosterol within a mixture of phytosterols used in the other three effective clinical trials [29–31]. Overall, there were no differences in withdrawal rates in the beta-sitosterol (7.8 %) compared to the placebo groups (8.0 %) [26]. Gastrointestinal side effects were the most common side effects and occurred in 1.6 % of men on beta-sitosterol compared to 0 % on placebo. Erectile dysfunction was reported in approximately 0.5 % of men on beta-sitosterol and none on placebo. The authors of this systematic review concluded that beta-sitosterol "improves urological symptoms and flow measures" but that more long-term studies and standardization of beta-sitosterol preparations were needed. The beta-sitosterols utilized in these studies were known by the names Harzol, Azuprostat, or WA184, usually derived from South African star grass (*Hypoxis rooperi* or from species of *Picea* or *Pinus*). Studies used purified extracts, and three studies used "nonglucosidic B-sitosterol," again from 60 to 195 mg/day (two of these studies used Azuprostat, 65 mg TID or 195 mg/day with a 70 % beta-sitosterol content). The preparation generally contained 50 % or higher amounts of B-sitosterol. The mean age of participants was 65 years (34–85 year range), mean baseline International Prostate Symptom Score (IPSS) was 15.2 points, maximum urinary flow rate (Q_{max}) of 10.2 mL/s, post-void residual urine volumes (PVR) of 73.3 mL, and a prostate size of 49.1 mL. Again, it is of interest that all three studies that used nonglucosidic B-sitosterol found significant improvements in urinary symptoms, Q_{max}, and PVR compared to placebo. The single study that used a purified B-sitosterol B-D-glucoside preparation (also known as WA184) found no improvement in Q_{max}, PVR, and prostate size.

The second review was published in 2000 and consisted of similar authors compared to the first review [27]. The results published in this review were identical to those published in the first review. However, there was a discussion of statistical significance and nocturia results in this review that mentioned one study that looked at this impact and found that the weighted mean difference (WMD) was approximately −1.00 times in favor of beta-sitosterol [27, 29]. Test for overall effect of the meta-analysis found a statistically significant impact in favor of beta-sitosterol compared to placebo for IPSS ($p<0.00001$, two studies), quality of life ($p<0.00001$, one study), patient evaluation of efficacy ($p<0.000011$, one study), physician evaluation of efficacy ($p<0.000019$, one study), nocturia ($p=0.0089$, one study), peak urinary flow ($p=0.011$, four studies), peak urinary flow sensitivity analysis ($p=0.00027$, three positive studies only included), residual volume ($p=0.000012$), residual volume sensitivity analysis ($p<0.00001$, three positive studies only included), but not prostate size ($p=0.18$, two studies). It is noteworthy that prostate size was reduced compared to placebo in two studies by a mean difference of −6.50 and −4.97 cc, favoring beta-sitosterol, but this was not enough to reach statistical significance, which is of interest because again there is some preliminary evidence that beta-sitosterol could mildly inhibit 5-alpha reductase [32]. The positive results observed in these trials compare with results from pharmaceutical agents. Although beta-sitosterol was considered the active ingredient in these clinical trials, this has not been definitively proven, but it is reasonable to conclude that it is the most likely or primary efficacious ingredient. The need for surgery, acute urinary retention rates, or the overall ability to prevent BPH complications are items that would be more helpful in a more long-term study of beta-sitosterol or any intervention.

The clinical question is why not just try beta-sitosterol, a heart-healthy ingredient with or without medications for BPH? The dosage recommended in cholesterol treatment guidelines is 2,000–3,000 mg a day to reduce LDL by 6–15 %, and in fact in these National Cholesterol Education Panel recommendations it states the following: "Plant stanol/sterol esters (2 g/day) are a therapeutic option to enhance LDL cholesterol lowering" [33]. Keep this in mind when consulting with patients about beta-sitosterol for BPH, because it is important to be able to discuss the efficacious dosages from the older 1990 studies (20–65 mg TID) compared to the heart-healthy guidelines of plant stanol/sterols to reduce LDL cholesterol (2,000–3,000 mg/day). Personally, I have few concerns about whether or not beta-sitosterol would interfere with any prescription BPH medications or cause any drug-supplement reactions, but again this is based on experience and not on any research.

Cernilton (Pollen Extract, *Secale cereale*) Dietary Supplements

Interestingly, cernilton is a fairly well known dietary supplement in urology because it has been shown to significantly improve quality of life and reduce pain in men with chronic prostatitis/chronic pelvic pain syndrome (CP/CPPS) compared to placebo [34–36]. However, it has not been shown in these patients to consistently improve urinary flow measures, and this should be kept in mind when trying to apply this data to the BPH/LUTS studies. Cernilton, the original phytotherapeutic extract, is currently a mixed pollen extract (see the chapter on chronic prostatitis for more detail), and it is generally composed of a water-soluble pollen fraction and an acetone-soluble extract fraction that contains some beta-sterols.

One past meta-analysis has been published on cernilton that included 444 men (163 in placebo-trials and 281 in comparative trials) from four clinical trials that were 12–24 weeks in duration; the mean age was 69 years old (range 42–89 years) [37]. Two studies were placebo-controlled and two were comparative trials against another supplement agent (*Pygeum africanum* or Paraprost = 265 mg of L-glutamic acid, 100 mg of L-alanine, and 45 mg of aminoacetic acid). Cernilton was not more effective compared to placebo or other comparative interventions in the area of objective measures, including urinary flow rates, residual volume, or prostate size. Cernilton did improve subjective symptoms, such as reduced nocturia compared to placebo, and WMD was −0.40 times per evening. Side effects were mild and rare, and the withdrawal rate was 4.8 % versus to 2.7 % ($p = 0.26$), and 5.2 % for Paraprost. In these studies, one dose of cernilton contained 60 mg of Cernitin T60, a water-soluble extract fraction, and 3 mg of an acetone-soluble extract fraction known as Cernitin GBX. Cernilton dosages were not reported in three studies, and it was not known if a standardized extract was utilized. In another trial of 12 weeks, men utilized 63 mg of cernilton twice daily. A recent similar review of this meta-analysis arrived at similar conclusions but appeared to be more of an advocate of the potential use of cernilton for BPH [38]. A primary mechanism of action is difficult to determine because an older laboratory study found that it may reduce prostate size [39], but this again was not found in the meta-analysis [37]. Interestingly in the CP/CPPS studies there were suggestive anti-inflammatory and muscle relaxation effects in the prostate and perhaps bladder and urethra [34–36], which could be occurring in the BPH studies.

Interestingly, a study from Shanghai, China, of 240 BPH patients with an IPSS >7 utilized 350 or 750 mg of cernilton twice a day for 4 years [40]. Improvement was more rapid in the high-dose group. The study itself was published in Chinese, but significant improvements for the high-dose (over the low-dose) form were found for IPPS (20–10), prostate volume (38–29 mL), PVR (42–15 mL), and Q_{max} (10–16 mL/s) and a significantly lower rate of urinary retention and surgery, and there were no significant prostate-specific antigen (PSA) changes. No toxicity or adverse effects were found. This is an interesting clinical trial because it at least raises the question of whether or not utilizing higher dosages of cernilton might make more clinical sense for BPH/LUTS or at least should be tested in a future clinical trial. A primary mechanism of action is difficult to determine because an older laboratory study found that it may reduce prostate size [40], but in the CP/CPPS studies there were suggestive anti-inflammatory and muscle relaxation effects in the prostate and perhaps bladder and urethra [34–36]. Regardless, although this agent certainly has data in chronic nonbacterial prostatitis (CP/CPPS) and could be utilized for this condition, it does not have consistent impressive data for BPH/LUTS, and further clinical research is needed in this area. Personally, I am not concerned about the use of this product with and without conventional medicine in terms of interactions, but again this is based on experience and not clinical research. My biggest concern is that this supplement simply has not received enough recent clinical data or attention.

Flaxseed and SDG Dietary Supplements

It is also of interest that a flaxseed-derived supplement made of purified lignan (phytoestrogen) extract (secoisolariciresinol diglucoside, or SDG) at 300 or 600 mg/day showed favorable and significant results compared to a placebo in a clinical trial of 87 participants over a 4-month period [41]. IPSS were reduced by approximately 7 points in the intervention arms compared to 3.5 points in the placebo group, with additional improvements in quality of life. Similar SDG derivatives of a variety of doses have also now been found to preliminarily and significantly reduce cholesterol and glucose values [42, 43]. Whether or not ingesting low-cost flaxseed as well as an SDG supplement will reduce BPH symptoms has not been studied, but it is worthy of an attempt for some individuals because these interventions are at least heart healthy. Dietary flaxseed is one of the largest dietary plant sources of omega-3 fatty acids, fiber, and phytoestrogens [44]. Most flaxseed dietary supplements do not contain fiber but at least are excellent sources of omega-3 and/or phytoestrogens. Regardless, whether the supplements provide some benefit beyond the cost-effective dietary sources (seeds and powder) is questionable, especially in terms of BPH, but this has not been studied. A preliminary clinical trial that examined tissue from BPH patients before and after three rounded tablespoons of ground flaxseed (30 g total per day for 6 months) were utilized daily along with a low-fat diet found significant reductions in PSA, cholesterol, and tissue proliferation rates [45]. A subsequent randomized trial from this same group found that proliferation rates were impacted more by flaxseed alone compared to a low-fat diet in men with prostate cancer [46]. These are encouraging dietary flaxseed studies, but again they were not compared to flaxseed supplements. Thus, one could argue right now that dietary flaxseed powder (2–3 tablespoons per day) and/or an SDG supplement from flaxseed could be utilized with and without conventional therapy. Despite minimal clinical data overall, I am an advocate of flaxseed for BPH and health simply because in the worst-case scenario it is a heart-healthy intervention [43, 44], which is a good "first do no harm" and beneficial approach. Other strong sources of phytoestrogens, such as soy products or soy supplements, have not accumulated positive data in BPH, but at least dietary (not soy dietary supplements) soy products are also heart healthy.

Pumpkin Seed Oil

The oil found in the pumpkin (*Cucurbita pepo*) seed is a commonly used salad oil in Austria, Hungary, and Slovenia, and it is produced by cleaned seeds that are dried, grounded, kneaded, roasted, and then pressed at 100–130 °C [47]. It is of interest that four fatty acids comprise 98 % of the total and include linoleic acid (C18:2, 36–61 %), oleic acid (C18:1, 21–47 %), palmitic acid (C16:0, 9.5–14.5 %), and stearic acid (C18:0, 3–7.5 %). Thus, the majority of the fatty acids in pumpkin seed are mono- and polyunsaturated. It is also high in alpha- and gamma-tocopherol and tocotrienol (vitamin E) and carotenoids, including lutein and zeaxanthin. It is also of interest that pumpkin seed oil contains a high content of plant sterols.

Pumpkin seed oil has preliminary past laboratory data to suggest that it may inhibit testosterone-induced hyperplasia of the rat prostate [48]. Basic science work suggests multiple potential mechanisms of action, including reducing prostate weight, protein content, and prostatic acid phosphatase levels, altering cholesterol metabolism, and increasing the testosterone-to-estradiol ratio [49]. This also suggests a potential preventive role for pumpkin seed oil and BPH.

A past small trial found that the combination of saw palmetto and pumpkin seed oil resulted in a significant increase in Q_{max} in BPH patients after 3 months [50]. Another older study of pumpkin seed for 12 months demonstrated an improved IPSS of at least 5 points and a 65 % overall improvement [51]. A more recent randomized, double-blind, placebo-controlled trial over 12 months of 47 BPH patients (mean age 53 years and IPSS >8) was published [52]. Subjects received placebo, 320 mg/day pumpkin seed oil, 320 mg/day saw palmetto oil, or the combination of these two nutraceuticals. None of the measurements significantly improved with the combination of pumpkin seed and saw palmetto compared to the single interventions. Prostate volume was not impacted in any group, but the baseline volumes were in the range of 21–27 mL. However, the IPSS scores were significantly reduced after 3 months in all intervention groups (−34 % change with pumpkin seed, −25 % with saw palmetto, and −33 % with combination vs. 10 % with placebo). After 12 months there was a −58 % impact in IPSS compared to baseline in the pumpkin seed group, −50 % with saw palmetto, −75 % with the combination, and −39 % with placebo. There were no significant differences after 12 months in IPSS between intervention groups. Quality of life improved after 3 months in the pumpkin seed or saw palmetto groups and improved after 6 months in the combination groups, but after 12 months there was approximately a 40 % positive change with pumpkin seed or saw palmetto and a 58 % with the combination. Serum PSA was reduced after 3 months in the combination arm and after 12 months was significantly reduced by 42 % (1.2–0.7 ng/mL) compared to baseline. Q_{max} significantly improved after 6 months in the pumpkin seed–only group (by 14 % or 14.8–16.9 mL/s) and after 12 months in the saw palmetto–only group (51 %, from 14 to 21.2 mL/s), and combination experienced only a 5 % change after 12 months from 20.1 to 21.2 mL/s. One obvious limitation of this study is that the placebo group consisted of only seven subjects and the largest intervention group was the pumpkin seed oil group, with only 16 subjects. Another critical examination of the protocol is that the participants needed to take two capsules in the morning and two capsules in the evening after meals (four total capsules a day) for 12 months, which is not a simplistic compliance-enhancing protocol. Basically, this small clinical trial of a long duration for a BPH supplement study did not demonstrate that the combination of pumpkin seed and saw palmetto was significantly better compared to pumpkin seed only, for example. It may have suggested that utilizing more than one nutraceutical in a regimen may reduce PSA, and it suggests that utilizing either pumpkin seed or saw palmetto or the combination is as safe as a placebo.

Pumpkin seed oil appears to be a safe intervention for BPH that can be utilized with and without conventional treatment options. It seems that 320 mg/day is an appropriate dosage, but there are not enough clinical data thus far to feel confident that it is an effective dietary supplement, but it appears to be a very safe dietary supplement. Regardless, pumpkin seed oil is an option, and it is rich in heart-healthy fatty acids, but if the number of pills daily from any manufacturer is more than one to two pills daily or if cost is an issue, then I would not be as excited to utilize this option for patients.

Pygeum africanum (African Plum Tree) Dietary Supplements

A 2002 meta-analysis of 18 *Pygeum africanum* clinical trials (17 were double blind) involving 1,562 men suggested a potential benefit with this supplement [53]. This compound(s) is an extract of the African prune tree. The majority of the studies utilized a standardized extract effective at approximately 75–200 mg per day. In terms of the placebo-controlled trials, one study utilized 75 mg per day, seven utilized 100 mg per day, and four used a 200 mg/day dosage; one study did not report dosage. Mean age was 66 years (range 42–89 years), and nocturia was three times per evening with four studies at baseline. Out of 13 placebo-controlled trials, a total of 12 reported a positive impact on at least one measure of effectiveness (overall symptoms, nocturia, peak urine flow, or residual volume). The mean duration of clinical studies was 64 days (range of 30–122 days), but men were more than two times as likely to report an improvement in overall symptoms, nocturia was reduced by 19 %, residual volume by 24 %, and peak urine flow increased by 23 %.

Again, all of the following providing statistical benefits with pygeum versus placebo:

- Overall symptom improvement (rating by doctor)
- Peak urinary flow
- Residual volume

Nocturia was reduced by almost one episode per night, but this failed to reach statistical significance. Whether or not pygeum actually reduces long-term complications of BPH, such as acute urinary retention, renal issues, or surgery, is not known. Pygeum has not been shown to shrink the prostate gland. The withdrawal rate was similar to placebo at 12 %. Adverse effects were similar to placebo, and the most frequently reported adverse effects were gastrointestinal.

It is also of interest that one of the main components of *Pygeum africanum* (similar to other nutraceuticals such as pumpkin seed and saw palmetto) consists of phytosterols that include beta-sitosterol [54, 55]. Most of the active substances in the *Pygeum* bark are lipid-soluble compounds triterpenes, ferulic acid esters, and phytosterols (Β-sitosterol, Β-sitosterone, and campesterol). However, the problem with pygeum is demand compared to precious supply, in that the bark is derived from an endangered tree [56]. This is not the case with most other BPH nutraceuticals, such as saw palmetto or pumpkin seed, which appear to be in abundance and have arguably a diverse number of heart-healthy compounds beyond beta-sitosterol, including the primary monounsaturated fat found in olive oil (oleic acid) and a variety of other potentially healthy dietary fats that may have the ability to increase HDL and lower cardiovascular events [57–60].

Pygeum africanum in reality has arguably the largest number of consistently positive clinical trials to date compared to almost any other nutraceutical product [53–56, 61], especially since the latest data on saw palmetto have not been impressive, even in moderate to higher dosages [62, 63]. Pygeum has been used in Europe since 1969 for the treatment of mild to moderate BPH. Multiple mechanisms of action have been proposed for pygeum, including the following [53–56, 61]:

- Anti-inflammatory activity
- Modulating bladder contractility
- Reduced production of leukotrienes
- Reduced production of other 5-lipoxygenase metabolites
- Inhibits fibroblast production
- Impact on adrenal androgens
- Restore secretory activity of the prostate epithelium

Again, an adequate dosage for pygeum for BPH is 75–200 mg of an extract usually standardized to 14 % sterol content or higher, including beta-sitosterol, and generally given in two divided daily doses [53]. One brand sold outside the United States is Tadenan (France), which has been the source for older and more recent laboratory studies that suggest a clinical benefit [61], but the problem of whether or not most other companies are selling the actual pygeum utilized from some past studies, from the endangered African plum tree, or a new or altered version of it is a matter of debate. In other words, in my experience pygeum is fraught with issues, especially quality control, so try to investigate where the actual pygeum was derived before recommending or using it. Should real pygeum even be recommended today because real pygeum is endangered? A final issue with pygeum is the lack of any recent studies that could further define the efficacy of this compound.

Saw Palmetto (*Serenoa repens*) Dietary Supplements

One of the largest past reviews of clinical studies of saw palmetto for BPH found some interesting results in 1998 [64]. This analysis reviewed a total of 18 randomized trials ($n=2{,}939$ men) and found that most of the studies were limited by their short duration and study design. However, the existing evidence suggested that this herbal product improves urologic symptoms and flow measures. Compared with the drug finasteride, saw palmetto produced similar improvement in urinary tract symptoms and urinary flow, with fewer side effects. However, saw palmetto had only been compared to current drug therapies for a maximum of approximately 12 months. More data are needed on this herbal product.

Interestingly, the dosage of saw palmetto used in most randomized trials at this point in time was 320 mg/day, and this dosage had no effect on PSA levels.

Four years after this notable 1998 review was published, another one by similar authors added three new trials with 230 additional male participants that translated into a meta-analysis of 21 randomized trials. The conclusions were similar, with the authors simply stating that "The results of this update are in agreement with our initial review" [65]. In other words, saw palmetto could be an option that works as well as some pharmacologic agents but with fewer side effects. The authors then updated their original meta-analysis again in 2009 and came to this conclusion: "*Serenoa repens* was not more effective than placebo for treatment of urinary symptoms consistent with BPH" [66]. In 2012 another follow-up review by similar authors concluded with the following: "*Serenoa repens* therapy does not improve LUTS or Q_{max} compared with placebo in men with BPH, even at double and triple the usual dose" [67]. What happened that caused such a reversal in a long-standing recommendation or endorsement for saw palmetto? In the more recent meta-analysis, for example, there were nine new trials added to the analysis that included 2,053 more men (about 65 % increase), and overall there were 5,222 subjects from 30 randomized trials of a 4- to 60-week duration utilized, for example [66].

However, the answer to the question of what caused such a reversal in the saw palmetto enthusiasm lies first in a US government-funded trial called STEP (The Saw Palmetto for Treatment of Enlarged Prostates) [62], followed by the results of a more recent trial called CAMUS (Complementary and Alternative Medicine for Urological Symptoms) [63].

The STEP trial was simply a very well-done clinical trial [62], and the researchers and participants in this study should be commended for being a part of one of the better herbal studies ever completed in urology and in medicine (in my opinion). Saw palmetto enjoys a tremendous amount of sales around the world. Some areas of Europe have made this herbal product a prescription, but in the United States there are literally hundreds of over-the-counter brands. Florida and several coastal states are some of the largest exporters of this herbal product. This herbal product is so well known that it continues to be one of the more popular supplements taken by men to prevent prostate cancer, despite having no relevant evidence that it prevents prostate cancer [68, 69]. However, this is the concerning part, because saw palmetto has never had any credible data that it reduces the risk of prostate cancer. All of the preliminary data were for the improvement of BPH symptoms. Some researchers suggest it has a finasteride (a drug approved for BPH)-type effect, but unlike finasteride (also known as Proscar, Merck & Co., Whitehouse Station, NJ), it has not been shown to have any impact on PSA levels. Regardless, there was an ample need to conduct a non-industry-supported clinical trial to determine if saw palmetto really does have some efficacy. The STEP trial was funded by the National Institute of Diabetes and Digestive and Kidney Diseases (NIDDK) and by the National Center for Complementary and Alternative Medicine (NCCAM) [62].

In the STEP trial a total of 225 men with moderate to severe BPH symptoms were randomized to saw palmetto extract at a dosage of 160 mg twice a day (320 mg a day total) or placebo [62]. The primary outcomes were the change in score on the American Urological Association Symptom Index (AUASI), a subjective measurement completed by patients, and the maximal flow rate (an objective measure completed by the physician). There were also a number of secondary outcomes, including change in the prostate size, urine volume left in the bladder after urinating, quality of life, laboratory values, and side effects. Some of the baseline characteristics of the men that participated in the STEP trial are found in Table 3.1.

When the trial ended after 12 months of treatment, there was no difference between saw palmetto and placebo in all the major areas of study, including:

- AUASI score (only 0.04 point difference)
- Maximal urinary flow rate (only 0.4-mL difference)
- Prostate size or volume (only 1.22-mL difference)

Table 3.1 Characteristics of the participants at the initiation of the saw palmetto versus placebo STEP trial [62]

Approximate characteristics of the 225 participants	Saw palmetto group (112 patients)	Placebo group (113 patients)
Average age	63 years	63 years
Percentage of nonwhite or minorities	16 %	21 %
Average AUASI score (scores run 0–35 with 0–7 = normal, 8–19 = moderate, and 20–35 = severe BPH)	15.5	15
Prostate volume	34.5 mL	34 mL
Maximal urinary flow rate	11.5 mL/s	11.5 mL/s
Residual urine or amount left in bladder after urinating	80 mL	84.5 mL
PSA	1.8	1.6

- Residual volume after urinating (only a 4.51-mL difference)
- No difference in quality of life, PSA, or side effects

Numerous criticisms have been raised about this trial when I would lecture to public and health care professional groups, but let me answer some of the most popular inquires to demonstrate just how well this trial was designed and conducted.

Why Didn't the Researchers Use a Higher Dose of Saw Palmetto?

They used 320 mg/day because this was by far the most common dosage used in the past clinical trials that demonstrated a consistent benefit [64, 65].

Why Didn't the STEP Trial Use a More Popular Brand of Saw Palmetto for the Study?

In my opinion, the researchers attempted to do this, but some companies did not want to be a part of this trial. They ended up using a soft gelatin product from Indena USA provided by Rexall-Sundown, but this product went through rigorous testing to make sure it fits all the standards [62]. Also, I believe more people should give Rexall-Sundown company credit for volunteering their product when it seems they had little to gain and a lot to lose financially by participating in this trial.

What Notable Standards Did the Saw Palmetto Product Adhere to in This Trial?

Many of the popular alternative medicine consumer books and Web sites had espoused for years the use of a saw palmetto with either 80–95 % combination of fatty acids and sterols or 85–95 % fatty acids and greater than 0.2 % sterols. The herbal extract used in this trial demonstrated consistent 90–92 % fatty acids and 0.33 % sterols [62], which means it was right on target or even above the standards of what has been recommended in the past for effectiveness. The placebo even had an odor similar to saw palmetto so that the participants could not tell the difference. The placebo contained polyethylene glycol-400, which is a bitter-tasting liquid with an oil makeup. It contained no free fatty acids, and a brown coloring agent was used in order to ensure no difference in appearance between saw palmetto and placebo.

Why Didn't the STEP Trial Test Primarily Men with Mild BPH Symptoms and Larger Prostate Volumes?

Perhaps including men with more mild BPH symptoms and not those with moderate to severe BPH would have been a better study, and perhaps men with larger prostates would have also been a better group. The reason for this is due to the suggestion that saw palmetto works similar to a drug (finasteride) that shrinks larger prostate glands.

However, in defense of the researchers in this trial, a study of only mild BPH would have had led to such problems as a large placebo effect, and encouraging medication of a condition that for many men needs no intervention. Regardless, when the researchers looked at the small number of men with more or fewer symptoms than the average or with smaller or larger prostate glands, there was still no difference between saw palmetto and placebo [62].

How Effective Is a Placebo for BPH, and Did the STEP Trial Give Any Indication of the Placebo Response Rate?

What did not seem to receive attention from this trial was the fact that all of the potential participants in this trial were first placed in a 1-month, single-blind, placebo run-in phase and were not permitted in the trial unless they took 75 % or more of the placebo capsules [62]. In other words, in order to really determine who was committed to being compliant with the pills throughout this entire trial, the participants had to take placebo pills for 1 month prior to the start of the official study. It is interesting that there was actually a significant small improvement (or decrease) in the AUASI during this 1-month period! This demonstrates the impressiveness of the placebo effect, especially with BPH, and it has to be accounted for, and the researchers made an excellent effort accounting for this issue.

Were Men on Prescription Drugs for BPH Allowed to Be a Part of This Trial?

Men were not allowed to be on a prescription drug for BPH during this trial [62]. If they stopped taking a prescription alpha-blocker at least 1 month before the trial or a prescription 5-alpha-reductase inhibitor at least 6 months before the trial, then they were allowed to participate. Men with a higher risk of complete urinary blockage or urinary retention, which was defined as a urinary flow rate of less than 4 mL per second or urine amount of 250 mL left in bladder after urinating, were not allowed in the trial because this would be too severe to be treated by medication. Other types of men not eligible for the trial included men with a history of prostate cancer, surgery for BPH, serious urethra or bladder conditions, high creatinine levels, PSA level greater than 4.0 ng/dL, and those on medications that impact urinary flow or those individuals with a serious disease of any type.

Was There a Difference in Any of the Side Effects Between Saw Palmetto and Placebo?

There was no difference, and in fact no side effect was reported at a significantly higher rate than placebo [62]. Perhaps this might also explain why saw palmetto had no effect, because there may not have been enough active ingredients or it may not work any better than placebo anyway. Whenever a pill or any medical intervention has a side effect profile identical to placebo, I am usually concerned that it really does not have an impact any better than the sugar pill (of course, there are exceptions). Personally, I like to observe some low rate of side effects when there is some efficacy with an intervention, which provides some proof of a mechanism of action for an acute condition. Only ten men in the saw palmetto group (five lost to follow-up and five stopped the medication because of other issues) and nine in the placebo group (four lost to follow-up and five stopped the medication) did not complete the entire study, which means a dropout rate of less than 10 %, which is outstanding for a clinical trial.

Why Was the Trial Only 1 Year Long, and Not 2 Years, for Example?

This trial was one of the longest saw palmetto trials in the history of medicine. The majority of the past trials were about 3 months or shorter [64, 65]. BPH trials of 6 months to 1 year or more are more than adequate to determine if a medication is effective. The researchers could have done this trial over

6 months, but in my opinion 1 year was the perfect duration to determine if saw palmetto was better than placebo. In fact, participants had eight clinic visits during the trial [62], which was also more than sufficient to determine the impact of saw palmetto.

Okay, So What Is Next for Saw Palmetto? Should Men Use This Herbal Product Ever Again?

Saw palmetto was arguably one of the ten top-selling herbal supplements in the United States and around the world. Permixon, a saw palmetto product from France, is one of the most studied saw palmetto products in the world with consistent positive data in BPH clinical trials [64, 65, 70, 71], but it was not a part of this trial and men cannot generally buy this product in the United States, for example. Whether or not Permixon mirrors the product utilized in the STEP trial is controversial, there were some similarities. Also, a very large herbal trial called CAMUS was completed that also found no benefit compared to placebo [63], and this is also discussed briefly in this chapter. Thus, if one is a scientific purist, so to speak, then saw palmetto has no current role in BPH, but some would argue that the safety, which is similar to placebo, and unpredictable first-do-no-harm efficacy and usually low cost compared to prescription agents still allow it to be an option for some men.

If the STEP trial results were a surprise, then the CAMUS results were arguably even more surprising, in my opinion, because of the higher doses of saw palmetto utilized [63]. Basically, the CAMUS researchers found that low (320 mg), moderate (640 mg), and high doses (960 mg) of saw palmetto given over 72 weeks did not work better than a placebo for BPH/LUTS. Saw palmetto was again as safe as a placebo, but not more effective than a placebo in the follow-up North American study to the STEP trial. CAMUS was a double-blind, multicenter, placebo-controlled randomized trial conducted at 11 North American clinics, including Ontario, Canada [63]. A total of 369 men, with approximate mean age of 61 years, AUASI of 14.5, peak urinary flow rate of 14.9 mL/s, and PVR of 41 mL, were given escalating doses of saw palmetto or placebo over 72 weeks. Multiple other prostate and health parameters were also measured at baseline and at 72 weeks. Men needed to be 45 years and older with a Q_{max} of at least 4 mL/s and an AUASI between 8 and 24 at two screening visits to qualify for this study. Men were also allowed to be on 5 alpha-reductase inhibitor if they had stopped this medication 3 or more months before the trial (not 6 or more months, as in the STEP trial). The intervention consisted of one to three chocolate-covered gelcaps (320 mg each), and the starting dosage was 320 mg/day, with a dose escalation at 24 (640 mg/day) and 48 weeks (960 mg/day), with the trial ending at 18 months of intervention compared to placebo. The saw palmetto used in CAMUS consisted of 85–95 % fatty acids, and it was a lipidic ethanolic extract of ripe, dried saw palmetto berries manufactured by Rottapharm/Madaus, Cologne, Germany, and sold as PROSTA-URGENIN UNO capsules. The placebo contained 375 mg of polyethylene glycol and a matched weight (475 mg), and participants were told to take all gelcaps at same time.

Again, in the CAMUS trial the baseline and 72-week results found no significant differences between saw palmetto and placebo for any parameter [63]. For example, no differences were found for the following: AUASI (primary outcome), BPH impact index, AUASI quality of life, nocturia, peak flow rate, postvoid residual, PSA, IIEF, sleep dysfunction scale, incontinence scale, or NIH CPSI. Many items actually favored placebo except for the difference in AUASI for non-Caucasian participants, which favored saw palmetto (nonsignificantly).

Was CAMUS the Final Verdict for Saw Palmetto?

The CAMUS trial was very well done, but it certainly will raise some questions that may speak more to the mindset of conventional and alternative medicine currently compared to anything else. Originally, this trial was suppose to compare a prescription drug to saw palmetto and placebo, but this did not occur for reasons that were not clear, except it is my opinion that no prescription medication manufacturers wanted their drugs to be tested against this or another herbal product or a placebo. For example, even some recent prescription medication FDA approvals for BPH in the United States have not included a placebo arm including the combination of dutasteride and tamsulosin [72]. One could argue that these medications already proved themselves against placebo in the past, but I would argue that the expectations of current participants in clinical trials are different compared to a decade ago. Regardless, it would have been interesting for saw palmetto to be compared to a conventional agent, as it was in the past in European trials that demonstrated equivalence [70, 71].

Additionally, the most notable saw palmetto supplement/drug in the world (Permixon) with the most positive clinical research (popular in Europe) apparently either did not or could not participate in this trial [70, 71]. Thus, the researchers were left with another agent from a different manufacturer in this trial, which again arguably demonstrated that rigorous North American saw palmetto studies do not demonstrate efficacy of this herbal product compared to placebo. However, should researchers discount the European studies? How about the 1-year study that showed saw palmetto (Permixon) equivalent or even superior to tamsulosin, one of the biggest-selling prescription medications for BPH around the world [70, 71]? Some European saw palmetto products have drug-like standardized fatty acids in large amounts that may have a slight impact on 5-alpha reductase. For example, in a study of seven European lipid/sterol saw palmetto products tested on a 10-day co-cultured epithelial and fibroblast cell by a 5-alpha-reductase activity assay, interestingly all of these interventions demonstrated some impact on the isoforms of 5-alpha reductase [73]. However, Permixon demonstrated the greatest potency against 5-alpha-reductase type 1 and type 2 compared to any other nutraceutical product. There are a variety of fatty acids in some nutraceutical products, such as lauric acid (e.g., C12 saturated fat found in coconut oil), which could inhibit type 1 and 2 5-alpha reductase; myristic acid (C14 saturated fat), which inhibits type 2 5-alpha reductase only; and oleic acid (e.g., C18 monounsaturated fat found in olive oil) and linoleic acid, which inhibit type 1, but palmitic acid (C16 saturated fat) and stearic acid (C18 saturated fat) have no activity against type 1 or type 2 [74–76]. It is interesting that Permixon contains a high concentration of free fatty acids, primarily lauric and oleic acid, and, to a smaller extent, linoleic and myristic acid [77], which could theoretically explain its potential ability to have greater activity compared to other saw palmetto products. However, it is also plausible that it has no greater activity compared to any other product, because neither PSA levels nor prostate volumes have been significantly and consistently impacted by Permixon [71, 72]. Or is it possible that Permixon has some intermediate activity between a pharmacologic agent and a placebo and has multiple mechanisms of action, including intraprostatic inhibition of 5-alpha reductase and specific growth factors such as epidermal growth factor (EGF) [78]? Only an adequate or definitive clinical trial similar to the STEP or CAMUS could answer these critical questions. It is also interesting that since saw palmetto may have some 5-alpha-reductase activity, it is commonly utilized in over-the-counter male and female hair-growing nutraceutical products with some minimal evidence of efficacy [79]. However, until some definitive trial of subjects with hair loss is completed, no one knows for sure if it is effective.

Saw palmetto is much lower in price compared to prescription drugs for BPH, so I believe some men will continue to use it regardless of the results, just because of price and the possibility of receiving some efficacy. In fact, some men may want to try it for mild symptoms, and if it does not help, they should use a prescription or have a procedure done. The bottom line is that the prescription drugs work well for most men, but the long-term side effects have become concerning for some clinicians and patients. The recent concern over long-term libido and erectile dysfunction and possibly depression and infertility is a serious concern with the 5-alpha-reductase inhibitors [80]. Additionally, prescription alpha-blockers also contain their own significant potential vascular risk factors for some patients, for example, dizziness, hypotension, and syncope, along with other issues such as the potential for retrograde ejaculation [81].

In conclusion, saw palmetto faired well in most past clinical trials [64, 65], until the STEP and CAMUS trials [62, 63]. The STEP and CAMUS trials were well designed with few major controversial issues in my opinion. The STEP trial used a carbon dioxide extraction procedure for their saw palmetto preparation [62], compared to an ethanolic extraction procedure in the CAMUS trial [63]. In other words, some Internet criticisms of the extraction procedure for saw palmetto after the STEP trial were addressed in the CAMUS trial and did not produce better results. This is a testament to the researchers for these trials. In my opinion, the only other information or controversial inquiry I would add to the STEP and CAMUS trials is why 5-alpha-reductase inhibitors with long half-lives and effects (especially dutasteride) were allowed to be used by a subject if it was stopped greater than 3 or even 6 months before recruitment? It would have been helpful for the researchers to mention the number of participants in the saw palmetto and placebo arm that fit this category of previously using a prescription 5-alpha-reductase inhibitor. And why did the more recent CAMUS trial allow a 5-alpha-reductase inhibitor to be used 3 or more months before the trial compared to 6 or more months before the STEP trial, when more recent 5-alpha-reductase inhibitors such as dutasteride have much longer half-lives (5 weeks plus)? In addition, it would have be helpful for the STEP and CAMUS researchers to explain the specific or precise difference or similarity between the saw palmetto products utilized in their studies and Permixon, the European saw palmetto product that has the most positive clinical research for any nutraceutical in the area of BPH [64, 65]. It seems that there might have been some similarities and some differences that should be specifically explained so that clinicians and patients can decide for themselves if STEP and CAMUS products represented most commercial saw palmetto products (or not) that their patients can access. It is interesting that in the CAMUS manuscript the authors wrote: "Do our findings apply to other saw palmetto extract preparations? We studied only one extract and because the potential active ingredients and mechanisms are not unknown, our findings may not be generalizable. Nevertheless, a recent series of negative trials using different saw palmetto extract preparations makes it increasingly unlikely a dose of some preparation will be identified that is better than placebo." The problem with this commentary is that although I agree with most of the statement, the researchers cannot tell their audience the exact difference between their products utilized and Permixon, for example. Thus, I decided to take a closer look at the CAMUS trial publication and the supplementary information provided, and it shows a gas chromatogram with the strongest peaks for lauric acid, and moderate or smaller peaks for myristic and oleic acid, which essentially suggests a similar product to Permixon (a product with 85–95 % fatty acids, arguably somewhat similar to the one used in the STEP trial). In other words, unless more clarification is provided, with some additional analysis it appears that the product used in CAMUS and possibly the one used in STEP were somewhat similar to the Permixon product. Still, there is some minimal controversy here that should be resolved in time, hopefully by the researchers themselves.

Another objective comment that should be considered is that some BPH agents are often tested for individuals dealing with some other prostate issues, such as chronic prostatitis/chronic pelvic pain syndrome (CP/CPPS). Currently, there is some recent evidence to suggest that saw palmetto (e.g., Permixon and other products) could have some efficacy against chronic prostatitis [82, 83], but there is also some older evidence that challenges these recent findings [84]. Until a more definitive clinical trial against placebo is initiated, the controversy in this area will continue with saw palmetto. This is arguably similar to the prescription alpha-blockers and chronic nonbacterial prostatitis issues that occurred until a more rigorous trial questioned their utilization for many patients with CP/CPPS [85, 86]. Hopefully, saw palmetto will not experience the same fate.

Stinging Nettle (*Urtica dioica*, Common Nettle) Dietary Supplements

There are plenty of laboratory data to suggest that this herbal product has activity in some aspects of medicine, such as arthritis and BPH [87, 88]. In fact, stinging nettle has been suggested as a treatment for LUTS for decades by some authors [89]. However, stinging nettle is plagued by a lack of high-quality clinical data, and this was reiterated by an older systematic review, which stated, "Evidence from randomized trials suggest combination preparations of Urticae appear to provide some benefits for treatment of lower urinary tract symptoms, although stinging nettle extracts alone do not appear to be beneficial" [90]. Still, multiple components of stinging nettle have been suggested to have some activity, including the following [87]:

- Isolectin mixture
- Polysaccharides
- Sterols
- Phenols
- Dimeric phenylpropane-lignans
- Triterpenoic acids
- Monoterpenoids and their respective glucosides
- Ceramides
- Scopoletin (coumarin)
- Phenylpropanes

Yet there are actually minimal quantities of phytosterols (<0.01 %) reported by some authors, so which components have activity and the true mechanism of action is poorly understood [87]. In fact, more recent publications suggest higher quantities of beta-sitosterol (20–30 %) in stinging nettle utilizing newer extraction procedures (ethanolic) compared to what was reported in the older literature [88]. Some authors have suggested that there are impacts on SHBG, inhibition of aromatase, growth factors, or prostate steroid receptors but that it is less likely that 5-alpha-reductase inhibition occurs [87], while other authors suggest 5-alpha-reductase inhibitory activity is a potential mechanism of action [90].

One of the last clinical trials of significance was published in 2005, and it was a 6-month randomized crossover trial of stinging nettle compared to placebo in 620 patients [91]. The following results were found for stinging nettle compared to placebo:

- A total of 81 % versus 16 % reported improved LUTS ($p<0.001$).
- IPSS was reduced from 19.8 to 11.8 versus 19.2 to 17.7 ($p=0.002$).
- Peak flow rate improved by 8.2 mL/s versus 3.4 mL/s ($p<0.05$). PVR was reduced from 73 to 36 mL ($p<0.05$).
- No changes in PSA or testosterone were found, but prostate size was slightly reduced (measured by TRUS) from 40.1 to 36.3 cc ($p<0.001$) versus no change with placebo.

There was no significant difference compared to placebo in prostate size by the end of the study. At the 18-month follow-up, only compliant patients that continued treatment had favorable responses, and no side effects were found compared to placebo. These results were initially interesting, but no relevant high-quality positive data have been published since this time to support or negate these findings. Studies such as this one and others have used a range of formulations including stinging nettle 120 mg per day in 18 drops TID or 300 mg BID or even as much as 600 mg BID. Most of the positive clinical data were from open older clinical trials that were not rigorous, but did use a common methanolic nettle root extract [87]. This may also be of concern because a majority of participants in clinical studies were treated with an extract derived from 20 % methanol. In addition, although the number of adverse events reported was approximately 2 % (in those trials that reported side effects), it is of interest that the most common side effects have been reduced libido or erectile dysfunction. This could have been due to the patient population used in these studies and/or the dietary supplement itself.

The majority of clinical efficacy data is in agreement with the past systematic review that suggests that if stinging nettle is efficacious, it has more data to suggest a benefit in combination with other herbal products, such as saw palmetto [92], compared to stinging nettle alone [90]. However, the question of whether or not saw palmetto is effective may have been answered by the STEP and CAMUS trials [62, 63], so whether or not stinging nettle is effective is also a matter of controversy.

Zinc

Dietary supplements that contain zinc have been utilized by approximately 15 % of the US population in past studies [93]. This should already be a concern because the actual current recommended government dietary intake of zinc is very low and may be a surprise to some individuals. The current intake levels are listed in Table 3.2 along with dietary levels of copper because large doses of zinc can actually reduce the concentration of copper in the body, so a proper balance or intake between the two is important [94].

The recommended daily allowance (RDA) is 11 mg/day for men, but it seems that some individuals consume far greater daily quantities than the RDA [95]. The reason for this discrepancy is not currently known but may include some highly publicized alternative medicine magazines/books that promote the regular use of zinc supplements for everything from the common cold to cancer. Greater zinc intake may also potentially be due to the findings from several laboratory studies that zinc may inhibit the growth and progression of prostate cancer [96–100].

Table 3.2 The current government guidelines for the recommended daily dietary allowance of zinc and copper (RDA)

Age	Zinc (mg)	Copper (μg)
0–6 months	2	200
7–12 months	3	220
1–3 years	3	340
4–8 years	5	440
9–13 years	8	700
14–18 years	11 (male) and 9 (female)	890
19 or older years	11 (male) and 8 (female)	900

The concentration of zinc in the prostate gland is higher than that in any other tissue in the human body [101]. Zinc levels in prostate cancer are dramatically reduced compared to normal prostate tissue, which again may lead some individuals to falsely believe that prostate cancer is actually a state of zinc deficiency that may be amenable or prevented by larger intakes of zinc.

Increased zinc consumption may also increase the risk of BPH. The impact of dietary zinc intake on subsequent intraprostatic zinc levels is not known. However, a case-control study from Greece of diet and BPH found that higher intakes of dietary zinc had the most significant correlation with the overall risk of BPH (OR = 1.89) [102]. In fact, in this investigation it appeared that zinc (from mostly meat and some seed sources) was more closely correlated with BPH risk than any other evaluated dietary nutrient and zinc also strongly confounded the relationship of saturated fat with the risk of BPH. Thus, the suggestion that meat consumption increases the risk of prostatic disease may be simplistic. Additionally, other factors in meat such as zinc may have a more profound impact. Interestingly, zinc concentration increases in BPH tissue [103–109]. Testosterone appears to be involved in the development of BPH and prostate cancer, and it significantly increases the concentration of cellular and mitochondrial zinc. Laboratory studies have also found that androgen uptake by the prostate was significantly increased by the addition of zinc [106]. Zinc also appears to impact the enzyme 5-alpha reductase in the prostate [110]. Whether or not this is a favorable or unfavorable impact has yet to be researched.

Perhaps studies initially completed outside of urology can provide some insight into high-dose zinc supplementation. The largest randomized trial ($n = 3{,}640$, four groups, called AREDS) of a combination daily dietary supplement (500 mg vitamin C + 400 IU vitamin E + 15 mg beta-carotene + 80 mg zinc + 2 mg copper) versus the combination without zinc, just 80 mg zinc, or placebo for age-related macular degeneration (AMD) found a significant reduction in the risk of disease progression and vision loss over the 6-year study in the combination supplement that included zinc [111]. However, the only individuals that benefited were those with intermediate to advanced stages of already diagnosed macular degeneration. Individuals at risk or with early-stage macular degeneration did not benefit from taking this supplement over the study period. In addition, the supplement did not have any effect on cataract development or risk.

This study was a landmark US clinical trial for eye health because it arguably advocated for this combination dietary supplement to be included as standard medicine for those with the dry form of macular degeneration [111]. However, there may have been an increased risk of urologic problems. A research group from the University of Wisconsin published an interesting follow-up study. In a further analysis from the original eye health study in 2001, they published the potential urologic side effects with this supplement [111, 112]. There was a significant increase in hospitalizations for urologic causes such as BPH, kidney stones, urinary tract infection, and kidney failure in patients on the high-dose zinc versus the non-zinc supplement from this study ($p = 0.0003$), and this risk was greater in male compared to female patients. However, there was a higher rate of urinary tract infections in females with high-dose zinc compared to men. There was no increased risk of prostate or any other type of cancer with high-dose zinc supplementation, and there may have even been a decreased risk of prostate cancer, but this only occurred in smokers who are also known to be very deficient in these compounds. Patients in this study were an average age of 69 years old and were followed for a little more than 6 years. Again, review how much 80 mg of zinc daily compares to the government's recommended daily intake of zinc, which is found in Table 3.2. Also, keep in mind that the recommended intake of copper is also listed here because one impacts the absorption of another. In other words, if an individual consumes too much zinc, it impacts copper absorption, which can cause a variety of problems, such as a type of anemia and overall immune suppression (neutropenia). In my opinion, if it is a matter of preserving your eyesight from AMD, there should be some allowance of zinc in an eye product, but keep in mind that the average multivitamin already contains 10–20 mg, and this has been found to be generally safe. In my experience, the vast majority of men and women on eye health supplements would not qualify for them based on the AREDS trial [111]; in other words, they do not have moderate to advanced forms of macular degeneration but are either just concerned about AMD or have early signs of AMD. In my opinion, these individuals should follow a heart-healthy lifestyle and continue to follow ongoing studies, because one of the best ways to prevent AMD currently is simply to keep your cardiovascular risk as low as possible [113].

Whether or not high doses of zinc from supplemental sources or even diet definitely raise the risk of prostate conditions including BPH is still controversial [114, 115]. However, what is not controversial is that zinc supplements do not have a plethora of positive data for prostate conditions and may be associated with an increased risk of prostate issues, as mentioned in this chapter. Some countries such as Canada have now limited the amount of zinc (40 mg or less) that can be sold in an individual tablet unless a specific purpose or indication for that dosage is demonstrated [116]. There is little doubt that the utilization of individual zinc supplements does have some merit for some medical conditions, but even in these mostly acute situations, (e.g., to reduce the duration of a common cold), there is an agreement that acute toxicities (bad taste, taste changes, nausea, etc.) are fairly common [117, 118].

Miscellaneous

A randomized trial of 40 patients receiving 15 mg per day of lycopene from a dietary supplement or a placebo for 6 consecutive months was published that garnered some interest in the use of this supplement for BPH [119]. A total of four visits were completed in this trial, which included baseline, after 1 month, after 3 months, and after 6 months. The mean age was 67 years, and body mass index was 26 (slightly overweight). PSA levels decreased significantly in the lycopene group after 6 months from 6.6 to 5.8 μg/L, and there was no PSA change in the placebo group. Progression of prostate enlargement did not occur in the lycopene group compared to placebo as assessed by trans-rectal ultrasonography (TRUS) and digital rectal examination (DRE). International Prostate Symptom Score questionnaire improvements significantly improved in both groups but to a greater degree with lycopene. However, the placebo group experienced significantly greater reductions in LDL cholesterol compared to the lycopene group.

The most impressive finding was not the reduction of PSA by lycopene but that both groups reduced their intake of overall calories to a large degree during this trial. In other words, is the lycopene supplement responsible for the favorable impact in this study or is it the fact that men reduced caloric intake, which may have also caused the LDL and PSA reductions? In the Prostate Cancer Prevention Trial (PCPT), men in the placebo arm with a reduced overall caloric intake also experienced significantly lower PSA velocity parameters [120]. Regardless, a subsequent meta-analysis of lycopene studies for BPH has not found overall support for this nutrient for BPH [121], and I am in agreement. Other recent studies of specific supplements, such as soy pills, have also not found a benefit over placebo [122], and others have questionable methodology such as amino acid mixture supplements [37]. Additionally, attempting to micro-dissect all of the BPH supplement studies that use a variety of herbal formulations was not the purpose of this chapter and ultimately does not provide much insight into which herbal components have clinical activity. Thus, I attempted to simply focus only on evidence-based medicine in this chapter and BPH/LUTS outcomes.

Conclusion

A summary of the dietary supplements or CAM interventions discussed in this chapter, along with some personal commentary, is provided in Table 3.3 for a quick but pithy review.

I find it interesting that after working for more than 25 years in the area of CAM and urology, most of the BPH supplements or lifestyle interventions that appear to have activity also appear to be heart healthy. In fact, this observation is reiterated by other authors, who have also summarized the data in this specific area of medicine [123, 124]. I think it is a shame that there has not been a major phase 3 clinical trial of aggressive heart-healthy lifestyle interventions with and versus dietary supplements and/or prescription BPH agents for men with mild to moderate or even severe BPH/LUTS. It is my belief that a profound result would be observed that would either match some of the effects of the oral over-the-counter or prescribed interventions or at least significantly enhance the results of these agents. For example, the finding from the PCPT finasteride trial that men following a heart-unhealthy lifestyle, such as excessive daily alcohol consumption, actually abolished the efficacy of their prescription BPH medication is fascinating, disturbing, and should be a major topic of discussion for patients dealing with BPH [125]. Thus, the primary recommendation should first be to follow numerous heart-healthy lifestyle changes and also discuss some of the treatment options. It is hoped that future CAM BPH studies will also focus on some potentially effective pharmacologic unique mechanisms of action that may also improve BPH/LUTS, such as the utilization of PDE-5 inhibitory or nitric oxide-enhancing activity [126, 127], which seems to be occurring now on a minimal scale [127].

Some researchers or clinicians require the so-called level 1 evidence to recommend a dietary supplement for BPH, and I could not disagree more. As mentioned earlier, despite several pharmacologic agents containing level 1 evidence, there also exists clear long-term toxicity and cost issues that must be addressed on an individual basis. As long as a dietary supplement is of low cost or is cost-competitive and has some adequate heart-healthy and BPH/LUTS data as an intervention, such as beta-sitosterol, why not try and utilize it for a 3- to 6-month period or with a conventional agent that is not providing maximum benefit (the natural history of BPH/LUTS is difficult to predict)? This approach may also motivate the patient to turn toward other cost-effective

Table 3.3 A summary of CAM interventions commonly touted to prevent or improve BPH/LUTS

CAM intervention and some scientific, common, and trade names	Commentary
Acupuncture	May have indirect benefits for some by reducing stress and anxiety, improving sleep, and reducing sympathetic hyperactivity (lowering blood pressure, heart rate, etc.). Otherwise, the direct impact or data on this intervention is weak for BPH/LUTS
Beta-sitosterol/other plant sterols (a mixture of phytosterols, phytosterol extract, *Hypoxis rooperi* = South African star grass, popular trade names of Azuprostat or Harzol in the literature)	No relevant recent data on this supplement. Data from over a decade ago suggest objective and subjective benefits, and this supplement may lower LDL cholesterol levels, especially in far greater dosages (2,000 mg/day). Dosages of 60–195 mg/day total (usually in divided doses throughout the day) have suggested benefits against BPH/LUTS in three clinical trials. May reduce the absorption of fat-soluble vitamins, so a low-dose multivitamin may be needed
Cernilton (*Secale cereale* = cereal rye pollen, but product today is a mixed pollen extract)	Older studies suggest no objective benefit, but subjective benefits were observed. A dosage of 63 mg bid was utilized in one positive trial, but a recent study suggests far greater dosages may be needed for some efficacy (350–750 mg bid). This supplement has more ample positive data in chronic bon-bacterial prostatitis (CP/CPPS), but again newer studies suggest higher dosages may have some minimal efficacy in BPH/LUTS. Check for gluten-free status
Flaxseed dietary supplements (SDG supplementation)	A purified lignan (phytoestrogen) extract from flaxseed known as SDG (300–600 mg/day) may have some minimal efficacy in BPH/LUTS for objective and subjective parameters, but dietary flaxseed may also be beneficial from a clinical study of 30 g per day (3 rounded tablespoons). Dietary flaxseed is a good source of fiber and plant omega-3 fatty acids (heart healthy), whereas SDG supplements are a large phytoestrogen source that could be beneficial
Pumpkin seed oil (*Cucurbita pepo*)	Dosage of 320 mg/day has some minimal clinical data to improve subjective and objective measures
Pygeum africanum (African plum tree, bark of the African plum tree, trade name of Tadenan)	Dosage of 75–200 mg per day was utilized in most of the effective studies. Arguably, *Pygeum* has the most positive data for a dietary supplement in the area of BPH/LUTS, or it is second to beta-sitosterol, but pygeum is slightly controversial because this herbal product is an endangered species in some areas of the world (check the manufacturer and source)
Saw palmetto (*Serenoa repens*, Sabal serrulata)	Dosages of 320–960 mg/day have now been tested in two rigorous phase 3-like studies (STEP and CAMUS) over 12–18 months and have found no efficacy beyond a placebo for men with moderate to severe BPH, but it is as safe as a placebo. Whether or not other European saw palmetto extract compounds such as Permixon (perhaps higher in free fatty acids such as lauric, oleic, myristic, linoleic, etc.) that continue to demonstrate positive data against some pharmacologic agents are still beneficial is a matter of controversy and opinion
Stinging nettle root (*Urtica dioica*, extracts of the root of stinging nettle)	Most clinical data suggest that in combination with other phytotherapies such as saw palmetto, it may have efficacy. However, most studies have poor methodology and outcomes, and no recent relevant studies have been published. There may also be a minority of men that experience sexual dysfunction from this intervention based on past studies. Whether or not this is an effective herbal product is controversial, and the dosage range has been wide (100–1,000+ mg per day)
Zinc	Zinc supplements in high dosages can cause toxicity (nausea, taste, and smell changes), and there is a hint that large supplemental dosages may actually increase the risk of BPH and other prostate issues. Utilizing zinc supplements chronically for BPH is NOT recommended
Miscellaneous category	The data for lycopene as a supplement are weak, but it appears safe, which is similar to other dietary supplements such as soy and amino acid mixtures. Otherwise, a BPH supplement should be heart healthy or positively influence some cardiovascular parameter before it is recommended. Novel mechanisms of action that mimic novel pharmacologic pathways (PDE-5 inhibition or nitric oxide enhancing) should be tested in clinical studies with supplements that have this potential ability, such as Panax ginseng ginsenosides, L-citrulline, L-arginine

Note: Keep in mind that some well-referenced trade names for BPH supplements in the medical literature generally consist of one or more of the ingredients found in this summary table. For example, Harzol or Azuprostat = South African star grass = *Hypoxis rooperi* = Beta-sitosterol; Permixon = saw palmetto extract; Prostagutt forte = *Serenoa repens* and *Urtica dioica* extract = saw palmetto and stinging nettle; Tadenan = *Pygeum africanum*; Paraprost = L-glutamic acid, L-alanine, glycine

heart-healthy measures, such as heart-healthy lifestyle changes, which has been my experience. If we can simultaneously improve heart and prostate health with lifestyle first and/or other cost-effective interventions, I believe this is the right path that would allow the patient and clinician to observe the forest over the single tree. It could also be argued that acute or chronic PSA increases (changes in velocity) are one of the most common triggers for a biopsy for prostate cancer, but it would be appropriate to first discern if the PSA rise is from BPH or cancer or both. Making heart-healthy lifestyle changes is one method of determining what might be truly contributing to this change in PSA.

References

1. Nickel CJ, Shoskes D, Roehrborn CG, Moyad M. Nutraceuticals in prostate disease: the urologist's role. Rev Urol. 2008;10:192–206.
2. Moyad MA, Lowe FC. Educating patients about lifestyle modifications for prostate health. Am J Med. 2008;121(8 Suppl 2):S34–42.
3. Ashamalla H, Jiang ML, Guirguis A, Peluso F, Ashamalla M. Acupuncture for the alleviation of hot flashes in men treated with androgen ablation therapy. Int J Radiat Oncol Biol Phys. 2011;79: 1358–63.
4. Emmons SL, Otto L. Acupuncture for overactive bladder: a randomized controlled trial. Obstet Gynecol. 2005;106:138–43.
5. Honjo H, Kawauchi A, Ukimura O, Soh J, Mizutani Y, Miki T. Treatment of monosymptomatic nocturnal enuresis by acupuncture: a preliminary study. Int J Urol. 2002;9:672–6.
6. Kim JH, Nam D, Park MK, Lee ES, Kim SH. Randomized control trial of hand acupuncture for female stress urinary incontinence. Acupunct Electrother Res. 2008;33:179–92.
7. Liu QG, Wang CY, Jlao S, Tang LX, Peng MH, Tlan LF, et al. Electroacupuncture at Zhongji (CV3) for treatment of benign hyperplasia of prostate: a multicentral randomized controlled study. Zhongguo Zhen Jiu. 2008;28:555–9.
8. Johnstone PA, Bloom TL, Niemtzow RC, Crain D, Riffenburgh RH, Amling CL. A prospective, randomized pilot trial of acupuncture of the kidney-bladder distinct meridian for lower urinary tract symptoms. J Urol. 2003;169:1037–9.
9. Flachskampf FA, Gallasch J, Gefeller O, Gan J, Mao J, Pfahlberg AB, et al. Randomized trial of acupuncture to lower blood pressure. Circulation. 2007;115: 3121–9.
10. Lee H, Kim SY, Park J, Kim YJ, Lee H, Park HJ. Acupuncture for lowering blood pressure: systematic review and meta-analysis. Am J Hypertens. 2009;22:122–8.
11. Chen HY, Shi Y, Ng CS, Chan SM, Yung KK, Zhang QL. Auricular acupuncture treatment for insomnia: a systematic review. J Altern Complement Med. 2007;13:669–76.
12. Jones PJ, AbuMweis SS. Phytosterols as functional food ingredients: linkages to cardiovascular disease and cancer. Curr Opin Clin Nutr Metab Care. 2009;12:147–51.
13. Berryman CE, Preston AG, Karmally W, Deckelbaum RJ, Kris-Etherton PM. Effects of almond consumption on the reduction of LDL-cholesterol: a discussion of potential mechanisms and future research directions. Nutr Rev. 2011;69: 171–85.
14. Aldemir M, Okulu E, Neselioglu S, Erel O, Kayigil O. Pistachio diet improves erectile function parameters and serum lipid profiles in patients with erectile dysfunction. Int J Impot Res. 2011;23:32–8.
15. Guardamagna O, Abello F, Baracco V, Federici G, Bertucci P, Mozzi A, et al. Primary hyperlipidemias in children: effect of plant sterol supplementation on plasma lipids and markers of cholesterol synthesis and absorption. Acta Diabetol. 2010;48:127–33.
16. Malinkowski JM, Gehret MM. Phytosterols for dyslipidemia. Am J Health Syst Pharm. 2010;67:1165–73.
17. Hamilton P. Role of ezetimibe in the management of patients with atherosclerosis. Coron Artery Dis. 2009;20:169–74.
18. Dujovne CA, Suresh R, McCrary Sisk C, Maccubbin D, Strony J, Veltri E. Safety and efficacy of ezetimibe monotherapy in 1624 primary hypercholesterolaemic patients for up to 2 years. Int J Clin Pract. 2008;62:1332–6.
19. Pelton K, Di Vizio D, Insabato L, Schaffner CP, Freeman MR, Solomon KR. Ezetimibe reduces enlarged prostate in an animal model of benign prostatic hyperplasia. J Urol. 2010;184:1555–9.
20. Mills IW, Crossland A, Patel A, Ramonas H. Atorvastatin treatment for men with lower urinary tract symptoms and benign prostatic enlargement. Eur Urol. 2007;52:503–9.
21. Stamatiou KN, Zaglavira P, Skolarikos A, Sofras F. The effects of lovastatin on conventional medical treatment of lower urinary tract symptoms with finasteride. Int Braz J Urol. 2008;34:555–61.
22. Hall SA, Chiu GR, Link CL, Steers WD, Kupelian V, McKinlay JB. Are statin medications associated with lower urinary tract symptoms in men and women? Results from the Boston Area Community Health (BACH) Survey. Ann Epidemiol. 2011;21: 149–55.
23. St Sauver JL, Jacobsen SJ, Jacobson DJ, McGree ME, Girman CJ, Nehra A, et al. Statin use and decreased risk of benign prostatic enlargement and lower urinary tract symptoms. BJU Int. 2011;107: 443–50.

24. Padayatty SJ, Marcelli M, Shao TC, Cunningham GR. Lovastatin-induced apoptosis in prostate stromal cells. J Clin Endocrinol Metab. 1997;82:1434–9.
25. Freeman MR, Solomon KR. Cholesterol and benign prostate disease. Differentiation. 2011;82:244–52.
26. Wilt TJ, Macdonald R, Ishani A. B-sitosterol for the treatment of benign prostatic hyperplasia: a systematic review. BJU Int. 1999;83:976–83.
27. Wilt TJ, Ishani A, MacDonald R, Stark G, Mulrow CD, Lau J. Beta-sitosterols for benign prostatic hyperplasia. Cochrane Database Syst Rev. 2000;2, CD001043.
28. Kadow C, Abrams PH. A double-blind trial of the effect of beta-sitosteryl glucoside (WA184) in the treatment of benign prostatic hyperplasia. Eur Urol. 1986;12:187–9.
29. Fischer A, Jurincic-Winkler CD, Klippel KF. Conservative treatment of benign prostatic hyperplasia with high-dosage b-sitosterol (65 mg): results of a placebo-controlled double-blind study. Uroscopy. 1993;1:12–20.
30. Berges RR, Windeler J, Trampisch HJ, Senge T. Randomised, placebo-controlled, double-blind clinical trial of beta-sitosterol in patients with benign prostatic hyperplasia. Beta-sitosterol Study Group. Lancet. 1995;345(8964):1529–32.
31. Kippel KF, Hiltl DM, Schipp B. A multicentric, placebo-controlled, double-blind clinical trial of b-sitosterol (phytosterol) for the treatment of benign prostatic hyperplasia. Br J Urol. 1997;80:427–32.
32. Cabeza M, Bratoeff E, Heuze I, Ramirez E, Sanchez M, Flores E. Effect of beta-sitosterol as inhibitor of 5 alpha-reductase in hamster prostate. Proc West Pharmacol Soc. 2003;46:153–5.
33. National Cholesterol Education Program (NCEP) Expert Panel on Detection, Evaluation, and Treatment of High Blood Cholesterol in Adults (Adult Treatment Panel III). Third Report of the National Cholesterol Education Program (NCEP) Expert Panel on Detection, Evaluation, and Treatment of High Blood Cholesterol in Adults (Adult Treatment Panel III) final report. Circulation. 2002;106:3143–421.
34. Murphy AB, Macejko A, Taylor A, Nadler RB. Chronic prostatitis: management strategies. Drugs. 2009;69:71–84.
35. Wagenlehner FM, Schneider H, Ludwig M, Schnitker J, Brahler E, Weidner W. A pollen extract (Cernilton) in patients with inflammatory chronic prostatitis-chronic pelvic pain syndrome: a multicentre, randomized, prospective, double-blind, placebo-controlled phase 3 study. Eur Urol. 2009;56:544–51.
36. Wagenlehner FM, Bschleipfer T, Pilatz A, Weidner W. Pollen extract for chronic prostatitis-chronic pelvic pain syndrome. Urol Clin North Am. 2011;38:285–92.
37. Wilt T, Mac Donald R, Ishani A, Rutks I, Stark G. Cernilton for benign prostatic hyperplasia. Cochrane Database Syst Rev. 2000;2, CD001042.
38. Kim TH, Lim HJ, Kim MS, Lee MS. Dietary supplements for benign prostatic hyperplasia: an overview of systematic reviews. Maturitas. 2012;73:180–5.
39. Talpur N, Echard B, Bagchi D, Bagchi M, Preuss HG. Comparison of saw palmetto (extract and whole berry) and Cernitin on prostate growth in rats. Mol Cell Biochem. 2003;250:21–6.
40. Xu J, Qian WQ, Song JD. A comparative study on different doses of cernilton for preventing the clinical progression of benign prostatic hyperplasia. Zhonghua Nan Ke Xue. 2008;14:533–7.
41. Zhang W, Wang X, Liu Y, Tian H, Flickinger B, Empie MW, et al. Effects of dietary flaxseed lignan extract on symptoms of benign prostatic hyperplasia. J Med Food. 2008;11:207–14.
42. Zhang W, Wang X, Liu Y, Tian H, Flickinger B, Empie MW, Sun SZ. Dietary flaxseed lignan extract lowers plasma cholesterol and glucose concentrations in hypercholesterolaemic subjects. Br J Nutr. 2008;99:1301–19.
43. Fukumitsu S, Aida K, Shimizu H, Toyoda K. Flaxseed lignan lowers blood cholesterol and decreases liver disease risk factors in moderately hypercholesterolemic men. Nutr Res. 2010;30:441–6.
44. Martinchik AN, Baturin AK, Zubtsov VV, Molofeev VLU. Nutritional value and functional properties of flaxseed. Vopr Pitan. 2012;81:4–10.
45. Denmark-Wahnefried W, Robertson CN, Walther PJ, Polascik TJ, Paulson DF, Vollmer RT. Pilot study to explore effects of low-fat, flaxseed-supplemented diet on proliferation on benign prostatic epithelium and prostate-specific antigen. Urology. 2004;63:900–4.
46. Demark-Wahnefried W, Polascik TJ, George SL, Switzer BR, Madden JF, Ruffin 4th MT, et al. Flaxseed supplementation (not dietary fat restriction) reduces prostate cancer proliferation rates in men presurgery. Cancer Epidemiol Biomarkers Prev. 2008;17:3577–87.
47. Procida G, Stancher B, Cateni F, Zacchigna M. Chemical composition and functional characterization of commercial pumpkin seed oil. J Sci Food Agric. 2013;93:1035–41.
48. Gossell-Williams M, Davis A, O'Connor N. Inhibition of testosterone-induced hyperplasia of the prostate of Sprague-dawley rats by pumpkin seed oil. J Med Food. 2006;9:284–6.
49. Tsai YS, Tong YC, Cheng JT, Lee CH, Yang FS, Lee HY. Pumpkin seed oil and phytosterol-F can block testosterone/prazosin-induced prostate growth in rats. Uro Int. 2006;77:269–74.
50. Carbin BE, Larsson B, Lindahl O. Treatment of benign prostatic hyperplasia with phytosterols. Br J Urol. 1990;66:639–41.
51. Bach D. Placebo-controlled, long-term therapeutic study of a pumpkin seed extract product in patients with micturition complaints from benign prostatic hyperplasia. Urologe B. 2000;40:437–43.
52. Hong H, Kim CS, Maeng S. Effects of pumpkin seed oil and saw palmetto oil in Korean men with symptomatic benign prostatic hyperplasia. Nutr Res Pract. 2009;3:323–7.

53. Wilt T, Ishani A, Mac Donald R, Rutks I, Stark G. *Pygeum africanum* for benign prostatic hyperplasia. Cochrane Database Syst Rev. 2002;1, CD001044.
54. McQueen CE, Bryant PJ. Pygeum. Am J Health Syst Pharm. 2001;58:120–3.
55. Suzuki M, Ito Y, Fujino T, Abe M, Umegaki K, Onoue S, et al. Pharmacological effects of saw palmetto extract in the lower urinary tract. Acta Pharmacol Sin. 2009;30:227–81.
56. Stewart KM. The African cherry (Prunus Africana): can lessons be learned from an over-exploited tree. J Ethnopharmacol. 2003;89:3–13.
57. Lopez-Miranda J, Perez-Jimenez F, Ros E, De Caterina R, Badimón L, Covas MI, et al. Olive oil and health: summary of the II international conference on olive oil and health consensus report, Jaen and Cordoba (Spain) 2008. Nutr Metab Cardiovasc Dis. 2010;20:284–94.
58. Mensink RP, Zock PL, Kester AD, Katan MB. Effects of dietary fatty acids and carbohydrates on the ratio of serum total to HDL cholesterol and on serum lipids and apolipoproteins: a meta-analysis of 60 controlled trials. Am J Clin Nutr. 2003;77:1146–55.
59. Kochikuzhyil BM, Devi K, Fattepur SR. Effect of saturated fatty acid-rich dietary vegetable oils on lipid profile, antioxidant enzymes and glucose tolerance in diabetic rats. Indian J Pharmacol. 2010;42:142–5.
60. Yamagishi K, Iso H, Yatsuya H, Tanabe N, Date C, Kikuchi S, JACC Study Group, et al. Dietary intake of saturated fatty acids and mortality from cardiovascular disease in Japanese: the Japan Collaborative Cohort Study for Evaluation of Cancer Risk. Am J Clin Nutr. 2010;92:759–65.
61. Larre S, Camparo P, Comperat E, Boulbes D, Haddoum M, Baulande S, et al. Biological effect of human serum collected before and after oral intake of Pygeum africanum on various benign prostate cell cultures. Asian J Androl. 2012;14:499–504.
62. Bent S, Kane C, Shinohara K, Neuhaus J, Hudes ES, Goldberg H, et al. Saw palmetto for benign prostatic hyperplasia (BPH). N Engl J Med. 2006;354:557–66.
63. Barry MJ, Meleth S, Lee JY, Kreder KJ, Avins AL, Nickel JC, Complementary and Alternative Medicine for Urological Symptoms (CAMUS) Study Group, et al. Effect of increasing doses of saw palmetto extract on lower urinary tract symptoms: a randomized trial. JAMA. 2011;306:1344–51.
64. Wilt TJ, Ishani A, Stark G, MacDonald R, Lau J, Mulrow C. Saw palmetto extracts for treatment of benign prostatic hyperplasia: a systematic review. JAMA. 1998;280:1604–9.
65. Wilt T, Ishani A, Mac Donald R. Serenoa repens for benign prostatic hyperplasia. Cochrane Database Syst Rev. 2002;3, CD001423.
66. Tacklind J, MacDonald R, Rutks I, Wilt TJ. Serenoa repens for benign prostatic hyperplasia. Cochrane Database Syst Rev. 2009;2, CD001423.
67. MacDonald R, Tacklind JW, Rutks I, Wilt TJ. Serenoa repens monotherapy for benign prostatic hyperplasia (BPH): an updated Cochrane systematic review. BJU Int. 2012;109:1756–61.
68. Bauer CM, Ishak MB, Johnson EK, Beebe-Dimmer JL, Cooney KA. Prevalence and correlates of vitamin and supplement usage among men with a family history of prostate cancer. Integr Cancer Ther. 2012;11:83–9.
69. Uzzo RG, Brown JG, Horwitz EM, Hanlon A, Mazzoni S, Konski A, et al. Prevalence and patterns of self-initiated nutritional supplementation in men at high risk of prostate cancer. BJU Int. 2004;93:955–60.
70. Debruyne F, Koch G, Boyle P, Da Silva FC, Gillenwater JG, Hamdy FC, et al. Comparison of a phytotherapeutic agent (Permixon) with an alpha-blocker (Tamsulosin) in the treatment of benign prostatic hyperplasia: A 1-year randomized international study. Eur Urol. 2002;41:497–507.
71. Debruyne F, Boyle P, Calais Da Silva F, Gillenwater JG, Hamdy FC, Perrin P, et al. Evaluation of the clinical benefit of permixon and tamsulosin in severe BPH patients-PERMAL study subset analysis. Eur Urol. 2004;45:773–9.
72. Roehrborn CG, Siami P, Barkin J, Damiao R, Becher E, Minana B, CombAT Study Group, et al. The influence of baseline parameters on changes in international prostate symptom score with dutasteride, tamsulosin, and combination therapy among men with symptomatic benign prostatic hyperplasia and an enlarged prostate: 2-year data from the CombAT study. Eur Urol. 2009;55:461–71.
73. Scaglione F, Lucini V, Pannacci M, Caronno A, Leone C. Comparison of the potency of different brands of Serenoa Repens extract on 5-alpha-reductase types I and II in prostatic co-cultured epithelial and fibroblast cells. Pharmacology. 2008;82:270–5.
74. Veeresh Babu SV, Veeresh B, Patil AA, Warke YB. Lauric acid and myristic acid prevent testosterone induced prostatic hyperplasia in rats. Eur J Pharmacol. 2010;626:262–5.
75. Arruzabala ML, Molina V, Mas R, Carbajal D, Marrero D, Gonzalez V, Rodriguez E. Effect of coconut oil on testosterone-induced prostatic hyperplasia in Sprague-Dawley rats. J Pharm Pharmacol. 2006;59:995–9.
76. Liang T, Liao S. Inhibition of steroid 5alpha-reductase by specific aliphatic unsaturated fatty acids. Biochem J. 1992;285:557–62.
77. Raynaud JP, Cousse H, Martin PM. Inhibition of type 1 and type-2 5alpha-reductase activity by free fatty acids, active ingredients of Permixon. J Steroid Biochem Mol Biol. 2002;82:233–9.
78. Di Silverio F, Monti S, Sclarra A, Varasano PA, Martini C, Lanzara S, et al. Effects of long-term treatment with Serenoa repens (Permixon) on the concentration and regional distribution of androgens and epidermal growth factor in benign prostatic hyperplasia. Prostate. 1998;37:77–83.
79. Prager N, Bickett K, French N, Marcovici G. A randomized, double-blind, placebo-controlled trial to determine the effectiveness of botanically derived inhibitors of 5-alpha reductase in the treatment of androgenetic alopecia. J Alt Comp Med. 2002;8:143–52.

80. Traish AM, Hassani J, Guay AT, Zitzmann M, Hansen ML. Adverse side effects of 5 alpha-reductase inhibitors therapy: persistent diminished libido and erectile dysfunction and depression in a subset of patients. J Sex Med. 2011;8:872–84.
81. Nickel JC, Sander S, Moon TD. A meta-analysis of the vascular-related safety profile and efficacy of alpha-adrenergic blockers for symptoms related to benign prostatic hyperplasia. Int J Clin Pract. 2008;62:1547–59.
82. Giulianelli R, Pecoraro S, Sepe G, Leonardi R, Gentile BC, Albanesi L, Cooperative Ur.O.P Group, et al. Multicentre study on the efficacy and tolerability of an extract of Serenoa repens in patients with chronic benign prostate conditions associated with inflammation. Arch Ital Urol Androl. 2012;84:94–8.
83. Morgia G, Mucciardi G, Gall A, Madonia M, Marchese F, Di Benedetto A, et al. Treatment of chronic prostatitis/chronic pelvic pain syndrome category IIIA with Serenoa repens plus selenium and lycopene (Profluss) versus S. repens alone: an Italian randomized multicenter-controlled study. Urol Int. 2010;84:400–6.
84. Kaplan SA, Volpe MA, Te AE. A prospective, 1-year trial using saw palmetto versus finasteride in the treatment of category III prostatitis/chronic pelvic pain syndrome. J Urol. 2004;171:284–8.
85. Wagenlehner FM, Weidner W. Prostatitis: no benefit of alpha-blockers for chronic prostatitis. Nat Rev Urol. 2009;6:183–4.
86. Nickel JC, Krieger JN, McNaughton-Collins M, Anderson RU, Pontari M, Shoskes DA, et al. Alfuzosin and symptoms of chronic prostatitis-chronic pelvic pain syndrome. N Engl J Med. 2008;359:2663–73.
87. Chrubasik JE, Roufogalis BD, Wagner H, Chrubasik S. A comprehensive review on the stinging nettle effect and efficacy profiles. Part II: urticae radix. Phytomedicine. 2007;14:568–79.
88. Nahata A, Dixit VK. Ameliorative effects of stinging nettle (Urtica dioica) on testosterone-induced prostatic hyperplasia in rats. Andrologia. 2012;44 (Suppl):396–409.
89. Alken CE. Konservative Behandlung des ProstataAdenoms und Stadien-Einteilung. Urologe B. 1973;13:95–8.
90. Wilt TJ, Ishani A, Rutks I, MacDonald R. Phytotherapy for benign prostatic hyperplasia. Public Health Nutr. 2000;3:459–72.
91. Safarinejad MR. Urtica dioica for treatment of benign prostatic hyperplasia: a prospective, randomized, double-blind, placebo-controlled, crossover study. J Herb Pharmacother. 2005;5:1–11.
92. Azimi H, Khakshur AA, Aghdasi I, Fallah-Tafti M, Abdollahi M. A review of animal and human studies for management of benign prostatic hyperplasia with natural products: perspective of new pharmacological agents. Inflamm Allergy Drug Targets. 2012;11: 207–21.
93. Briefel RR, Bialostosky K, Kennedy-Stephenson J, McDowell MA, Ervin RB, Wright JD. Zinc intake of the US population: findings from the third National Health and Nutrition Examination Survey, 1988–1994. J Nutr. 2000;30(5S Suppl):1367S–73.
94. Food and Nutrition Board, National Academy of Sciences. Dietary reference intakes for vitamin A, vitamin K, arsenic, boron, chromium, copper, iodine, iron, manganese, molybdenum, nickel, silicon, vanadium, and zinc. Washington, DC: National Academy Press; 2001. p. 177–204. 351–98.
95. Leitzmann MF, Stampfer MJ, Wu K, Colditz GA, Willett WC, Giovannucci EL. Zinc supplement use and risk of prostate cancer. J Natl Cancer Inst. 2002;95:1004–7.
96. Ishii K, Usui S, Sugimura Y, Yamamoto H, Yoshikawa K, Hirano K. Inhibition of aminopeptidase N (AP-N) and urokinase-type plasminogen activator (uPA) by zinc suppresses the invasion activity in human urological cancer cells. Biol Pharm Bull. 2001;24:226–30.
97. Ishii K, Usui S, Sugimura Y, Yoshida S, Hioki T, Tatematsu M, et al. Aminopeptidase N regulated by zinc in human prostate participates in tumor cell invasion. Int J Cancer. 2001;92:49–54.
98. Iguchi K, Hamatake M, Ishida R, Usami Y, Adachi T, Yamamoto H, et al. Induction of necrosis by zinc in prostate carcinoma cells and identification of proteins increased in association with this induction. Eur J Biochem. 1998;253:766–70.
99. Feng P, Liang JY, Li TL, Guan ZX, Zou J, Franklin R, Costello LC. Zinc induces mitochondria apoptogenesis in prostate cells. Mol Urol. 2000;4: 31–6.
100. Liang JY, Liu YY, Zou J, Franklin RB, Costello LC, Feng P. Inhibitory effect of zinc on human prostatic carcinoma cell growth. Prostate. 1999;40:200–7.
101. Zaichick V, Sviridova TV, Zaichick SV. Zinc in the human prostate gland: normal, hyperplastic and cancerous. Int Urol Nephrol. 1997;29:565–74.
102. Lagiou P, Wuu J, Trichopoulou A, Hsieh CC, Adami HO, Trichopoulos D. Diet and benign prostatic hyperplasia: a study in Greece. Urology. 1999;54:284–90.
103. Dunzendorfer U, Drahovsky D. C-peptide, testosterone, estrogen, cortisol and zinc in patients with benign prostatic hyperplasia of the prostate. Urol Int. 1980;35:369–74.
104. Wilden EG, Robinson MR. Plasma zinc levels in prostatic disease. Br J Urol. 1975;47:295–9.
105. Tisell LE, Fjelkegard B, Liessner KH. Zinc concentration and content of the dorsal, lateral and medial prostatic lobes and of periurethral adenomas in man. J Urol. 1982;128:403–5.
106. Leake A, Chrisholm GD, Busuttil A, Habib FK. Subcellular distribution of zinc in the benign and malignant human prostate: evidence for a direct zinc androgen interaction. Acta Endocrinol (Copenh). 1984;105:281–8.

107. Feustel A, Wenrich R. Zinc and cadmium in cell fractions of prostatic cancer tissues of different histological grading in comparison to BPH and normal prostate. Urol Res. 1984;12:147–50.
108. Lahtonen R. Zinc and cadmium concentrations in whole tissue and in separated epithelium and stroma from human benign hypertrophic glands. Prostate. 1985;6:177–83.
109. Brys M, Nawrocka AD, Miekos E, Zydek C, Foksinski M, Barecki A, Krajewska WM. Zinc and cadmium analysis in human prostate neoplasms. Biol Trace Elem Res. 1997;59:145–52.
110. Leake A, Chrisholm GD, Habib FK. The effect of zinc on the 5 alpha-reduction of testosterone by the hyperplastic human prostate gland. J Steroid Biochem. 1984;20:651–5.
111. Age-Related Eye Disease Study Research Group. A randomized, placebo-controlled, clinical trial of high-dose supplementation with vitamins C and E, beta-carotene, and zinc for age-related macular degeneration and vision loss: AREDS Report Number 8. Arch Ophthalmol. 2001;119:1417–36.
112. Johnson AR, Munoz A, Gottlieb JL, Jarrard DF. High dose zinc increases hospital admissions due to genitourinary complications. J Urol. 2007;177:639–43.
113. Chakravarthy U, Wong TY, Fletcher A, Plault E, Evans C, Zlateva G, et al. Clinical risk factors for age-related macular degeneration: a systematic review and meta-analysis. BMC Ophthalmol. 2010;10:31.
114. Kristal AR, Arnold KB, Schenk JM, Neuhouser ML, Goodman P, Penson DF, Thompson IM. Dietary patterns, supplement use, and the risk of symptomatic benign prostatic hyperplasia: results from the prostate cancer prevention trial. Am J Epidemiol. 2008;167:925–34.
115. Tavani A, Longoni E, Bosetti C, Maso LD, Polesel J, Montella M, et al. Intake of selected micronutrients and the risk of surgically treated benign prostatic hyperplasia: a case-control study from Italy. Eur Urol. 2006;50:549–54.
116. Health Canada Website. Multi-vitamin/Mineral Supplements. http://www.hc-sc.gc.ca/dhp-mps/prodnatur/applications/licen-prod/monograph/multi_vitmin_suppl-eng.php. Accessed on 10 Nov 2012.
117. Lazzerini M, Ronfani L. Oral zinc for treating diarrhoea in children. Cochrane Database Syst Rev. 2012;6, CD005436.
118. Science M, Johnstone J, Roth DE, Guyatt G, Loeb M. Zinc for the treatment of the common cold: a systematic review and meta-analysis of randomized controlled trials. CMAJ. 2012;184:551–61.
119. Schwarz S, Obermuller-Jevic UC, Hellmis E, Koch W, Jacobi G, Biesalski HK. Lycopene inhibits disease progression in patients with Benign Prostate Hyperplasia. J Nutr. 2008;138:49–53.
120. Kristal AR, Chi C, Tangen CM, Goodman PJ, Etzioni R, Thompson IM. Associations of demographic and lifestyle characteristics with prostate-specific (PSA) concentration and rate of PSA increases. Cancer. 2006;106:320–8.
121. Ilic D, Misso M. Lycopene for the prevention and treatment of benign prostatic hyperplasia and prostate cancer: a systematic review. Maturitas. 2012;72:269–76.
122. Wong WC, Wong EL, LI H, You JH, Ho S, Woo J, Hui E. Isoflavones in treating watchful waiting benign prostate hyperplasia: a double-blinded, randomized controlled trial. J Altern Complement Med. 2012;18:54–60.
123. Sebastiano C, Vincenzo F, Tommaso C, Giuseppe S, Marco R, Ivana C, et al. Dietary patterns and prostatic diseases. Front Biosci (Elite Ed). 2012;4:195–204.
124. Poon KS, McVary KT. Dietary patterns, supplement use, and the risk of benign prostatic hyperplasia. Curr Urol Rep. 2009;10:279–86.
125. Gong Z, Kristal AR, Schenk JM, Tangen CM, Goodman PJ, Thompson IM. Alcohol consumption, finasteride, and prostate cancer risk: results from the Prostate Cancer Prevention Trial. Cancer. 2009;115:3661–9.
126. Porst H, Kim ED, Casabe AR, Mirone V, Secrest RJ, Xu L, et al. Efficacy and safety of tadalafil once daily in the treatment of men with lower urinary tract symptoms suggestive of benign prostatic hyperplasia: results of an international randomized, double-blind, placebo-controlled trial. Eur Urol. 2011;60:1105–13.
127. Jang HA, Cho S, Kang SG, Ko YH, Kang SH, Bae JH, et al. The relaxant effect of ginseng saponin on the bladder and prostatic urethra: an in vitro and in vivo study. Urol Int. 2012;88:463–9.

Complementary and Alternative Medicine Interventions for Male Infertility/Subfertility: First Do No Harm

4

Introduction

Authoritative medical reviews have suggested for some time that antioxidant supplement treatment could be considered a primary treatment with conventional therapy, or at least an option for some male fertility issues [1], but more clinical evidence was needed [2, 3]. Yet, it is difficult to at least argue with the consistent suggestion that up to 80 % of male factor subfertility cases are believed to be the result of "oxidative stress" [4]. Perhaps some of the evidence to espouse the use of dietary supplements for male infertility has now been fulfilled.

A Cochrane systematic review was arguably one of the most extensive ever published in male fertility and dietary supplements, as it reviewed 34 randomized clinical trials with 2,876 couples in total [5]. Studies used in this analysis were for couples undergoing ART, for example, in vitro fertilization (IVF), intrauterine insemination (IUI), or intracyclic sperm injection (ICSI). The inclusion criteria were randomized controlled trials that included only men who were part of a couple with unexplained subfertility or subfertility and who were using ART with their own gametes. Excluded trials were nonrandomized and included men taking any other fertility-enhancing medications or men who had used chemotherapy treatment. The primary outcome was the live birth rate per couple, randomized, as well as these multiple secondary outcomes:

- Pregnancy rate per couple
- Miscarriage rate per couple or spontaneous abortion
- Stillbirth rate per couple
- Level of sperm DNA damage after treatment
- Sperm concentration and sperm motility
- Side effects associated with dietary supplements and withdrawals

The overall findings continue to surprise a number of healthcare professionals and patients, in my opinion, by concluding that antioxidant supplementation in males appears to have a positive role in improving the outcomes of live birth and pregnancy rates in couples participating in ART [5]. In fact, for live births the p-value was 0.0008 and for pregnancy rates it was $p<0.00001$. Critics of this analysis on "live births" will also arguably point toward the small number of such events: 20 live births that occurred from a total of 214 couples in only three studies were used in this part of the analysis, or the "pregnancy rates," which actually were derived from 96 pregnancies in 15 trials that included 964 couples. However, it is still remarkable that this is a viable minimal or moderate option for some men, given the low cost of most "antioxidants" utilized in these studies. Additionally, acute side effects were similar to a placebo with no serious adverse events reported in any trial.

Some of the antioxidants/complementary and alternative medicine (CAM) that may have demonstrated some impact (positive or negative) from this large analysis and from my experience include:

- Acupuncture and other CAM
- Astaxanthin
- Combined unique formula antioxidants

M.A. Moyad, *Complementary & Alternative Medicine for Prostate and Urologic Health*,
DOI 10.1007/978-1-4614-8492-9_4, © Springer Science+Business Media New York 2014

- Coenzyme Q10
- DHEA (and other prohormone supplements)
- Folic acid
- Glutathionine
- L-arginine
- L-carnitine
- Lycopene
- Magnesium
- Multivitamin
- *N*-acetylcysteine (NAC)
- Omega-3 fatty acids
- Plant estrogens
- Selenium
- Tongkat ali (*Eurycoma longifolia*)
- Vitamin C
- Vitamin D
- Vitamin E
- Zinc

The common question that will result from this or any other positive analysis for male fertility and antioxidants is, which specific dietary supplements and at what dosage and frequency? Interestingly, this extensive Cochrane review could not identify one superior individual antioxidant or combination product from these trials [5], so readers and patients are left with multiple questions. Thus, an overview of antioxidant supplements used in past, well-designed placebo-controlled trials is needed with an overall cost, safety, and health perspective to determine which products should be recommended and perhaps avoided by patients. This was the primary weakness of the Cochrane review and other reviews in male fertility [5]; the overall lack of specific recommendations based on overall safety and efficacy of these agents long-term for overall health and fertility maintenance.

This chapter will attempt to provide clarity on this issue of which supplements to recommend, and which ones should be avoided, based on heart healthy and overall health sensitivity recommendations. The endpoints of past, current, and future studies also matter, so clinicians need to constantly ask themselves in which of the following areas does this supplement impact:

- Oxidative stress reduction/markers
- Total sperm number
- Sperm concentration
- Sperm morphology
- Sperm motility (% motility and/or forward progression)
- Pregnancy rate
- Live births
- Short- and long-term safety
- Miscellaneous (ejaculate volume, pH, viscosity, sperm agglutination, other parameters)

Obviously, the impact on pregnancy and live birth rates along with overall safety are the more important variables and are in desperate need of more results in these areas for all of the dietary supplements mentioned in this chapter. And it is also of interest that if some supplements may improve male infertility when dealing with ART, then can it also be said that for those with motility issues (asthenospermia) or idiopathic oligoasthenoteratozoospermia (OAT), there may also be some benefit because of the overlap in those who use ART and men with this condition.

Dietary Supplements

Coenzyme Q10

CoQ10 (also known as "ubiquinone") appears to be a safe dietary supplement that requires a low dose for male fertility preservation. CoQ10 supplements have an excellent overall safety profile and actually have some clinical data to suggest that they may reduce blood pressure, but primarily in those with some form of hypertension. These supplements might also have some role in reducing myalgia from statin therapy [6, 7], but these results have been inconsistent, yet still proven to be safe at a variety of dosages [8]. The role of CoQ10 in the respiratory pathway as a method to improve energy production and reduce oxidative stress is well known in basic human physiology. It is for this reason that there should be some interest in utilizing this dietary supplement for the reduction of oxidative stress.

Seminal fluid also contains a measurable quantity of CoQ10 that appears to be associated with sperm count and motility. Patients with idiopathic asthenozoospermia may benefit in terms of spermatozoa motility when consuming 200 mg/day of CoQ10 for 6 months [9]. Another study of 212 infertile men taking 300 mg/day over 26 weeks found significant improvements in multiple parameters including sperm density, motility, and acrosome reaction [10]. Serum levels of FSH (follicle-stimulating hormone) and LH (luteinizing hormone) were significantly reduced by the supplement by the end of the study. But in a randomized trial of men with oligoasthenoteratozoospermia at a dosage of 200 mg/day compared to placebo, it appeared to reduce markers of oxidative stress, but did not demonstrate significant impacts on sperm concentration, motility, and morphology [11].

CoQ10 can be a costly supplement, so patients should be encouraged to compare prices from multiple commercial resources to determine the most cost-effective product. I have not observed in the medical literature profound differences in clinical effects with low-cost CoQ10 products compared to high-cost products. CoQ10 appears to be a heart-healthy or safe supplement [6], except it does have the rare potential to reduce the impact of warfarin because it has vitamin K-like properties [12], but ironically its slight antiplatelet effects may increase bleeding when combined with aspirin or clopidogrel. Regardless, it is a supplement that could be encouraged for fertility improvement in most men at a dosage of 200–300 mg/day.

My biggest reservation about CoQ10 is not side effects, or finding a low-cost product, but in its true efficacy over time. The reason I make this statement is due to the initial promise and then slight to moderate disappointment in this product in other areas of medicine. For example, the impact on statin-induced myalgia reduction was interesting initially [7], but is not a clear solution [8], and this is also true for the product in terms of its antihypertensive [13] effects and its role in Parkinson's disease research [14]. Still, the benefit outweighs the risk, so it should be part of the potential dietary supplement regimen approach for men with subfertility.

Folic Acid

Folic acid (vitamin B_9) is not an ideal antioxidant for male fertility in my opinion and should not be used at this time in certain patients, for example, those with a personal history or strong family history of cancer, especially prostate cancer. Folate is a water-soluble B vitamin, which is also known as vitamin B_9, and it occurs naturally in many healthy foods and multiple diverse beverages and foods [15]. Folic acid is the synthetic, human-produced, or manufactured form of folate that is found in dietary supplements and added to a variety of grain products, which are also known as "fortified foods."

Folate from foods and folic acid both assist in the production of DNA, RNA, and other items that are critical for the production and maintenance of cells, especially ones involved in rapid cell division and growth, such as in pregnancy and infancy [16]. Humans of all ages need folate to produce normal red blood cells and to prevent macrocytic anemia. Folate is also critical for metabolizing an amino acid known as "homocysteine," which may cause cellular damage in abnormally high amounts and is important for the synthesis of methionine. Folate has diverse roles in the development of a human being, which is why this compound is probably best known for preventing neural tube defects (NTDs) [15].

Green leafy vegetables, fruits, and legumes (beans, peas, lentils) are just some of the natural sources of folate. Still, due to the importance of folate in the prevention of NTDs, the Food and Drug Administration (FDA) required the addition of folic acid to grain products like breads, cereals, corn, flours, meals, pastas, and rice. In 1998, the USA and Canada officially began fortifying grain products with folic acid [15]. The recommended daily allowance (RDA) is only 400 micrograms (μg) a day [17]. A partial listing of food and other sources of folate and folic acid appears in Table 4.1 [17]. It is important to keep in mind that folic acid is generally added to foods that are labeled "enriched" and/or "fortified" in the USA and other countries. For this reason, it is easy to find recommended daily allowances of folate on products like breakfast cereals.

Synthetic folic acid was believed to be more bioavailable compared to folate from food, which may have been one of the many reasons to fortify foods around the world, along with the fact that a deficiency of folate in women of reproductive age can have devastating consequences. Research has

Table 4.1 A partial list of beverage/food and other sources of folate and folic acid

Food/beverage or other	Micrograms (μg)
100 % fortified breakfast cereals	400
Multivitamin (on average 1 pill)	400
B-complex vitamin (on average 1 pill)	400–800
Brewer's yeast (1 tablespoon)	250
Beef liver (cooked, 3 oz)	185
Spinach (cooked, 1/2 cup)	100
Asparagus (4 spears)	85
Rice (white, enriched, 1/2 cup)	65
Beans (baked, 1 cup)	60
Green peas (boiled, 1/2 cup)	50
Avocado (1/2 cup)	45
Broccoli (2 spears)	45
Lettuce (1/2 cup)	40
Peanuts (dry roasted, 1 oz)	40
Orange or orange juice (6 oz)	30–35
Tomato Juice (6 oz)	35
Bread (white, whole wheat, enriched, 1 slice)	25
Egg (whole)	25
Banana (medium)	20
Wheat germ (1 tablespoon)	20
Rice (brown, 1/2 cup)	5–10

now suggested that folate from foods may be only slightly less absorbable (about 20 %) compared to what was previously believed [18].

Other more critical issues with the overall safety and impact of folic acid on male health now exist. A large-scale meta-analysis has reviewed all of the randomized trial data on folic acid and other B-vitamin supplementation to reduce the risk of cardiovascular disease and cancer, or impact all-cause mortality [19]. It concluded that there was minimal to no impact of these supplements in reducing the risk of these conditions. In other words, currently it does not seem to impact the risk of most chronic diseases, despite the fact that it can reduce blood homocysteine levels by at least 25 %. Still, folic acid supplements may increase or encourage the growth of a variety of common tumors and precancerous lesions or polyps in high-risk individuals [20]. The cancer that receives the most attention in terms of a potential increased risk is prostate cancer [21, 22]. Serum levels of folic acid also appear to be increasing in the elderly such that unmetabolized folic acid (UMFA) has become a concern in men [23].

Still, the controversy over the clinical significance of a potential increased risk of prostate cancer will and should continue without any resolution in the near future. A meta-analysis of randomized trials found a significant increased risk of prostate cancer [24]. Arguably, another larger meta-analysis of randomized trials in cancer suggested that there was no risk and that past meta-analyses were influenced by a higher rate of cancer from one clinical trial [21], where prostate cancer incidence in the folic acid arm was probably increased due to chance [25]. Although these researchers make a compelling argument for this case, the problem with this theory is that most of the major trials looking at prostate cancer incidence still found at least nonsignificant increases in risk that cannot be disregarded due to chance, and this is confirmed by other recent meta-analysis [26], including population studies [27]. In other words, the sum of the data is not showing a neutral or reduced effect, only an increased risk overall, and the argument is whether or not it is statistically or clinically significant.

This argument tends to miss the forest for the trees in men's health, and until the risk is justified there is no sound benefit for most men in taking higher doses of supplemental folic acid for overall health and wellness. Thus, clinicians should not encourage supplemental folic acid use, especially in men with a history of cancer who are concerned about fertility, despite some minimal positive or just non-impressive data in the area of fertility itself [28, 29], because other supplements are safer, just as effective, and do not appear to require megadosage (like folic acid) for a clinical impact. Some of the early and only clinical trials that involved folic acid were using dosages such as 5 mg/day (along with zinc), which is 12.5 times the recommended daily intake [28]. Only sperm concentration, but not motility or morphology, was improved.

There is a dearth of studies, a question of safety in some men, and the potential need to utilize very high dosages of supplemental folic acid. Granted, the time periods that men need to be on these supplements are variable, but it is still not unusual in my experience to observe men taking these pills for several years. Food sources of folate can be recommended, because these have not been concerning overall, but the concentrated nutraceuticals do not follow the mantra right now of benefit exceeding risk.

L-Carnitine

L-Carnitine is a potential amino acid supplement for male fertility, but large dosages may be needed, and it is not a low-cost product in comparison to many other supplements mentioned in this chapter. L-Carnitine is an amino acid that transports fatty acids from the cytosol to the mitochondria for energy production in each cell of the body [30]. Humans can produce carnitine de novo in the liver from lysine and methionine (25 %), but dietary intake is the primary source of carnitine (75 %). Foods high in carnitine include dairy and meat; a plant-based diet is, in general, a poor source of carnitine. Excretion of carnitine occurs from the kidneys, but reabsorption is also efficient so that vegans are still able to maintain close to normal blood levels of this amino acid despite consuming 10 % less carnitine than omnivores.

Some preliminary research suggests that carnitine may slightly reduce fatigue in some cancer patients in higher dosages, but a phase III trial demonstrated 2,000 mg/day worked no better than a placebo for this specific situation over a 4-week testing period [31]. Even subset analysis revealed that those individuals who had lower blood levels of carnitine at baseline did not benefit. The future of L-carnitine in terms of energy production for patients with fatigue is now questionable, but there is still adequate data in other areas of medicine, for example, the ability of this product to increase the body weight or nutritional status of high-risk cachectic patients [32] and improve peripheral artery disease [33], and the impact of this supplement on male fertility—primarily motility [30].

It is of interest that vitamin C (ascorbic acid) is needed to synthesize carnitine in the human body [30]. The highest concentration of carnitine apart from supplements occurs in red meat and dairy products, so vegetarians who are trying to maintain fertility would potentially be better candidates for this supplement.

There are several minimally different forms of L-carnitine available for purchase that have been used in clinical trials, including L-carnitine, acetyl-l-carnitine (ALC), and propionyl-l-carnitine (PLC). These other types of L-carnitine have been tested because L-carnitine itself tends to be unstable. Yet these other forms of L-carnitine do not necessarily have better fertility data, especially when compared to each other at 3,000 mg/day [34], and they are more costly for the patient. Some clinical trials have suggested that the combination of these supplements may improve motility [35], but again this is not what I am deriving from these same studies with similar authors [35, 36]. Thus, multiple clinical trials have demonstrated the ability of L-carnitine, or other forms of carnitine, to improve primarily sperm motility and, potentially, pregnancy rates [34–42]. Yet there has been inconsistent or minimal evidence that it can impact sperm concentration and morphology.

A small US randomized, double-blind placebo-controlled study in men with idiopathic asthenospermia has challenged the potentially positive results with carnitine [43]. Male patients with sperm motility of 10–50 % were utilized, and over 24 weeks 2,000 mg/day of L-carnitine and 1,000 mg/day of acetyl-L-carnitine were ingested compared to placebo ($n=12$ vs. $n=9$). No significant differences in motility or total motile sperm counts occurred at 12 weeks or 24 weeks. These researchers called into question the clinical significance of the effect of L-carnitine for infertile men. They also reviewed past studies and suggested several methodology issues, such as exclusion of some patients from final analysis, as an issue [36], and also found carnitine to cause statistical significance in the past, but the clinical significance of the results are questionable. Another concern is lack of improvement in seminal plasma or sperm carnitine levels following supplementation [36, 43], which could be the result of adequate baseline levels or simply no ability to improve these concentrations with these supplements [43].

After this critical publication, a systematic review of nine clinical trials was published by independent researchers on the impact of L-CARNITINE for male infertility [44]. A significant improvement was shown in pregnancy rates ($p<0.0001$), total and forward sperm motility ($p=0.04$), and atypical sperms cell ($p<0.00001$), but no impact was found for sperm concentration or semen volume. Therefore, again clinicians are left to decide on this controversial supplement. L-carnitine causes an unpredictable change or minimal to moderate increase in sperm motility without a consistent change in sperm morphology and concentration, nor increase in seminal plasma carnitine levels, but there is a potential increase in pregnancy without any current safety issues. Is this enough to endorse the utilization of high doses of carnitine for male infertility? It should not be endorsed for preventive measures to preserve fertility, but its other features (especially safety) make it a controversial option at least.

Adverse events using L-carnitine or serious drug interactions have not been identified. Doses of 2–4 g (2,000–4,000 mg/day, divided doses two to three times a day) on average have been used in clinical trials. L-carnitine or acetyl-L-carnitine or the combination was used in these past studies. There was no commentary as to whether L-carnitine was ingested with or without a meal, so it seems there is flexibility with regard to this issue.

Omega-3 Fatty Acids

Recommending dietary sources of omega-3 should be encouraged in most individuals. There are numerous marine or fish sources that contain high levels of omega-3 fatty acids, vitamin D, protein, and selenium, including salmon, tuna, and sardines. A variety of other baked, broiled, raw, but not fried, fish are potentially beneficial [45]. Variety should be encouraged to increase compliance and exposure.

The benefit of fish consumption to reduce the risk or progression of cancer is preliminary, but its positive role in reducing a cardiovascular event or impacting all-cause mortality is a more definitive conclusion based on older clinical trials encouraging fish consumption [46] and other later selective clinical trials utilizing fish oil consumption [47, 48] in patients with a history of heart disease. Still, the overall and most up-to-date clinical trial data with fish oil supplementation on primary endpoints has been minimal to controversial and discouraging [49] and in perfectly healthy individuals does not currently espouse the use of these supplements [50]. Thus, fish oil supplements should probably be reserved for patients who want to reduce triglycerides [45], where they are FDA approved for this purpose.

The data on fish oil for male subfertility are minimal and controversial because there have not been enough studies. For example, in a randomized trial of DHA (docosahexaenoic acid) at 400 or 800 mg/day compared to placebo over 3 months for 28 asthenozoospermic (50 % or less motility) men, the omega-3 supplement did appear to increase serum and potentially seminal plasma DHA levels. However, it did not impact DHA into the spermatozoa phospholipid, which may have explained why it did not impact sperm motility compared to placebo [51]. A later trial of men with idiopathic oligoasthenoteratospermia (OAT) randomized to 1,840 mg of total omega-3 (EPA [eicosapentaenoic acid] and DHA) product compared to placebo over 32 weeks found a significant increase in sperm count, concentration, morphology, and motility, which may have been associated with the reductions in markers of oxidative stress [52]. Several cases of reflux, itching, and diarrhea occurred in the omega-3 group, which are known rare side effects of these supplements [45]. Again, until more research is conducted taking one to two omega-3 supplements that equate to 1,000–1,840 mg/day of EPA and DHA could be of benefit, but this is speculative.

Still, dietary sources of healthy fish can be encouraged. Mercury concentrations in specific fish have been reported by the FDA and in the overall medical literature, but the preliminary data are controversial and it is not known at this time what kind of clinical impact these mercury levels may have on the individual [45]. Four types of larger predatory fish have been most concerning because these fish (king mackerel, shark, swordfish, and tilefish) have the ability to retain greater amounts of methylmercury. Moderate consumption (two to three times/week) of most fish should have minimal impact on overall human mercury serum levels, but more ongoing research in this area should soon provide better clarity.

The positive impact of consuming fish seems to outweigh the negative impact in the majority of individuals, with the exception of women considering pregnancy or who are pregnant. A variety of fish have consistently demonstrated low levels of mercury, as summarized here [45]:

- Anchovies
- Catfish
- Cod
- Crab
- Flounder/sole
- Haddock
- Herring
- Lobster
- Mahi-mahi
- Ocean perch
- Oysters
- Rainbow trout
- Salmon (farmed and wild)
- Sardines
- Scallops
- Shrimp
- Spiny lobster
- Tilapia
- Trout (farmed)
- White fish (Great Lakes)

It should be kept in mind that approximately two servings per week of fatty, oily low-mercury fish is the equivalent to ingesting approximately one 250- to 500-mg fish oil pill per day. Clinicians who still desire to recommend high dosages of fish oil supplements must keep in mind that these supplements could increase the risk of internal bleeding at higher dosages and in combination with other blood thinners [12]. Although the risk of bleeding events is extremely rare, it has been observed in some clinical trials of healthy individuals and in combination with statins at a dosage of only 1,800 mg/day [48].

Some fish are low in mercury levels, but also low in omega-3 fatty acid concentration. Tilapia, which is high in protein, is a classic example. On the other hand, it is interesting that low-cost, small, and short-lived fish—such as anchovies and sardines—are low in mercury and have some of the highest concentrations of omega-3 oils and are used more than any other fish in the manufacturing of fish oil pills utilized by the public and in many clinical trials [45]. Patients who cannot eat fish or do not want to utilize fish oil because of an allergy or a personal belief could be recommended the newer algae-based omega-3 oils or encouraged to regularly consume the largest plant-based source of omega-3 fatty acids, which are found in plant oils (canola and soy), flaxseed, and chia seed.

Plant Estrogens or Phytoestrogens

It is easy to presume that weak plant estrogens found in foods, such as flaxseed, red clover, and soy, and in supplements could increase the risk of male infertility. This will be discussed in greater detail in the dietary section. There is simply no tangible evidence that these foods alter testosterone, or other parameters that would cause impairments in fertility [53–55]. The arguably largest two reviews of soy isoflavone supplements or foods and nine clinical trials and a review examining 15 placebo-controlled treatment groups all found no evidence to indicate any feminizing effects in men, including reduction in testosterone or changes in sperm or semen parameter [56, 57]. Although most clinical trials were less than 3 months in length, I do believe there is the potential for some plant estrogen supplements (not foods), such as red clover or any other plant estrogen supplements in excess, to cause some harm, and even have the potential to reduce DHT, so it should not be promoted in infertile men until proved otherwise.

A 1-year trial of 20 older men (mean age of 65 years) found significant increases in liver transaminases at a dosage of only 60 mg/day of red clover, and there was a suggestion of a 5-alpha reductase inhibition [58]. Other isoflavone studies using 60 mg/day of a concentrated supplement also appeared to significantly reduce DHT in a study of 28 healthy men [59], or free testosterone when tested for a 1-year period in a separate group of 20 men [60]. If there is even the slightest probability that consuming plant estrogen dietary supplements may reduce DHT levels, then there could be a potential and profound impact on libido and fertility. This is due to the ongoing concerns with more potent prescription drug DHT reducers, such as finasteride and dutasteride, that do not benefit sexual health or fertility, especially in cases of subfertility [61–66].

There is simply no reason to utilize these concentrated dietary plant estrogen supplements to improve male fertility or overall health. Instead, dietary sources are safe and can be recommended for general health. Soy and flaxseed have minimal calories, ample fiber, and omega-3 fatty acids and are low caloric foods that can improve lipid profiles and be utilized in most weight-loss interventions, in my opinion. These heart-healthy changes could theoretically improve fertility by also improving androgen levels and normalization of these hormones, especially if it helps those men in need of weight loss [67–70].

Selenium and Vitamin E

Selenium or vitamin E supplements should not be recommended to improve fertility in subfertile men strictly based on their overall safety issues and not on efficacy. For example, the initiation and even the final results of the Selenium and Vitamin E Cancer Prevention Trial (SELECT), trial of selenium and/or vitamin E, to prevent prostate cancer were concerning for a multitude of reasons [71, 72]. Both agents failed to prevent prostate cancer, and there were multiple past and current safety issues with these nutritional supplement agents. Selenium had a history of potentially increasing the risk of skin cancer recurrence [73], and there were concerns over an increased risk of type 2 diabetes [74]. Interestingly, SELECT observed a nonsignificant increased risk of type 2 diabetes when the trial was stopped [71]. And, there was a nonsignificant increase in the risk of aggressive (Gleason score 7–10) prostate cancer with vitamin E and/or selenium [72].

Vitamin E supplements were also replete with some similar but even more concerning issues compared to selenium during the SELECT. Past meta-analyses of other clinical trials found a potential increased risk of all-cause mortality with higher doses of vitamin E supplements [75]. Other large clinical trials found a significant increased risk of heart failure in those with vascular disease or diabetes [76]. A significant increased risk of hemorrhagic stroke was found for vitamin E supplements in another major chemoprevention trial of healthy physicians (Physicians' Health Study II) that was concurrently being conducted during the time of SELECT [77]. And, again SELECT found a nonsignificant ($p = 0.06$) increased risk of prostate cancer in the vitamin E arm when the study was terminated and a significantly higher risk with more follow-up after termination [71, 72]. Thus, both of these supplements have no impressive overall or heart-health research unless there is a profound deficiency in these compounds [78–82], and multiple past and ongoing concerns abound [83, 84], as outlined earlier.

There needs to be more clinician and patient awareness over the multiple serious safety issues with vitamin E and selenium, and these supplements should not be encouraged for any healthy individual attempting to improve fertility, despite past trials in infertility demonstrating some benefit [85–87]. It is also interesting that all of the past trials of vitamin E and/or selenium that have suggested benefit in male subfertility have also been at dosages equivalent or actually larger than past clinical trials in other areas of health that found large concerns [71, 72, 75–77]. And, since these supplements have not been found to have profound benefits beyond what has been observed with other supplements discussed in this chapter [5], then it would be prudent again to not recommend this particular compound, which has such a negative and nebulous history.

Tongkat Ali

This is a dietary supplement extract derived from a common shrub (*Eurycoma longifolia*, also known as "Malaysian ginseng" but is not in the ginseng family) found along the slopes of hilly areas in the Malaysian rainforest. It has preliminary human data that shows it might improve various aspects of male health—including sex drive—normalize testosterone in men with age-related androgen deficiency, and improve sperm quality and quantity at 200–300 mg/day [88–90].

Multiple laboratory studies have shown an ability of this herbal product to potentially improve male fertility status [91–94]. I also learned from multiple visits with healthcare professionals in this region that there is a history of using this product in Malaysia and other nearby locations to enhance fertility and male sexual health.

The one open-label study involved 75 men with idiopathic infertility who utilized the supplement for at least the first 3 months, and also followed pregnancy rates and improved semen measurements [90]. Significant improvement in all semen parameters occurred and 11 (14.7 %) spontaneous pregnancies occurred, although multiple methodologic issues still need to be resolved in a placebo-controlled trial. For example, the authors claim that 350 men started the trial and only 75 completed one full cycle of supplementation (3 months) and fulfilled the inclusion criteria, and only 17 men completed all 9 months of supplementation. This is a concerning exclusion and/or noncompliance rate that needs further investigation. The authors also point toward the possibility of a "bioactive peptide" that can increase testosterone levels in animals and humans and may reduce oxidative stress.

The product that has the most research and the only one with real clinical data is the standardized water-soluble extract (Physta) of *E. longifolia* root from the company Biotropics Malaysia Berhad, Kuala Lumpur, Malaysia. The company has also financially supported most of these studies. Their proprietary standardized water-soluble extract from the root of the plant and other Tongkat ali studies shows that this root has multiple diverse ingredients, such as [88–95]:

- Amino acid isoleucine
- Calcium, magnesium, and potassium
- Glycoproteins mucopolysacchrides
- High-molecular-weight polysaccharides
- Quassinoid alkaloids
- Tannins

It is theorized that this product may produce benefits in the area of male health because it may have a prohormone effect or DHEA mimic (yet, DHEA supplementation has not been adequately researched for its impact on male fertility), or perhaps because it is acting more like a diverse multivitamin for men. It could be that this product is no better than a really low-cost source or another supplement of Tongkat ali, but the problem is that other brands or just generic Tongkat ali do not have adequate clinical trials or quality control testing (for lead, arsenic, etc.).

Therefore, Tongkat ali does not have enough clinical evidence to recommend its use in men with idiopathic infertility, but few herbal supplements have even received adequate laboratory and clinical testing in this area with quality control and standardization measures. Thus, it could be utilized for a trial period if other less costly products appear not to be efficacious.

Vitamin C

There is enough indirect information and long-term safety of vitamin C that this supplement may have a small role in improving male subfertility [5]. Some positive preliminary data exists for improving fertility in men consuming 200–1,000 mg/day of vitamin C supplements in combination with other antioxidants [5]. Whether or not vitamin C alone can perform as well as the combination supplement treatments is not adequately known.

Vitamin C utilization for potentially improving male fertility has a long history, but there is a lack of good placebo-controlled trials [96, 97]. One small placebo-controlled trial of vitamin C (1,000 mg) in combination with high-dose vitamin E (800 mg) for 31 patients with asthenospermia showed no difference compared to placebo for 56 days and no pregnancies [98]. Interestingly, prolonged abstinence increased sperm count, concentration, total number of motile spermatozoa, and ejaculate volume. This highlights the difficulty in truly identifying what is working to improve fertility in some of these antioxidant studies. Yet, it is known that supplementation improves seminal plasma vitamin C in nonsmokers and smokers and could be correlated with improved morphology [99–101].

Seminal plasma has concentrations of vitamin C that are several orders of magnitude higher than that found in the bloodstream. Smoking has the ability to profoundly reduce vitamin C concentration [102]. A placebo-controlled trial of smokers found improvements in sperm quality at 200 and 1,000 mg/day [103]. Therefore, for smokers, ex-smokers, or those who have recently quit or are on smoking cessation regimens and trying to improve subfertility, including vitamin C, supplementation up to 1,000 mg/day seems logical. Whether or not it is needed outside of this population is questionable. Perhaps this is why there was also such interest in vitamin C years ago as opposed to recently, because such a large percentage of the population were smokers. It is also possible that the low cost of this supplement does not lead to much industry support for this product and fertility. Regardless of the reason, it still seems appropriate for all patients to be encouraged to eat a healthy diet high in vitamin C.

Some of the best dietary sources of vitamin C are listed in Table 4.2 [45, 104], but keep in mind that although these foods are healthy, one should be careful about getting an excessive amount of calories from them. It is also possible that with the stasis in fruit and vegetable consumption and the growing popularity of the low-carbohydrate dietary programs for weight loss, a consequence of this behavioral change may be a lower intake of citrus fruits, which could lead to lower vitamin C blood levels. Regardless, being able to achieve vitamin C concentrations from diet that are similar to the dosage utilized in clinical trials of supplementation is simply unrealistic. Still, a combination of regular vitamin C intake from food and daily dietary supplementation may be one of the best methods of maintaining adequate ascorbic acid and antioxidant blood levels that could improve fertility.

Table 4.2 Food/beverage sources of vitamin C

	Portion size	Vitamin C amount (mg)
Fruit		
Guava	1 medium	100
Strawberry	1 cup	95
Papaya	1 cup	85
Kiwi	1 medium	75
Orange	1 medium	70
Cantaloupe	1/4 medium	60
Mango	1 cup	45
Cantaloupe melon	1 cup	40
Grapefruit	1/2 fruit	40
Honeydew melon	1/8 medium	40
Lemon	1 medium	40
Tangerine or tangelo	1 medium	25
Watermelon	1 cup	15
Apple	1 medium	10
Avocado	1 medium	10
Apricot	1 medium	10
Banana	1 medium	10
Blueberry	1 cup	10
Crabapple	1 medium	10
Grape	1 cup	10
Pawpaw	1 medium	10
Pineapple	1 cup	10
Plum	1 medium	10
Juice		
Grape juice	1/2 cup	120
Apple juice	1/2 cup	50
Orange (fortified) juice	1/2 cup	50
Cranberry juice	1/2 cup	45
Grapefruit juice	1/2 cup	35
Tomato juice	6 oz	35
Vegetables		
Pepper (raw red or green)	1/2 cup	65
Broccoli (cooked)	1/2 cup	60
Kale (cooked)	1 cup	55
Brussels sprouts (cooked)	1/2 cup	50
Snow peas (fresh, cooked)	1/2 cup	40
Mustard greens (cooked)	1 cup	35
Potato (sweet or regular, baked)	1 medium	25–30
Cauliflower (raw or cooked)	1/2 cup	25
Cabbage (red, raw or cooked)	1/2 cup	20–25
Plantains (sliced, cooked)	1 cup	15
Tomato (raw)	1/2 cup	15
Cabbage (raw or cooked)	1/2 cup	10–15
Asparagus (cooked)	1/2 cup	10

There is some small concern about oxalate increases with plain vitamin C supplements, especially in those with a history of oxalate stones, and low-cost buffered vitamin C or calcium ascorbate may be a safer alternative for these specific patients [105]. The most practical criticism or real concern I hear from colleagues today about vitamin C is that sperm spends minimal time in seminal secretions before ejaculation. Thus, any true DNA injury would occur before entry in the seminal vesicle and ejaculatory ducts. In other words, vitamin C is more of a protective antioxidant after ejaculation and during transit time in the female reproductive tract. This makes sense, but in my opinion it is still an endorsement for using vitamin C for male subfertility and for trying to improve at least pregnancy probability. Overall, the safety of vitamin C at dosages of 200–1,000 mg on general health is outstanding [45], and as good as any supplement mentioned in this chapter. Smokers or those who have recently quit make an ideal group to consider using vitamin C for fertility.

Zinc

The excitement for the use of zinc alone or with other supplements is supported by some older clinical trials. For example, more than 100 subfertile and fertile men experienced a large improvement in sperm counts (74 % significant increase) over 24 weeks, which was not observed in the placebo group [28]. The problem with this study is that it was published in 2002 and 66 mg of zinc sulfate (six times the recommend daily dietary intake) was used alone or combined with 5 mg of folic acid (over 12 times the recommend dietary intake). Additionally, there was no difference in the serum or seminal plasma level of zinc between the subfertile and fertile men in this study, zinc supplements did not increase those levels, and the study did not include pregnancy as a clinical endpoint.

Another even older clinical trial of 100 men with asthenozoospermia was randomized to 250 mg twice daily (over 45 times the recommended dietary intake) of zinc for 3 months compared to no treatment [106]. Significant improvement in sperm quality, sperm count, motility, fertilizing capacity, and the incidence of antisperm antibodies were observed in the zinc group. After 12 months of follow-up, there were 11 pregnancies (22.5 %) in the zinc group and two (4.3 %) in the control group ($p<0.03$). There were no hormonal differences found between the groups.

Other studies have methodology issues, including a lack of controls or short treatment periods [107].

The problem with zinc is that the recommended dietary intake is only 11 mg/day [108], and megadoses of zinc supplements are replete with issues, especially in urology [109]. For example, one of the largest prospective studies to look at high-dose zinc supplement intake found an increased risk of advanced prostate cancer [110]. And in arguably the largest dietary supplement study to use high-dose zinc (Age-Related Eye Disease Study for macular degeneration) found an increased risk of hospital admissions in regard to genitourinary complications (BPH, stones, and UTI) in the 80-mg zinc arm [111, 112]. Whether or not this will be further confirmed is not the issue, because at this time zinc supplements in high doses like the ones needed in the fertility trials are too concerning short- and long-term. In fact, some countries such as Canada now discourage the sale of high-dose zinc supplements (40 mg or more) unless research suggests a specific benefit otherwise and proven safety simply because of these issues [113]. Some major clinical trials (AREDS 2) are now testing lower zinc dosages compared to the older effective higher dosage based on this history of adverse events [114].

Miscellaneous and Combination Products

Multiple individual antioxidants have just not garnered data through the years. Magnesium orotate given to ten males for idiopathic infertility over 90 days at a dosage of 3,000 mg/day compared to a ten-male control group did not improve sperm parameters or pregnancy rates [115]. One case of severe diarrhea occurred that required treatment to be discontinued in the magnesium group. This is the primary reason it would be difficult to ever endorse high dosages of magnesium supplements for infertility because of this well-known toxicity and the potential for severe harm from electrolyte disturbances that can cause neurologic and cardiovascular problems [116, 117].

It is plausible that low levels of magnesium are associated with a higher rate of infertility [118], but food sources (almonds, other nuts, spinach, soybeans, oatmeal, and so on) should be encouraged because they are so heart healthy and the recommended intake is only 350–400 mg/ day.

Astaxanthin is a carotenoid that can be found in microalgae, some red yeast, and krill oil [119]. Astaxanthin is a fairly new supplement that has one clinical trial at 16 mg/day for 3 months compared to placebo in 30 men with infertility. There was a significant increase in pregnancy rate and questionable impacts on sperm parameters (zona-free hamster oocyte test) that do not account for the pregnancy rate differences [120]. There were only 11 men in the intervention group, and three of them were on tamoxifen and neither morphology, motility, nor volume increased compared to placebo, but reactive oxygen species were reduced. This supplement receives enormous hype on the Internet, but studies need to catch up to the advertising because it is not cost-effective and long-term toxicity still needs to be researched. In my opinion, this type of advertising and highlighting of its antioxidant capacity reminds me of long ago when the common thinking was that vitamin E supplements could provide multiple benefits in similar patient populations.

Other supplements that are commonly brought up in some reviews also suffer from a similar fate of lacking consistent impressive data. *N*-acetylcysteine (NAC) at 600 mg/day in 120 infertile men compared to placebo found reductions in oxidative stress and significant improvements in semen volume, motility, and viscosity, but no change in sperm number or morphology [121]. This is at least an encouraging data, but these results somewhat challenge the results of another positive trial using the same dose of NAC [87]; however, this study used high-dose selenium with NAC, which could have explained the difference.

Since NAC is used to increase or restore glutathione levels for acetaminophen toxicity [122], then why not utilize it for male infertility because it is a safe option? Why not just give the supplement glutathione directly because it is the most potent precursor to glutathione itself, which reduces oxidative stress? The problem is that glutathione has known weak bioavailability and needs to be given intravenously or as an intramuscular injection [123–125]. Thus, it really does not have a role as a dietary supplement right now, but NAC has potential for use.

L-arginine may be a precursor of nitric oxide, but megadoses are needed to really observe any potential impact, which is arguably why lower doses were not initially effective [126], but 9 g or 18 g might have value [127]. This represents an unusually high and potentially unsafe amount in some patients [128]. It would be better to research a more potent nitric oxide producer, such as L-citrulline, at smaller and more realistic dosages that do not get extensively removed by first-pass metabolism or intestinal arginases, as is the case with L-arginine [129].

Other individual supplements, such as lycopene, just need more data [130], and their moment of extensive attention has passed, so I am skeptical that further definitive studies will be conducted. And, although vitamin D receptors have been found on sperm cells [131], there are no clinical data to espouse its use for male subfertility beyond the recommended daily intake (600–800 IU/day) at the current time [132].

ProXeed® (Sigma-Tau, Gaithersburg, MD, USA) is a popular combination dietary supplement for male infertility in some parts of the world, and in my opinion it has no unsafe amounts of any ingredients. It is a combination of L-carnitine (145 mg), acetyl-L-carnitine (64 mg), fructose (250 mg), citric acid (50 mg), selenium (50 mcg), coenzyme Q10 (20 mg), zinc (10 mg), vitamin C (90 mg), B_{12} (1.5 mcg), and folic acid (200 mcg) taken once a day [133]. In an open trial of 114 men with idiopathic asthenoteratozoospermia (96 men completing the trial) for at least 18 months, the mean sperm progressive motility significantly increased from 18.3 to 42.1 and 16 patients "achieved pregnancy." No significant improvement was noted for sperm density and the rate of morphologically normal forms.

The real question with this commercialized product and many others is whether or not it works the same, better, or worse compared to other less costly supplements mentioned in this chapter. It will be difficult to get clarity from this anytime soon because these comparison trials are lacking, and I cannot visualize how manufacturers of these products will ever be motivated to conduct such head-to-head studies. Of course, they would be welcomed and provide a unique perspective, but personally I am just not optimistic these will occur. In the meantime, it would make sense to follow the plethora of the data. I could argue that using the lower-cost individual or combined supplements for a trial period is completely logical and, if not effective, then switching to a more commercial combination product would be the next step. I believe the one advantage to these commercial combination products used by healthcare professionals is quality control, but the downside is cost and the lack of impressive research beyond what has already been potentially observed with other antioxidants.

I could further argue that the simplest compounds used in most studies do not have concerning quality-control issues overall. Part of the reason for this is that no herbal products (more notorious for quality control because of the need for standardization) are utilized to any extent in past studies and only single-ingredient vitamins, minerals, and other simplistic compounds have been used. The only recent exception to this list is *E. longifolia* (Tongkat Ali).

Why not just encourage the use of a daily multivitamin? It has good long-term safety data in men and is heart healthy, safe, and may provide cancer preventive impacts when only one pill is used per day [134, 135], and there are also some minimal infertility data [136]. These logical approaches are for clinicians and their patients to decide.

I am often asked about other areas of CAM that have minimal research, such as acupuncture or meditation, because these are utilized in a minority of patients [137]. The data in this area are mixed for women and men [138, 139], especially with acupuncture (other CAM have virtually no consistent or adequate studies) [139]. Some believe and have tested the possibility that scrotal hyperthermia can be normalized with acupuncture for those who qualify for this condition [140], and perhaps this has some future merit. My concern with acupuncture is not the safety but the combination of efficacy and costs with multiple treatments. Many acupuncturists also give or recommend herbal medicines, but patients should be told about all of the non-herbal supplements that have data to potentially improve male subfertility.

Conclusion

It is time to view male subfertility supplements with a wider perspective because a plethora of research has been performed on numerous antioxidants. Large and authoritative meta-analyses have actually endorsed the utilization of multiple products for men attempting to maintain or improve fertility [5]. However, before endorsement of a specific supplement becomes logical, it would seem imperative to teach clinicians and patients about the overall safety and efficacy of each proposed intervention outside of fertility. What is the impact of these agents on general health and specific conditions that have the largest toll on morbidity and mortality in men and women, such as heart disease and cancer?

When this is kept in mind, the so-called "forest over the tree" approach that benefits all our patients will have been exercised. This is the first do-no-harm approach that seems the most logical, because CAM including supplements has been used at a high rate for couples who want to become pregnant [137, 141], and there is a need for good, objective information right now. Therefore, an extensive summary of the supplements/CAM options discussed in this chapter is described in Table 4.3.

Critics of dietary supplements for infertility may point to the lack of extremely rigorous long-term clinical trials in this area and the lack of correction for multiple confounding factors in these studies such as dietary intake [142], and these are valid points. Like many critics, I do not believe there are data to support the use of dietary supplements to maintain normal fertility; in fact, prooxidant activity or DNA damage could theoretically occur in this setting. Yet, when critics mention and emphasize every possible side effect ever reported with a specific dietary supplement, even if that risk is almost improbable or rare, this does not make for a compelling argument against the use of dietary supplements for male subfertility.

Table 4.3 A summary of most supplements/cam with some level of evidence in the area of male subfertility[a]

CAM/supplement option (quick clinical recommendation)	Advantages	Disadvantages
Acupuncture and other CAM, such as meditation (no)	Usually safe and commonly utilized by couples from surveys of infertility clinics. May be advantageous for those seeking stress relief or other holistic benefits	Minimally researched and can be expensive. Herbal recommendations are commonly offered with these procedures
Combination low-dose supplements with vitamins, minerals (maybe)	Safe and has some data (e.g., ProXeed), and some companies can ensure good quality control	Whether this offers a benefit beyond a multivitamin or a single-ingredient supplement is controversial
CoQ10 (maybe)	Preliminary evidence suggests a positive impact on sperm motility at 200–300 mg/day. Minimal safety issues overall	Only preliminary clinical evidence, questionable impacts on sperm concentration, and morphology and pregnancy rate. Not a low-cost supplement. Patients on blood thinners could experience further antiplatelet effects, and those on warfarin could paradoxically experience vitamin K–like effects or reduced efficacy
DHEA and other prohormones (no)	May improve testosterone levels in those with androgen deficiency	Has no adequate research in male infertility and could also increase estradiol levels and theoretically worsen infertility
Folic acid (vitamin B_9) (no)	A more efficiently absorbed form compared to dietary sources. Preliminary research suggests some role in male fertility	Doses utilized in preliminary trials are extremely high, and the safety of these dosages in men with a history of cancer is concerning and unresolved. Minimal direct evidence and some safety issues
Glutathione (no)	Future research should be able to improve the absorption of these pills	Precursors to glutathione such as NAC make more sense because of the poor absorption from oral doses, and injections or IV need to be given for efficacy
L-arginine (no)	Has some scientific evidence when used in very large dosages (9–18 g)	Megadoses needed for potential efficacy, which gets eliminated on first-pass metabolism and has questionable safety. Using L-citrulline at lower doses has greater potential
L-carnitine and/ or acetyl-L-carnitine (maybe)	2,000–4,000 mg individually or in combination does not appear to have any serious safety issues, and there is some evidence for increased sperm motility and pregnancy rate	No consistent increase in seminal plasma carnitine levels and no consistent impact on sperm concentration and morphology. Sperm motility results have also been questioned
Lycopene (no)	Good safety	No preliminary adequate clinical research.
Magnesium (no)	Can be found in heart-healthy foods, and a few hundred milligrams has been safe in most clinical trials	Research is poor overall, and side effects such as diarrhea can occur at low doses; higher doses can cause severe electrolyte changes that can be serious
Multivitamin (yes)	Preliminary research indicates improved semen parameters One pill a day in men now has short- and long-term safety based on the PHS2 randomized trial. This 11-year general health trial in men used Centrum Silver (low-cost option) compared to placebo	Only one pill a day should be encouraged; there is suggestion of potential harm from taking two pills a day long-term

(continued)

Table 4.3 (continued)

CAM/supplement option (quick clinical recommendation)	Advantages	Disadvantages
N-acetylcysteine (NAC) (maybe)	600 mg/day. Improvements shown in volume, motility, and viscosity of semen, and possibly concentration and morphology Arguably one of the best precursors of glutathione as a dietary supplement. Used already in medicine to improve glutathione at prescription dosages—e.g., for acetaminophen overdose	Strong research on pregnancy rates is lacking from clinical trials
Omega-3 fatty acids (maybe, but food sources should be emphasized over pills)	Minimal research suggests it may improve multiple parameters in those with OAT. Overall good safety at 800–1,840 mg total of EPA and DHA per day	Minimal to no impact on asthenospermia and no confirmed impact on OAT. Suffers from a lack of high-quality clinical research
Plant estrogen–flaxseed, red clover, soy–supplements (no)	Dietary sources may improve heart health and fertility	Supplements are not beneficial or harmful, but red clover supplements may increase liver enzymes and may have 5-alpha reductase inhibitory activity, which could theoretically reduce male fertility
Selenium and/or vitamin E (no, not a current option as individual high-dose supplements)	Multiple clinical trials have been completed with these supplements with positive potential impacts on semen parameters and good short-term safety	Selenium at high dosages has a history of increasing the risk of type 2 diabetes and recurrent nonmelanoma skin cancer. Minimal data in human fertility. Vitamin E has been found to increase the risk of prostate cancer at 400 IU; also, there are minimal data regarding its use for male fertility
Tongkat ali (*E. longifolia*) (no)	One product from Malaysia (200 mg proprietary extract) has a good safety record and an open clinical trial that suggests it may improve semen parameters. Arguably one of the only herbals that could be used if other options are not working or cannot be utilized	Needs more research and overall; herbals for infertility have a risk-greater-than-benefit profile
Vitamin C (maybe—especially in ex-smokers, smokers, and those on smoking cessation regimens)	1,000 mg/day does not appear to have overt safety issues, is low cost, and now comes in a buffered (calcium ascorbate) option to reduce gastrointestinal effects for those who cannot tolerate the acidity of this supplement	Increases in oxalate may be a minimal to moderate concern for some high-risk kidney stone patients. Minimal research in the area of male infertility
Vitamin D (no)	Low cost and plays a research-based role in the male reproductive tract to potentially enhance a variety of outcomes	Needs blood testing to determine if deficiency or insufficiency exists, and then patient would need to be monitored and dosed based on continuing these blood tests
Zinc (no)	May improve a variety of semen parameters	High dosages of zinc (80 mg or higher) show a potential for higher rates of urologic risks that require treatment, including BPH, prostate cancer, stones, and UTI from a large randomized trial (AREDS)

[a]Note: Past clinical trials have shown that any recommended product can be taken with or without food, and the dosage should ideally be divided into half and utilized in the morning and evening, with or after a meal, to reduce gastrointestinal side effects. Whether or not to take more than one recommended product at a time is not known and has not been adequately researched

If this same argument was also done for prescription medications or procedures, then I could argue no one would ever attempt to take a single pill or be the subject of any inpatient or outpatient maneuvers.

Until a large randomized trial is conducted by experts in this field that can provide more clarity, the question remains as to the potential downside of recommending low-cost safe supplements for couples spending enormous amounts of money already on conventional treatments to enhance pregnancy and the chance for a live birth. Conventional medicine can profoundly improve the chances of pregnancy for struggling couples, yet clinicians have to be honest with themselves about the costs, time, side effects, and overall success rate associated with current regimens as stand-alone answers to infertility. Compliance (e.g., with ART) is not the issue [143]; cost and success rate are the issues. Thus, if a safe and affordable CAM product has the potential to improve conventional medicine and does not reduce efficacy, clinicians have to ask themselves this question: If they were in the same position as their patient, would they take a dietary supplement? In my experience, this has already been answered by the plethora of clinicians who are now working in the area of infertility all around the world.

References

1. Agarwal A, Sekhon LH. The role of antioxidant therapy in the treatment of male infertility. Hum Fertil (Camb). 2010;13:217–25.
2. Agarwal A, Nallella KP, Allamaneni SS, Said TM. Role of antioxidants in treatment of male infertility: an overview of the literature. Reprod Biomed Online. 2004;8:616–27.
3. Ghanem H, Shamloul R. An evidence-based perspective to the medical treatment of male infertility: a short review. Urol Int. 2009;82:125–9.
4. Tremellen K. Oxidative stress and male infertility-a clinical perspective. Hum Reprod Update. 2008;14:243–58.
5. Showell MG, Brown J, Yazdani A, Stankiewicz MT, Hart RJ. Antioxidants for male subfertility. Cochrane Database Syst Rev 2011; Jan 19;(1):CD007411.
6. Littarru GP, Tiano L. Clinical aspects of coenzyme Q10: an update. Nutrition. 2010;26:250–4.
7. Wyman M, Leonard M, Morledge T. Coenzyme Q10: a therapy for hypertension and statin-induced myalgia? Cleve Clin J Med. 2010;77:435–42.
8. Bogsrud MP, Langslet G, Ose L, Arnesen KE, Sm Stuen MC, Malt UF, et al. No effect of combined coenzyme Q10 and selenium supplementation on atorvastatin-induced myopathy. Scand Cardiovasc J. 2013;47(2):80–7.
9. Balercia G, Buldreghini E, Vignini A, Tiano L, Paggi F, Amoroso S, et al. Coenzyme Q10 treatment in infertile men with idiopathic asthenozoospermia: a placebo-controlled randomized trial. Fertil Steril. 2009;91:1785–92.
10. Safarinejad ME. Efficacy of coenzyme Q10 on semen parameters, sperm function and reproductive hormones in infertile men. J Urol. 2009;182: 237–48.
11. Nadjarzadeh A, Sadeghi MR, Amirjannati N, Vafa MR, Motevalian SA, Gohari MR, et al. Coenzyme Q10 improves seminal oxidative defense but does not affect on semen parameters in idiopathic oligoasthenoteratozoospermia: a randomized double-blind, placebo-controlled trial. J Endocrinol Invest. 2011;34:e224–8.
12. Mousa SA. Antithrombotic effects of naturally derived products on coagulation and platelet function. Methods Mol Biol. 2010;663:229–40.
13. Young JM, Florkowski CM, Molyneux SL, McEwan RG, Frampton CM, Nicholis MG, et al. A randomized, double-blind, placebo-controlled crossover study of coenzyme Q10 therapy in hypertensive patients with the metabolic syndrome. Am J Hypertens. 2012;25:261–70.
14. National Institute of Neurological Disorders and Stroke. Statement on the termination of QE3 Study. http://www.ninds.nih.gov/disorders/clinical_trials/CoQ10-Trial-Update.html. Accessed on 15 Feb 2013.
15. Obican SG, Finnell RH, Mills JL, Shaw GM, Scialli AR. Folic acid in early pregnancy: a public health success story. FASEB J. 2010;24:4167–74.
16. Zeisel SH. Importance of methyl donors during reproduction. Am J Clin Nutr. 2009;89:673S–7.
17. Institute of Medicine. Food and Nutrition Board. Folate. Dietary Reference Intakes for Thiamin, Riboflavin, Niacin, Vitamin B6, Folate, Vitamin B12, Pantothenic Acid, Biotin, and Choline. Washington, DC: National Academy Press; 2000. p. 196–305.
18. Winkels RM, Brouwer IA, Siebelink E, Katan MB, Verhoef P. Bioavailability of food folates is 80 % of that of folic acid. Am J Clin Nutr. 2007;85:465–73.
19. Clarke R, Halsey J, Lewington S, Lonn E, Armitage J, Manson JE, Bønaa KH, B-vitamin Treatment Trialists' Collaboration, et al. Effects of lowering homocysteine levels with B vitamins on cardiovascular disease, cancer, and cause-specific mortality. Meta-analysis of 8 randomized trials involving 37,485 individuals. Arch Intern Med. 2010;170:1622–31.

20. Cole BF, Baron JA, Sandler RS, Halle RW, Ahnen DJ, Bresaller RS, et al. Polyp Prevention Study Group. Folic acid for the prevention of colorectal adenomas: a randomized clinical trial. JAMA. 2007;297:2351–9.
21. Figueriredo JC, Grau MV, Haile RW, Sandler RS, Summers RW, Bresalier RS, et al. Folic acid and risk of prostate cancer: results from a randomized clinical trial. J Natl Cancer Inst. 2009;101:432–5.
22. Collin SM, Metcalfe C, Refsum H, Lewis SJ, Zuccolo L, Smith GD, et al. Circulating folate, vitamin B12, homocysteine, vitamin B12 transport proteins, and risk of prostate cancer: a case–control study, systematic review, and meta-analysis. Cancer Epidemiol Biomarkers Prev. 2010;19:1632–42.
23. Balley RL, Millis JL, Yetley EA, Gahche JJ, Pfeiffer CM, Dwyer JT, et al. Unmetabolized serum folic acid and its relation to folic acid intake from diet and supplements in a nationally representative sample of adults aged > or =60 y in the United States. Am J Clin Nutr. 2010;92:383–9.
24. Wien TN, Pike E, Wisloff T, Staff A, Smeland S, Klemp M. Cancer risk with folic acid supplements: a systematic review and meta-analysis. BMJ Open. 2012;2(1):e000653.
25. Vollset SE, Clarke R, Lewington S, Ebbing M, Halsey J, Lonn E, et al. Effects of folic acid supplementation on overall and site-specific cancer incidence during the randomized trials: meta-analyses of data on 50,000 individuals. Lancet. 2013;381:1029–36.
26. Qin X, Cui Y, Shen L, Sun N, Zhang Y, Li J, et al. Folic acid supplementation and cancer risk: a meta-analysis of randomized controlled trials. Int J Cancer. 2013;133:1033–41.
27. Bassett JK, Severi G, Hodge AM, Baglietto L, Hopper JL, English DR, et al. Dietary intake of B vitamins and methionine and prostate cancer incidence and mortality. Cancer Causes Control. 2012;23:855–63.
28. Wong WY, Merkus HM, Thomas CM, Menkveld R, Zielhuis GA, Steegers-Theunissen RP. Effects of folic acid and zinc sulfate on male factor subfertility: a double-blind, randomized, placebo-controlled trial. Fertil Steril. 2002;77:491–8.
29. Murphy LE, Mills JL, Molloy AM, Qian C, Carter TC, Strevens H, et al. Folate and vitamin B12 in idiopathic male infertility. Asian J Androl. 2011;13:856–61.
30. Acetyl-L-carnitine. Monograph. Altern Med Rev 2010;15:76–83.
31. Cruciani RA, Zhang JJ, Manola J, Cella D, Ansari B, Fisch MJ. L-carnitine supplementation for the management of fatigue in patients with cancer: an eastern cooperative oncology group phase III, randomized, double-blind, placebo-controlled trial. J Clin Oncol. 2012;30:3864–9.
32. Kraft M, Kraft K, Gartner S, Mayerle J, Simon P, Weber E, et al. L-carnitine-supplementation in advanced pancreatic cancer (CARPAN)-a randomized multicentre trial. Nutr J. 2012;11:52.
33. Goldenberg NA, Krantz MJ, Hiatt WR. L-carnitine plus cilostazol versus cilostazol alone for the treatment of claudication in patients with peripheral artery disease: a multicenter, randomized, double-blind, placebo-controlled trial. Vasc Med. 2012;17:145–54.
34. Balercia G, Regoli F, Armeni T, Koverech A, Mantero F, Boscaro M. Placebo-controlled double-blind randomized trial on the use of L-carnitine, L-acetylcarnitine, or combined L-carnitine and L-acetylcarnitine in men with idiopathic asthenozoospermia. Fertil Steril. 2005;84:662–71.
35. Lenzi A, Sgro P, Salacone P, Paoli D, Gillio B, Lombardo F, et al. A placebo-controlled double-blind randomized trial of the use of combination L-carnitine and L-acetyl-carnitine treatment in men with asthenozoospermia. Fertil Steril. 2004;81:1578–84.
36. Lenzi A, Lombardo F, Sgro P, Salacone P, Caponecchia L, Dondero F, et al. Use of carnitine therapy in selected cases of male factor infertility: a double-blind crossover trial. Fertil Steril. 2003;79:292–300.
37. Li Z, Chen GW, Shang XJ, Bal WJ, Han YF, Chen B, et al. A controlled randomized trial of the use of combined L-carnitine and acetyl-L-carnitine treatment in men with oligoasthenozoospermia. Zhong Hua Nan Ke Xue. 2005;11:761–4.
38. Cavallini G, Ferraretti AP, Gianaroli L, Biagiotti G, Vitali G. Cinnoxicam and L-carnitine/acetyl-l-carnitine treatment for idiopathic and varicocele-associated oligoasthenospermia. J Androl. 2004;25:761–70.
39. Moncada ML, Vivari E, Cimino C, Calogero AE, Monglol A, D' Agata R. Effect of acetylcarnitine treatment in oligoasthenospermic patients. Acta Eur Fertil. 1992;23:221–4.
40. Costa M, Canale D, Filicori M, D'lddio S, Lenzi A. L-carnitine in idiopathic asthenozoospermia: a multicenter study. Italian Study Group on carnitine and male infertility. Andrologia. 1994;26:155–9.
41. Vitali G, Parente R, Melotti C. Carnitine supplementation in human idiopathic asthenospermia: clinical results. Drugs Exp Clin Res. 1995;21:157–9.
42. Vicari E, Calogero AE. Effects of treatment with carnitines in infertile patients with prostato-vesciculo-epididymitis. Hum Reprod. 2001;16:2338–42.
43. Sigman M, Glass S, Campagnone J, Pryor JL. Carnitine for the treatment of idiopathic asthenospermia: a randomized, double-blind, placebo-controlled trial. Fertil Steril. 2006;85:1409–14.
44. Zhou X, Liu F, Zhai S. Effect of L-carnitine and/or L-acetyl-carnitine in nutrition treatment for male infertility: a systematic review. Asia Pac J Clin Nutr. 2007;16 Suppl 1:383–90.
45. Moyad MA. Dr. Moyad's no bogus science health advice. Ann Arbor, MI: Ann Arbor Editions Publishing; 2009.
46. Burr ML, Fehlly AM, Gilbert JF, Rogers S, Holliday RM, Sweetnam PM, et al. Effects of changes in fat, fish, and fibre intakes on death and myocardial reinfarction: Diet and Reinfarction Trial (DART). Lancet. 1989;2:757–61.

47. Marchioli R, Barzi F, Bomba E, Chieffo C, Di Mascio R, Franzosi MG, et al. Early protection against sudden cardiac death by n-3 polyunsaturated fatty acids after myocardial infarction: time-course analysis of the results of the Gruppo Italiano per lo Studio della Sopravvivenza nell'Infarto Miocardico (GISSI)-Prevenzione. Circulation. 2002;105:1897–903.
48. Matsuzaki M, Yokoyama M, Saito Y, Origasa H, Ishikawa Y, Oikawa S, JELIS investigators, et al. Incremental effects of eicosapentaenoic acid on cardiovascular events in statin-treated patients with coronary artery disease. Circ J. 2009;73:1283–90.
49. Mozaffarian D, Marchioli R, Macchia A, Silleta MG, Ferrazzi P, Gardner TJ, OPERA Investigators, et al. Fish oil and postoperative atrial fibrillation: the Omega-3 Fatty Acids for Prevention of Post-operative Atrial Fibrillation (OPERA) randomized trial. JAMA. 2012;308:2001–11.
50. Rizos EC, Ntzani EE, Bika E, Kostapanos MS, Elisaf MS. Association between omega-3 fatty acid supplementation and risk of major cardiovascular disease events: a systematic review and meta-analysis. JAMA. 2012;308:1024–33.
51. Conquer JA, Martin JB, Tummon I, Watson L, Tekpetey F. Effect of DHA supplementation on DHA status and sperm motility in asthenozoospermic males. Lipids. 2000;35:149–54.
52. Safarinejad MR. Effect of omega-3 polyunsaturated fatty acid supplementation on semen profile and enzymatic anti-oxidant capacity of seminal plasma in infertile men with idiopathic oligoasthenoteratospermia: a double-blind, placebo-controlled, randomized study. Andrologia. 2011;43:38–47.
53. Nagata C, Takatsuka N, Shimizu H, Hayashi H, Akamatsu T, Murase K. Effect of soymilk consumption on serum estrogen and androgen concentrations in Japanese men. Cancer Epidemiol Biomarkers Prev. 2001;10:179–84.
54. Habito RC, Montalto J, Leslie E, Ball MJ. Effects of replacing meat with soyabean in the diet on sex hormone concentrations in healthy adult males. Br J Nutr. 2000;84:557–63.
55. Dillingham BL, McVeigh BL, Lampe JW, Duncan AM. Soy protein isolates of varying isoflavone content exert minor effects on serum reproductive hormones in healthy young men. J Nutr. 2005;135:584–91.
56. Messina M. Soybean isoflavone exposure does not have feminizing effects on men: a critical examination of the clinical evidence. Fertil Steril. 2010;93:2095–104.
57. Hamilton-Reeves JM, Vazquez G, Duval SJ, Phipps WR, Kurzer MS, Messina MJ. Clinical studies show no effects of soy protein or isoflavones on reproductive hormones in men: results of a meta-analysis. Fertil Steril. 2010;94:997–1007.
58. Riedl CR, Engelhardt PF. Effects of one-year treatment with isoflavone extract from red clover on prostate, liver function, sexual function and quality of life in men with elevated PSA levels and negative prostate biopsy findings. Urology. 2008;71:185–90.
59. Tanaka M, Fujimoto K, Chlhara Y, Torimoto K, Yoneda T, Tanaka N, et al. Isoflavone supplements stimulated the production of serum equol and decreased the serum dihydrotestosterone levels in healthy male volunteers. Prostate Cancer Prostatic Dis. 2009;12:247–52.
60. Pendleton JM, Tan WW, Anal S, Chang M, Hou W, Shiverick KT, et al. Phase II trial of isoflavone in prostate-specific antigen recurrent prostate cancer after previous local therapy. BMC Cancer. 2008; 8:132.
61. Garcia PV, Barbieri MF, Perobeli JE, Consonni SR, Mesquita Sde F, Kempinas Wde G, et al. Morphometric-stereological and functional epididymal alterations and a decrease in fertility in rats treated with finasteride after a 30-day post-treatment recovery period. Fertil Steril. 2012;97:1441–51.
62. Chiba K, Yamaguchi K, Li F, Ando M, Fujisawa M. Finasteride-associated male infertility. Fertil Steril. 2011;95:1786.e9–e11.
63. Amory JK, Wang C, Swerdloff RS, Anawalt BD, Matsumoto AM, Bremner WJ, et al. The effect of 5alpha-reductase inhibition with dutasteride and finasteride on semen parameters and serum hormones in healthy men. J Clin Endocrinol Metab. 2007;92:1659–65.
64. Liu KE, Binsaleh S, Lo KC, Jarvi K. Propecia-induced spermatogenic failure: a report of two cases. Fertil Steril. 2008;90:849.e17–e19.
65. Gur S, Kadowitz PJ, Hellstrom WJ. Effects of 5-alpha reductase inhibitors on erectile function, sexual desire, and ejaculation. Expert Opin Drug Saf. 2013;12:81–90.
66. Traish AM, Hassani J, Guay AT, Zitzmann M, Hansen ML. Adverse side effects of 5alpha-reductase inhibitors therapy: persistent diminished libido and erectile dysfunction and depression in a subset of patients. J Sex Med. 2011;8:872–84.
67. Hakonsen LB, Thulstrup AM, Aggerholm AS, Olsen J, Bonde JP, Andersen CY, et al. Does weight loss improve semen quality and reproductive hormones? Results from a cohort of severely obese men. Reprod Health. 2011;8:24.
68. Hammiche L, Laven JS, Twigt JM, Boellaard WP, Steegers EA, Steegers-Theunissen RP. Human Reprod. 2012;27:2365–72.
69. Cabler S, Agarwal A, Flint M, du Plessis SS. Obesity: modern man's fertility nemesis. Asian J Androl. 2010;12:480–9.
70. Du Plessis SS, Cabler S, McAlister DA, Sabanegh E, Agarwal A. The effect of obesity on sperm disorders and male infertility. Nat Rev Urol. 2010;7:153–61.
71. Lippman SM, Klein EA, Goodman PJ, Lucia MS, Thompson IM, Ford LG, et al. Effect of selenium and vitamin E on risk of prostate cancer and other cancers: the Selenium and Vitamin E Cancer Prevention Trial (SELECT). JAMA. 2009;301:39–51.
72. Klein EA, Thompson Jr IM, Tangen CM, Crowley JJ, Lucia MS, Goodman PJ, et al. Vitamin E and the risk of prostate cancer: the Selenium and Vitamin E

Cancer Prevention Trial (SELECT). JAMA. 2011; 306:1549–56.
73. Duffield-Lillico AJ, Slate EH, Reid ME, Turnbull BW, Wilkins PA, Combs Jr GF, Nutritional Prevention of Cancer Study Group, et al. Selenium supplementation and secondary prevention of non-melanoma skin cancer in a randomized trial. J Natl Cancer Inst. 2003;95:1477–81.
74. Stranges S, Marshall JR, Natarajan R, Donahue RP, Trevisan M, Combs GF, et al. Effects of long-term selenium supplementation on the incidence of type 2 diabetes: a randomized trial. Ann Intern Med. 2007;147:217–23.
75. Miller 3rd ER, Pastor-Barriuso R, Dalal D, Riemersma RA, Appel LJ, Guallar E. Meta-analysis: high-dosage vitamin E supplementation may increase all-cause mortality. Ann Intern Med. 2005;142:37–46.
76. Lonn E, Bosch J, Yusuf S, Sheridan P, Pogue J, Arnold JM, HOPE and HOPE TOO Trial Investigators, et al. Effects of long-term vitamin E supplementation on cardiovascular events and cancer: a randomized controlled trial. JAMA. 2005;293:1338–47.
77. Sesso HD, Buring JE, Christen WG, Kurth T, Belanger C, MacFadyen J, et al. Vitamins E and C in the prevention of cardiovascular disease in men: the Physicians' Health Study II randomized controlled trial. JAMA. 2008;300:2123–33.
78. Stranges S, Marshall JR, Trevisan M, Natarajan R, Donahue RP, Combs GF, et al. Effects of selenium supplementation on cardiovascular disease incidence and mortality: secondary analyses in a randomized clinical trial. Am J Epidemiol. 2006;163: 694–9.
79. Neve J. Selenium as a risk factor for cardiovascular diseases. J Cardiovasc Risk. 1996;3:42–7.
80. Moyad MA. Selenium and vitamin E supplements for prostate cancer: evidence or embellishment? Urology. 2002;59(4 Suppl 1):9–19.
81. Pearson P, Lewis SA, Britton J, Young IS, Fogarty A. The pro-oxidant activity of high-dose vitamin E supplements in vivo. BioDrugs. 2006;20:271–3.
82. Rayman MP. Selenium and human health. Lancet. 2012;379:1256–68. Arch Intern Med 2010;170:256–61.
83. MacFarquhar JK, Broussard DL, Melstrom P, Hutchinson R, Wolkin A, Martin C, et al. Acute selenium toxicity associated with a dietary supplement. Arch Intern Med. 2010;170(3):256–61.
84. Diskin CJ, Tomasso CL, Alper JC, Glaser ML, Fliegel SE. Long-term selenium exposure. Arch Intern Med. 1979;139:824–6.
85. Keskes-Ammar L, Feki-Chakroun N, Rebai T, Sahnoun Z, Ghozzi H, Hammae S, et al. Sperm oxidative stress and the effect of an oral vitamin E and selenium supplement on semen quality in infertile men. Arch Androl. 2003;49:83–94.
86. Kessopoulou E, Powers HJ, Sharma KK, Pearson MJ, Russell JM, Cooke ID, et al. A double-blind randomized placebo cross-over controlled trial using the antioxidant vitamin E to treat reactive oxygen species associated with male infertility. Fertil Steril. 1995;64:825–31.
87. Safarinejad MR, Safarinejad S. Efficacy of selenium and/or N-acetyl-cysteine for improving semen parameters in infertile men: a double-blind, placebo controlled, randomized study. J Urol. 2009;181: 741–51.
88. Tambi MI, Imran MK, Henkel RR. Standardized water-soluble extract of Eurycoma longifolia, Tongkat ali, as testosterone booster for managing men with late-onset hypogonadism. Andrologia. 2012;44 Suppl 1:226–30.
89. Ismall SB, Wan Mohammad WM, George A, Nik Hussain NH, Musthapa Kamal ZM, Liske E. Randomized clinical trial on the use of PHYSTA freeze-dried water extract on Eurycoma longifolia for the improvement of quality of life and sexual well-being in men. Evid Based Complement Alternat Med. 2012;2012:429268.
90. Tambi MI, Imran MK. Eurycoma longifolia Jack in managing idiopathic male infertility. Asian J Androl. 2010;12:376–80.
91. Low BS, Das PK, Chan KL. Standardized quassinoid-rich Eurycoma longifolia extract improved spermatogenesis and fertility in male rats via the hypothalamic-pituitary-gonadal axis. J Ethnopharmacol. 2013;13(145):706–14.
92. Erasmus N, Solomon MC, Fortuin KA, Henkel RR. Effect of Eurycoma longifollia Jack (Tongkat ali) extract on human spermatozoa in vitro. Andrologia. 2012;44:308–14.
93. Wahab NA, Mokhtar NM, Halim WN, Das S. The effect of eurycoma longifolia Jack on spermatogenesis in estrogen-treated rats. Clinics (Sao Paulo). 2010;65:93–8.
94. Chan KL, Low BS, The CH, Das PK. The effect of Eurycoma longifolia on sperm quality of male rats. Nat Prod Commun. 2009;4:1331–6.
95. Chua LS, Abdul-Rahman N, Rosidi B, Lee CT. Plant proteins, minerals and trace elements of Eurycoma longifolia (Tongkat ali). Nat Prod Res. 2013;27: 314–8.
96. Abel BJ, Carswell G, Elton R, Hargreave TB, Kyle K, Orr S, et al. Randomised trial of clomiphene citrate treatment and vitamin C for male infertility. Br J Urol. 1982;54:780–4.
97. Hargreave TB, Kyle KF, Baxby K, Rogers AC, Scott R, Tolley DA, et al. Randomised trial of mesterolone versus vitamin C for male infertility. Scottish Infertility Group. Br J Urol. 1984;56:740–4.
98. Rolf C, Cooper TG, Yeung CH, Nieschlag E. Antioxidant treatment of patients with asthenozoospermia or moderate oligoasthenozoospermia with high dose vitamin C and vitamin E: a randomized, placebo-controlled, double-blind study. Hum Reprod. 1999;14:1028–33.
99. Colagar AH, Marzony ET. Ascorbic acid in human seminal plasma: determination and its relationship to sperm quality. J Clin Biochem Nutr. 2009;45: 144–9.

100. Fraga CG, Motchnik PA, Shigenaga MK, Helbock HJ, Jacob RA, Ames BN. Ascorbic acid protects against endogenous oxidative DNA damage in human sperm. Proc Natl Acad Sci USA. 1991;88:11003–6.
101. Dawson EB, Harris WA, Powell LC. Relationship between ascorbic acid and male fertility. World Rev Nutr Diet. 1990;62:1–26.
102. Mostafa T, Tawadrous G, Roala MM, Amer MK, Kader RA, Aziz A. Effect of smoking on seminal plasma ascorbic acid in infertile and fertile males. Andrologia. 2006;38:221–4.
103. Dawson EB, Harris WA, Teter MC, Powell LC. Effect of ascorbic acid supplementation on the sperm quality of smokers. Fertil Steril. 1992;58:1034–9.
104. Vitamin C content in foods. http://www.vitaminc-foundation.org/usda.html. Accessed 10 Feb 2013.
105. Moyad MA, Combs MA, Baisley JE, Evans M. Vitamin C with metabolites: additional analysis suggests favorable changes in oxalate. Urol Nurs. 2009;29:383–5.
106. Omu AE, Dashti H, Al-Othman S. Treatment of asthenozoospermia with zinc sulphate: andrological, immunological and obstetric outcome. Eur J Obstet Gynecol Reprod Biol. 1998;79:179–84.
107. Netter A, Hartoma R, Nahoul K. Effect of zinc administration on plasma testosterone, dihydrotestosterone, and sperm count. Arch Androl. 1981;7:69–73.
108. Food and Nutrition Board, National Academy of Sciences. Dietary reference intakes for vitamin A, vitamin K, arsenic, boron, chromium, copper, iodine, iron, manganese, molybdenum, nickel, silicon, vanadium, and zinc. Washington, DC: National Academy Press; 2001. p. 177–204. 351–398.
109. Moyad MA. Zinc for prostate disease and other conditions: a little evidence, a lot of hype, and a significant potential problem. Urol Nurs. 2004;24:49–52.
110. Leitzmann MF, Stampfer MJ, Wu K, Colditz GA, Willett WC, Giovannucci EL. Zinc supplement use and risk of prostate cancer. J Natl Cancer Inst. 2003;96:1004–7.
111. Age-Related Eye Disease Study Research Group. A randomized, placebo-controlled, clinical trial of high-dose supplementation with vitamins C and E, beta-carotene, and zinc for age-related macular degeneration and vision loss: AREDS Report Number 8. Arch Ophthalmol. 2001;119:1417–36.
112. Johnson AR, Munoz A, Gottlieb JL, Jarrard DF. High dose zinc increases hospital admissions due to genitourinary complications. J Urol. 2007;177:639–43.
113. Health Canada Website. Multi-vitamin/Mineral Supplements. http://www.hc-sc.gc.ca/dhp-mps/prodnatur/applications/licen-prod/monograph/multi_vitmin_suppl-eng.php. Accessed on 10 Nov 2012.
114. AREDS2 Research Group, Chew EY, Clemons T, SanGiovanni JP, Danis R, Domalpally A, McBee W, et al. The Age-Related Eye Disease Study 2 (AREDS2): study design and baseline characteristics (AREDS2 report number 1). Ophthalmology. 2012;119:2282–9.
115. Zavaczki Z, Szollosi J, Kiss S, Koloszar S, Fejes I, Kovacs L, Pal A. Magnesium-orotate supplementation for idiopathic infertile male patients: a randomized, placebo-controlled clinical pilot study. Magnesium Res. 2003;16:131–6.
116. Fine KD, Santa Ana CA, Fordtran JS. Diagnosis of magnesium-induced diarrhea. N Engl J Med. 1991;11(324):1012–7.
117. Office of Dietary Supplements-National Institutes of Health. Dietary Supplement Fact Sheet: Magnesium. http://www.ods.od.nih.gov/factsheets/Magnesium-HealthProfessional/. Accessed on 25 Feb 2013.
118. Deger O, Akkus I. Semen magnesium levels in fertile and infertile subjects. Magnesium. 1988;7:6–8.
119. Yuan JP, Peng J, Yin K, Wang JH. Potential health-promoting effects of astaxanthin: a high-value carotenoid mostly from microalgae. Mol Nutr Food Res. 2011;55:150–65.
120. Comhaire FH, El Garem Y, Mahmoud A, Eertmans F, Schoonjans F. Combined conventional/antioxidant "Astaxanthin" treatment for male infertility: a double blind, randomized trial. Asian J Androl. 2005;7:257–62.
121. Ciftci H, Verit A, Savas M, Yeni E, Erel O. Effects of N-acetylcysteine on semen parameters and oxidative/antioxidant status. Urology. 2009;74:73–6.
122. Heard K, Green J. Acetylcysteine therapy for acetaminophen poisoning. Curr Pharm Biotechnol. 2012;13:1917–23.
123. Witschi A, Reddy S, Stofer B, Lauterburg BH. The systemic availability of oral glutathione. Eur J Clin Pharmacol. 1992;43:667–9.
124. Irvine DS. Glutathione as a treatment for male infertility. Rev Reprod. 1996;1:6–12.
125. Lenzi A, Lombardo F, Gandini L, Culasso F, Dondero F. Glutathione therapy for male infertility. Arch Androl. 1992;29:65–8.
126. Pryor JP, Blandy JP, Evans P, Chaput De Saintonge DM, Usherwood M. Controlled clinical trial of arginine for infertile men with oligozoospermia. Br J Urol. 1978;50:47–50.
127. De Aloysio D, Mantuano R, Mauloni M, Nicoletti G. The clinical use of arginine aspartate in male infertility. Acta Eur Fertil. 1982;13:133–67.
128. Schulman SP, Becker LC, Kass DA, Champion HC, Terrin ML, Forman S, et al. L-arginine therapy in acute myocardial infarction: the vascular interaction with AGE in myocardial infarction (VINTAGE MI) randomized clinical trial. JAMA. 2006;295: 58–64.
129. Schwedhelm E, Maas R, Freese R, Jung D, Lukacs Z, Jambrecina A, et al. Pharmacokinetic and pharmacodynamic properties of oral L-citrulline and L-arginine: impact on nitric oxide. Br J Clin Pharmacol. 2008;65:51–9.
130. Gupta NP, Kumar R. Lycopene therapy in idiopathic male infertility—a preliminary report. Int Urol Nephrol. 2002;34:369–72.
131. Corbett ST, Hill O, Nangia AK. Vitamin D receptor found in human sperm. Urology. 2006;68:1345–9.

132. Ramlau-Hansen CH, Moeller UK, Bonde JP, Olsen J, Thulstrup AM. Are serum levels of vitamin D associated with semen quality? Results from a cross-sectional study in young healthy men. Fertil Steril. 2011;95:1000–4.
133. Busetto GM, Koverech A, Messano M, Antonini G, De Berardinis E, Gentile V. Prospective open-label study on the efficacy and tolerability of a combination of nutritional supplements in primary infertile patients with idiopathic asthenoteratozoospermia. Arch Ital Urol Androl. 2012;84:137–40.
134. Gaziano JM, Sesso HD, Christen WG, Bubes V, Smith JP, MacFadyen J, et al. Multivitamins in the prevention of cancer in men: the Physicians' Health Study II randomized controlled trial. JAMA. 2012;308:1871–80.
135. Sesso HD, Christen WG, Bubes V, Smith JP, MacFadyen J, Schvartz M, et al. Multivitamins in the prevention of cardiovascular disease in men: the Physicians' Health Study II randomized controlled trial. JAMA. 2012;308:1751–60.
136. Singh AK, Tiwari AK, Singh PB, Dwivedi US, Trivedi S, Singh SK, et al. Multivitamin and micronutrient treatment improves semen parameters of azoospermic patients with maturation arrest. Indian J Physiol Pharmacol. 2010;54:157–63.
137. Smith JF, Eisenberg ML, Millstein SG, Nachtigall RD, Shindel AW, Wing H, et al. The use of complementary and alternative fertility treatment in couples seeking fertility care: data from a prospective cohort in the United States. Fertil Steril. 2010;93: 2169–74.
138. Andersen D, Lossi K, Nyboe Andersen A, Furbringer J, Bach H, Simonsen J, et al. Acupuncture on the day of embryo transfer: a randomized controlled trial of 635 patients. Reprod Biomed Online. 2010;21: 366–72.
139. Dieterie S, Li C, Greb R, Bartzsch F, Hatzmann W, Huang D. A prospective randomized placebo-controlled study of the effect of acupuncture in infertile patients with severe oligoasthenozoospermia. Fertil Steril. 2009;92:1340–3.
140. Sliterman S, Eltes F, Schechter L, Malmon Y, Lederman H, Bartoov B. Success of acupuncture treatment in patients with initially low sperm output is associated with a decrease in scrotal skin temperature. Asian J Androl. 2009;11:200–8.
141. Zini A, Fischer MA, Nam RK, Jarvi K. Use of alternative and hormonal therapies in male infertility. Urology. 2004;63:141–3.
142. Ko EY, Sabanegh Jr ES. The role of over-the-counter supplements for the treatment of male infertility—fact or fiction. J Androl. 2012;33:292–308.
143. Health Canada Website. Multi-vitamin/Mineral Supplements. http://www.hc-sc.gc.ca/dhp-mps/prodnatur/applications/licen-prod/monograph/multi_vitmin_suppl-eng.php. Accessed on 10 Nov 2012.

5 Lifestyle Changes, Erectile Dysfunction, and Female Sexual Dysfunction: Heart Health and Sexual Health

Introduction

Patients tend to construe that when a diet and exercise are not effective at ameliorating a common condition such as hypertension or dyslipidemia, then prescription medications are available as the next logical course of potential action. This protocol appears to be well placed in cardiovascular medicine as well as for multiple aspects of preventive health [1, 2]. For example, if lifestyle changes such as dietary changes, including the consumption of more plant sterols and fiber, do not lower cholesterol levels, then statins are a plausible option [1]. If lifestyle changes and dietary or supplemental calcium and vitamin D were not able to reduce the risk of bone loss or osteoporosis, then most clinicians would arguably recommend a bone mineral density prescription medication [2]. Interestingly, some conventional medical recommendations evolved long ago to adopt this type of lifestyle-first philosophy, as evidenced by guidelines from a plethora of specialty groups [1, 2].

Two areas in which lifestyle and over-the-counter recommendations appear to be missing, or at least are not emphasized or fully endorsed, despite ample research, are erectile dysfunction (ED) and female sexual dysfunction (FSD). The omission of these recommendations from urology-based guidelines should be reevaluated on the basis of the current quantity, quality, and duration of the data and the overall health changes these safe and cost-effective lifestyle changes options could immediately provide for patients.

One notable and laudable exception to the omission of lifestyle recommendations in urology, for example, are the European Association of Urology (EAU) guidelines that state "lifestyle changes and risk factor modification must precede or accompany ED treatment," and that classify the level of evidence as "1b" with a grade of "A," which essentially is tantamount to almost any other conventional treatment available in sexual medicine [3]. Yet, despite all other medical treatments being thoroughly discussed in the European guidelines, lifestyle changes received no further discussion beyond the recommendation. Clinicians need to be able to cite some specific studies and lifestyle recommendations to communicate sincere credibility and interest with their patients and to improve compliance and enthusiasm for these lifestyle changes. In addition, there are generally no recommendations or mention of lifestyle changes for FSD in most medical guidelines, and this also needs to change.

Weight and Waist Gain and Loss and Diet or Caloric Reduction for ED and FSD

The maintenance of a healthy weight, or reductions in weight or waist size, to reduce morbidity and mortality is well known from international investigations. One of the largest prospective studies ever conducted was the European Prospective Investigation into Cancer and Nutrition (EPIC), which included a total of

DOI 10.1007/978-1-4614-8492-9_5, © Springer Science+Business Media New York 2014

359,387 participants, ages 25–70 years, from nine countries [4]. The mean follow-up in that study was 9.7 years, and a total of 14,723 participants died during this time period. The lowest risk of death was associated with a body mass index (BMI; in kg/m^2) of approximately 24–25 for men and women. However, after adjustment for BMI, larger waist circumference (WC) measurements were also strongly associated with all-cause and disease-specific mortality, but both BMI and WC measurements provided better correlation than did one or the other measurement alone. Both measurements offer synergistic value for the patient attempting to lose weight [5]. Still, regardless of BMI, WC is becoming a significant predictor of mortality risk in men and women, as witnessed in the United States NIH-AARP Diet and Health Study of 154,776 men and 90,757 women aged 51–72 years at baseline [6]. A twofold or higher risk of mortality in men and women, regardless of BMI, was observed in the smaller US Cancer Prevention Study II Nutrition Cohort of 48,500 men and 56,343 women [7]. These and other studies provide the most accurate and realistic glimpse of the risk associated with BMI and WC and mortality. The only time I find that other studies question these findings that lower weight or waist is not associated with lower mortality is when a study does not adequately and precisely correct for specific smoking status and more specific comorbidity issues because reverse causation can occur in these studies [8]. In other words, it is not the low body weight that leads to morbidity and mortality, but morbidity (cancer, pulmonary disease) that leads to lower body weight and then mortality. Thus, it is critical to explain why there will always be some outliers in terms of the data on obesity and mortality risk, but overall the association of weight and waist increase and morbidity and mortality increase has become clear, regardless of race and ethnicity examined [9]. The correlation with BMI and WC and the increased risk of a variety of male and female cancers is also striking and has existed for some time [10, 11]. Table 5.1 summarizes the basic interpretation of the BMI and WC ranges of values for men and women [5].

Table 5.1 Body mass index (BMI) and waist circumference (WC) values for men and women[a]

	Interpretation
BMI value	
<18.5	Underweight
18.5–24.9	Normal
25–29.9	Overweight
≥30	Obese
30.0–34.9	Class I obesity
35.0–39.9	Class II obesity
≥40.0	Class III obesity
WC value in men	
<89 cm	Normal
89–100 cm	Overweight
≥101 cm	Obese
WC value in women	
<83 cm	Normal
83–92 cm	Overweight
≥94 cm	Obese

[a]Note: Some research methods also use a waist-to-hip ratio (WHR), for which lower values (smaller waist and larger hip) indicate lower risk of future disease outcomes

Most men reporting ED symptoms (up to 70–80 %) are overweight or obese, and men who carry abnormal amounts of weight have a consistently higher risk of sexual dysfunction than do men with a normal BMI, especially with aging [12–16]. Interestingly, this correlation, albeit not as strong, is also observed in a large minority of women in terms of obesity and FSD [17]. Regardless, it is no longer difficult to conclude that in both sexes obesity is a risk factor for sexual dysfunction and that cardiovascular disease risk factors are predictive of sexual function and vice versa [18–20].

In the placebo group of the Prostate Cancer Prevention Trial (PCPT), men with incident or prevalent ED had a significant ($p<0.001$) 45 % increased risk of a subsequent cardiovascular event during the study follow-up [19]. This risk was noted to be similar to the risk of a current smoker or that of a man with a family history of myocardial infarction. The average participant in the PCPT study was overweight (BMI 27.5), and increases in BMI were significantly associated with ED during the clinical trial and a subsequent cardiovascular event in the final multivariate statistical analysis. In women, the correlation between and FSD and obesity appeared to be greater in those with metabolic syndrome, which places postmenopausal women at a higher risk for a future cardiovascular event [21].

How strong is the correlation between weight gain and sexual function for men? In one of the largest meta-analyses ($n=6,800$ men, 31 studies) of hormonal changes and obesity, researchers found that 18 of 20 studies measuring testosterone, 15 of 16 measuring sex hormone binding globulin (SHBG), and 10 of 12 investigating free testosterone found an inverse correlation between BMI and these parameters [22]. A total of 4 of 10 studies found a direct relationship between BMI and estradiol. The conclusion of this unique meta-analysis was the profound and unambiguous observation: "There was strong evidence of a negative relationship for testosterone, SHBG and free testosterone with increased BMI." Studies continue to find significant inverse relationships between weight and testosterone and increases in estradiol in men [23, 24]. Additionally, a potential reduction in pregnancy rates with higher BMI is plausible because of sexual dysfunction, higher scrotal temperatures, and adipose hormone contributions [25]. Of concern, there is also recent evidence that this correlation is just as strong in boys aged 14–20 years with as much as a 40–50 % reduction in total testosterone compared to those with normal BMIs [26]. However, obesity in women increases androgen levels and also can result in hirsutism and reduced fertility [27, 28].

Patients are often surprised to learn that exercise is not needed to lose weight. Of course, it should be encouraged to promote overall and cardiovascular health, but weight loss can be achieved in men and women with strict caloric restriction. Weight loss-only studies of short- and/or long-term duration that do not include a rigid exercise component (again only caloric modification or restriction) are demonstrating increases in testosterone and sexual function in men. A pilot study of 43 obese men followed for just 14 weeks on a weight-loss program found significant ($p=0.02$), graded improvements in total testosterone with weight loss [29]. Median baseline testosterone was approximately 7–9 nmol/L, and men losing 3.5–12.1 %, 12.2–17.1 %, and 17.2–25.4 % of their body weight experienced adjusted mean increases in testosterone levels of 0.7, 3.3, and 3.7 nmol/L, respectively. The free androgen index (FAI) also increased significantly in the group with the largest weight reduction. Total sperm count, semen volume, and anti-Müllerian hormone significantly increased.

Bariatric surgical series of women demonstrate significant reductions in androgen levels and cardiovascular markers in pre- and postmenopausal women [30]. Significant reductions were also observed for DHEA-S in premenopausal women. These changes are also found in dietary restriction studies of obese women when following a high-protein (30 %+ of daily energy) and low glycemic index diet [31] or by adhering to a low-calorie diet (500–600 cal per day) over an 8-week period [32]. The hormonal benefits of weight loss in women are occurring in those with and without polycystic ovarian syndrome (PCOS) [31, 32].

Rapid weight loss also appears to be an effective method for rapidly improving lower urinary tract symptoms (LUTS), libido, and/or ED [33]. An 8-week low-calorie diet (approximately 900 cal per day) was given to nondiabetic and diabetic men with a BMI ≥30 and a WC ≥102.1 cm versus a control group. This was a nonrandomized intervention study and a dietitian communicated with these men and monitored their progress throughout the study period. A total of 68 men completed the study, and the mean age of the participants was 50 years. Weight loss of approximately 10 % or greater was correlated with significant improvements in insulin sensitivity, testosterone, erectile function, and sexual desire, as well with decreases in WC and LUTS, in both diabetic and nondiabetic men. Improvement in LUTS was associated with a significant increase in erectile function, sexual desire, and testosterone. Similar improvements were noted in nondiabetic and diabetic individuals on the sexual function score of the International Index of Erectile Function (IIEF-5) but not in the International Prostate Symptom Score (IPSS)

(−6.4 vs. −2.1). In the nondiabetic men, the mean weight and waist losses in 8 weeks were over 12 kg and approximately 12.5 cm. Thus, profound weight loss is plausible in motivated individuals utilizing severe caloric restriction without any initial change in physical activity levels. Reductions in LUTS with weight loss could be another mechanism of action that improves erectile function, similar to what is touted in conventional medicine with pharmacologic agents [34, 35].

A study that analyzed short- and long-term data and different caloric modifications or diet options continues to espouse the notion that weight loss can be achieved with diverse programs and more practical changes [36]. An 8-week study of 31 obese (mean BMI of 35 and WC of 122 cm) men with type 2 diabetes (mean age 60 years) who received a 1,000 cal/day meal replacement low-calorie (LC) diet ($n=19$) or a high-protein (HP), low-fat, reduced-carbohydrate ($n=12$) diet reduced total daily energy or caloric consumption by approximately 600 cal per day. After 8 weeks, all subjects were then placed on the HP (600 cal per day reduction) diet for an additional 44 weeks. After 8 weeks, the total weight and waist size of men in the LC diet group was reduced by 10 % compared with 5 % for men in the HP diet group. Both diets resulted in significant improvements in glucose, LDL, SHBG, IIEF-5, sexual desire inventory (SDI), IPSS, and endothelial function. ED, sexual desire, and urinary symptoms improved by approximately equal amounts with both diets. C-reactive protein (CRP) and interleukin-6 (IL-6) were lowered with the HP diet. At 52 weeks, the metabolic benefits were maintained, and sexual and urinary parameters continued to improve. Men switching to a more moderate diet after an 8-week caloric restriction challenge showed that results and compliance were sustainable up to 52 weeks. Mean weight loss after 1 year was approximately 9 kg, and mean reductions in the IPSS from 9 to 4 occurred after 52 weeks. The mean SDI score increased over 20 points. The IIEF-5 was 11 and improved to 18. Changes in total and free testosterone were not significant, but men were eugonadal at baseline.

Arguably, one of the more overt arguments to consistently demonstrate to healthcare professionals and patients that weight loss is critical to immediate overall and sexual health in men and women are the short- and long-term data on bariatric surgery [37–39]. This is not used to advocate for more bariatric procedures in obese men and women, but to provide a tangible example of how weight loss alone can profoundly and rapidly change disease risk and multiple health parameters over short and long time periods. Past studies evaluating bariatric surgery and changes in male sex hormones found improvements in sexual health or testosterone levels in almost every investigation completed. Testosterone increases would have been tantamount to receiving prescription androgen replacement therapy in some cases for men [38]. A notable study by Hammoud et al. found a mean significant increase in total testosterone of 15.3–47.6 ng/mL (increase of 310 ng/dL) and free testosterone (45.2 pg/mL) 2 years after a Roux-en-Y gastric bypass [40]. Dissatisfaction with sexual quality of life was associated with increases in obesity, and difficult sexual performance and low libido were inversely correlated with total and free testosterone. Other series demonstrate improvements in IIEF-5 scores 2 years after bariatric surgical weight loss of 30 % [41]. Significant improvements in all domains (drive, erectile, ejaculatory, problem assessment, and satisfaction) of the Brief Sexual Function Inventory (BSFI) were also demonstrated in a 2-year study of bariatric weight loss [42]. Mean age in this study was 48 years (range 19–75 years), and multivariate analysis demonstrated that the amount of weight loss was predictive of the amount of improvement in every BSFI domain. Few studies of women and bariatric surgery outcomes with a focus on sexual health have been completed, but the preliminary results also suggest the potential for noteworthy benefits. A US case series of reproductive-aged women ($n=29$) not utilizing confounding medications and followed up to 12–24 months found a significant increase in the Female Sexual Function Index (FSFI) by 28 % [39]. In a study from Greece, 59 obese females were given an FSFI 1 week before surgery and again at 1 year postoperatively [43]. Significant reductions in depression and sexual pain levels ($p=0.01$) and improvements in sexual desire ($p=0.005$), arousal ($p=0.001$), lubrication ($p=0.003$), satisfaction ($p=0.01$), and total sexual function ($p=0.003$) were observed. A US study of 54 sexually active women (mean age 43 years) with a FSFI and 6 months postoperatively found women with FSD ($n=34$) actually resolved in 68 % of these participants [44]. All domains of the FSFI significantly ($p<0.05$) improved and in regression analysis marriage, younger age, and worse preoperative sexual issues were associated with greater improvements in sexual function. The improvements in sexual function in women with FSD to that of the level of women without FSD in this study again suggest that improvements in women can be as notable as what is observed in men with sexual dysfunction. This is important because in some surgical series the rate of FSD is as high as 60 % and any domain of the FSFI, for example, can be impacted (desire, arousal, lubrication, orgasm, satisfaction, and pain) [45].

Critics of lifestyle changes may focus on a few select studies of men and women that demonstrated no benefit or even negative impacts on sexual health with significant weight loss regardless of the method used to accomplish that weight loss (diet, surgery, etc.) [46–48]. Yet, what needs to be highlighted is that these rare negative studies found other diverse quality-of-life benefits with weight loss [49]. An inability to improve some aspect of sexual health via lifestyle should be just another clinical indicator to begin to introduce other conventional medicine options to improve sexual function [46], which is no different than what is suggested in other medical specialties, such as cardiology, rheumatology, or orthopedics [1, 2].

It appears that weight loss alone of 5–10 % that does not include aerobic or resistance exercise in overweight or obese nondiabetic or diabetic men and women can result in improvements in sexual, reproductive, and urinary function in a short period of time. One of the first meta-analyses to review the correlation between weight loss and endocrine health in men was published and reviewed data from the past 40+ years [50]. A total of 24 studies met the inclusion criteria that examined diet or bariatric surgery. Researchers found that both low-calorie diets and bariatric surgery were associated with statistically significant ($p<0.001$) increases in SHBG and unbound total testosterone. Bariatric surgery was significantly more effective compared to caloric-restriction diets in raising testosterone (8.73 nmol/or 252 ng/dL vs. 2.87 nmol/L or 83 ng/dL; $p<0.001$) in men. Androgen levels were increased by greater amounts in those that lost more weight, and more so in younger patients and nondiabetics. Reductions in estradiol and an increase in gonadotropins also occurred with weight loss. I look forward to being able to cite a similar meta-analysis for women in the near future; again, there is a paucity of data for women, but I am optimistic that it will be profoundly positive.

Exercise: A Prevention and Treatment Option by Itself

One of the only meta-analyses of exercise and ED included seven cross-sectional studies, and there was an estimate of a 40–60 % reduction in ED risk with moderate to higher levels of exercise [51]. Another meta-analysis of randomized controlled trials and ED of arteriogenic origin identified five ($n=385$) randomized controlled studies utilizing the International Index of Erectile Function (IIEF) and found significant improvement of ED with aerobic activity [52].

Younger sedentary men (<40 years of age) appear to experience a significantly increased risk of ED in the domains of erectile function, orgasm function, and intercourse satisfaction. Increased amounts of exercise improve sexual function in younger men even after control for multiple confounding variables [53]. Sedentary lifestyles have also been associated with an increased risk of ED in multiple well-known, diverse prospective epidemiologic studies regardless of age or age range, such as the Massachusetts Male Aging Study [54], the Health Care

Professionals' Follow-up Study [55], and a Vienna Health Screening Project [56]. Cardiovascular fitness and exercise frequency also appear to provide reductions in risk or severity of ED of 40–50 % and even higher in men with diabetes and in men with hypertension and other comorbidities [57, 58].

There are a dearth of studies overall for the risk of FSD and lifestyle changes but especially in terms of exercise as an isolated intervention. Still, in populations with higher rates of FSD, such as diabetics, a large sampling of 595 women found a 10 % lower risk in those that reported greater amounts of physical activity [59]. This may not seem impressive, but the average age of the study participants (58 years) and the mean duration of diabetes was 5 years, which is still a noteworthy benefit. Just 20 min of exercise before sexual stimuli has been shown to increase genital arousal in women reporting antidepressant sexual arousal issues ($n=47$) and appeared to do this by increasing sympathetic nervous system activity [60].

How much exercise should be recommended, or is needed for some form of tangible impact? A population-based cross-sectional study of ED in Hong Kong that included 1,506 men aged 26–70 years found that being physically active by expending at least 1,000 kcal/week or more reduced the risk of ED in obese men [61]. Moderate-intensity exercise of 150 min/week or more was associated with maintaining healthy erectile function, and both a low physical activity level and a high WC were independently associated with ED in an analysis of 3,941 men [62]. A smaller study of 674 men aged 45–60 years found an 83 % reduction in severe ED in those who engaged in at least 3,000 kcal/week of physical activity compared with those doing less [63]. A metabolic syndrome comparative case–control study found a significant 88 % reduction in the risk of ED for middle-aged men who engaged in greater than 400 kcal/day of exercise [64].

Lifestyle changes could also significantly enhance the benefits of conventional medical prescription ED pill options [65] and perhaps other therapies if they were tested. One unique randomized, open-label study of 60 patients with ED allowed half of the participants on PDE-5 inhibitors alone, and the other half combined the pill with regular exercise for 3 months. Men were overall inactive at baseline and were instructed to choose any form of exercise and to include intensity and duration information. Men with a history of radical pelvic surgery were excluded. The mean age and BMI of the participants were 50 years and 27 (overweight), respectively. A significant improvement was observed in all aspects of the IIEF-15 except the orgasm domain for men who exercised 3 or more hours a week compared with the non-exercise, pill-only group. Erectile function, confidence, sexual desire, intercourse satisfaction, and total satisfaction were all significantly improved in the exercise group over the PDE-5 alone group. No significant difference in testosterone levels occurred between the groups, but within the exercise group only, there was an increase in testosterone. Intercourse frequency was nonsignificantly greater in the exercise group than in the pill-alone group. It is interesting that no single PDE-5 inhibitor has ever demonstrated a consistent benefit on libido [66, 67], but when combined with exercise, this precise benefit occurred [65]. And the synergism that has occurred in women's studies of adding caloric reduction to exercise has demonstrated more profound health benefits in terms of the potential for favorable hormonal changes and disease reduction [68]. Thus, recommending at least 30 min of aerobic exercise per day on average with a minimum of 300–500 cal utilized during each physical activity session should be discussed with patients. If any intervention had this kind of preliminary data to reduce or improve ED, would it be included in sexual health guidelines or recommended in most medical clinics as a legitimate treatment option for ED?

A variety of mechanisms of action have been suggested as to how exercise could improve sexual function, and these benefits revolve around heart-healthy parameters [55, 64, 66, 69–71]. Improved cardiovascular fitness, endothelial function, and neurotransmitter release reduced sympathetic overdrive, but improved sympathetic tone, inflammatory response, and fibrinogen and psychological benefit have all been demonstrated with exercise in laboratory and human studies.

Improved resting heart rate and heart rate recovery may also be novel factors associated with ED [72, 73]. Increases in resting heart rate over time may also be associated with a higher rate of mortality from heart disease and all causes in non-, former, and current smokers [74, 75]. Novel cardiovascular risk marker reductions that may improve erectile function appear to get adequate attention [76, 77], but more simplistic markers, such as resting heart rate, are low cost and appear to be needed to monitor the success of an exercise program. Patients should be encouraged to include daily exercise that is adequate to maintain a healthy sexual function, weight, WC, and heart rate.

Depression and other psychological issues and their conventional treatments have been correlated with sexual dysfunction [78, 79]. Approximately 60–70 % of patients (men and women) on antidepressants experience adverse sexual effects [79]. Yet, meta-analyses have demonstrated that exercise reduces depressive scores with and without conventional medicine [80–82]. A Cochrane review evaluated 32 randomized controlled trials in 1,858 patients diagnosed with Major Depressive Disorder (MDD) and found a potential clinical impact on depression scores that in some cases mirrored the impact with conventional drug treatment and behavioral therapies, but the pooled effect in more rigorous trials was smaller [81]. There appear to be no age limits on the impact of exercise and mood. A meta-analysis of nine randomized trials in older individuals (approximately 60–90 years of age, majority were female) found that exercise was correlated with significantly lower depression severity regardless if the individual was clinically diagnosed or identified based on a symptom checklist [83]. These results suggest that 63 % of those that engaged in exercise had a lower severity of depression compared to the average control participant. The pooled impact of exercise on depression severity was actually comparable to the effects predicted for different classes of antidepressant medication and psychotherapy.

A multitude of mechanisms as to how exercise reduces depression have been postulated: cortisol reduction, favorable neurotransmitter alterations, diversion from negative thoughts, social contact, improved sleep quality, and reductions in sympathetic overload that can reduce anxiety and agitation [80–82, 84]. Still, limitations with exercise and depression are arguably compliance, more strict methodology of trials, whether or not tachyphylaxis can occur in the short- or long-term and negative effects of excessive physical activity. An emerging limitation may simply be the lack of this treatment to be embraced and emphasized in clinical practice as an acceptable form of ancillary therapy.

Exercise is recommended to only one in three patients during a visit with a healthcare professional [85]. Psychological interventions, at the very minimum, without even considering physical health changes, appear to be effective for the treatment of certain forms of ED [86]. This must be kept in mind with any patient who seeks treatment for ED or who is trying to prevent ED. When exercise is truly considered, a standard treatment in most major ED and FSD clinical recommendation guidelines, enhancing medication compliance and treatment, improving quality of life, and reducing sexual dysfunction should be the standard expected outcomes of the patient and the clinician.

Other Individual Lifestyle Changes

Polypharmacy/Too Many Supplements

The list of potential prescription and over-the-counter medications, including dietary supplements, in my opinion, that have some potential risk of further negatively impacting ED and FSD is concerning [87–91]. Polypharmacy should be addressed by clinicians and could be considered a lifestyle modification itself. Hair-loss remedies and some benign prostatic hyperplasia products [89], pain medications [90, 91], and other commonly used medications may reduce sexual function, and these should be discussed with patients [87]. This should provide some motivation to utilize lifestyle changes to potentially reduce the risk of ED caused by these medications or to be judicious about adding medications, including dietary supplements, unless there is a careful analysis of risk versus benefit. I have always found it interesting that even BPH dietary supplement meta-analysis reported low rates of ED that were nonsignificantly increased compared to placebo [92–94], but this rarely receives attention. This is not to imply that these dietary supplements are significant risk enhancers for ED and FSD, but many supplements that claim to work in a somewhat similar fashion to prescription drugs that are known to increase the risk of sexual dysfunction also appear to slightly increase the risk of sexual issues themselves to some degree and should at least be mentioned.

Tobacco

Other lifestyle products that can impact sexual function are more overt but still deserve attention. For example, a meta-analysis of 19 studies found a consistently higher rate of ED for smokers than for nonsmokers [95]. Tobacco and ED continue to be correlated in recent studies, and this includes both the direct use of tobacco and second-hand smoke exposure [96, 97]. Over 20 % of the cases of ED in some countries may be due to tobacco use [98]. Lung cancer is still the number-one cause of cancer deaths globally [99], which should provide patients some impetus to quit along with the relationship of smoking with common morbidities such as sexual dysfunction. Clinicians should be willing to provide tobacco users with effective avenues for medical cessation, because involvement of a healthcare professional increases the probability of cessation from 3 to 5 % over a 1-year period to approximately 25 % [100]. There is ample room for improvement in most countries around the world. For example, 20 % of the US population smoke cigarettes and over 443,000 US adults now die annually from smoking-related morbidities [101]. One negative impact of smoking cessation that needs to be appreciated is significant weight gain that occurs immediately after quitting. Approximately 80 % of individuals experience rapid and significant weight gain [102, 103], with an average of 10 pounds (4–5 kg) in 12 months [103]. In terms of FSD, the impact of tobacco on sexual function is more controversial [104, 105], but the overall health benefits for women who quit smoking are unambiguous [106]. There is some association between intakes of other drugs such as hashish or marijuana and an increased risk of anorgasmia in women that needs more studies [107], but obviously the negative health impacts of drug use (illegal or not) are well known.

Alcohol

Excessive alcohol consumption, especially when combined with other heart-unhealthy risk factors, such as tobacco use, increases ED [107, 108]. However, this is a J-shaped risk curve arguably, and alcohol in moderation or infrequent consumption may provide some protection against ED [109, 110]. Clinicians should emphasize moderate (1 drink a day for women or 1–2 for men) or no intake for adequate sexual health because chronic excessive alcohol ingestion can inhibit Leydig and Sertoli cell function and reduce gonadotropins (LH and FSH) [111]. Whether or not alcohol in excess impacts various aspects of FSD is not well studied [112], but the finding that alcohol is becoming a major caloric contributor for men and women [113] suggests that it is contributing to the obesity epidemic that ultimately can increase the risk of sexual dysfunction in men and women.

Sleep

One of the largest production time intervals and release of testosterone for men during a 24-h period occurs during sleep [114]. Middle-aged men produce and secrete less testosterone during sleep than do younger men [115]. If sleep appears to be disrupted, there is evidence that testosterone levels can be suppressed. Sleep apnea is correlated with reduced testosterone levels, but obesity is a confounding variable [116]. Still, sleep deprivation could also be a risk factor for androgen deficiency, even in younger-aged men.

A study of ten men with a mean age of 24 years and BMI of 23.5 was conducted to determine the impact of voluntary sleep restriction [117]. The protocol allowed for 1 week of 8 h a day of sleep at home, and then these individuals were allowed 10 h a night for 3 days in a sleep laboratory followed by eight straight nights of 5 h of sleep. Blood samples were drawn every 15–30 min after a specific 10-h sleep night and after a 5-h sleep night. During waking hours (8 A.M.–10 P.M.), testosterone levels were significantly lower ($p=0.05$) after sleep restriction, and the impact was most apparent between 2 P.M. and 10 P.M. ($p=0.02$). The mean reduction in testosterone was 18.4–16.5 nmol/L (530–475 ng/dL) or approximately 10–15 % in most participants. Cortisol levels were not significantly different, but there was a significant ($p=0.002$) reduction in vigor scores with sleep restriction.

Should Fasting Be Required for Testosterone Testing?

Numerous other lifestyle changes that could impede sexual function in men and women are further discussed in detail from other sources [66]. For example, something as simple as a small caloric meal or even glucose or sugar before a testosterone blood test could cause short-term and, at times, profound (15 % of men becoming temporarily hypogonadal, or up to 47 % drop) reductions in total testosterone [118], which can last from 30 min to 2 h after consumption [118, 119]. This is due to insulin release that can acutely reduce pulsatile LH and then testosterone levels. Overnight fasting has been shown to be associated with higher testosterone levels in men 40 years and older [120]. Collectively, these findings could profoundly impact a sexual dysfunction work-up or evaluations and should be discussed with male patients. It is well known that chronic hyperglycemia (or hypoglycemia) or long-term fasting (several days) inhibits the male gonadal axis [118], but soon it should be well known that caloric intake also could block the same path acutely, which I could now argue should result in the requirement for fasting before drawing male testosterone blood levels. Other dietary factors also could impact hormone levels and more gender-specific disease risk. For example, low-fat and high-fiber diets may also acutely and slightly suppress testosterone levels [121], and similar healthy diets can reduce estradiol in women [122]. Again, more intensive research on lifestyle changes and sexual health markers are needed, but in the meantime fasting before androgen level determination makes sense. Other factors, such as lean muscle mass, strength, and frailty, that can be associated with lifestyle changes are just beginning to receive adequate attention in the area of sexual health [123].

Comprehensive, Simultaneous, and Diverse Lifestyle Changes

A truly novel and rare 2-year randomized trial of regular exercise and multiple dietary changes, which followed a Mediterranean diet, to improve ED in obese men should receive more clinical attention, discussion, and awareness, despite being initially published in 2004 [124]. A total of 110 obese men with a mean BMI of 36–37, waist-to-hip ratio (WHR) of 1.01–1.02, and age of 43 years were included. The mean IIEF score at baseline ranged from 13 to 14 out of 25, and men in this trial were without diabetes, high cholesterol, or high blood pressure. A total of 55 men were included in an intensive intervention group that reduced calories and increased physical activity via personalized dietary counseling, exercise advice, dietary changes, and regular appointments with a nutritionist and personal trainer. Another group of 55 men were in the control group and received basic and general information about exercise and healthy food choices. After 2 years, multiple, diverse, and significant mean changes occurred in the intervention group compared with the placebo group. These are summarized in Table 5.2 [124] in regard to the profound changes observed in the intervention arm. This should give the clinician and patient an overview of what may be needed comprehensively to achieve adequate or tangible effects in the area of ED improvement or even prevention.

Table 5.2 Significant changes in the lifestyle intervention group: results of a randomized controlled trial of the effect of lifestyle changes on ED[a]

Health parameter	Baseline (mean)	After 2 years (mean)
BMI	36.9	31.2
Waist-to-hip ratio (WHR)	1.02	0.93
Weight (kg)	103	88
HDL cholesterol (mmol/L)	1.01	1.24
Triglycerides (mmol/L)	1.91	1.69
Glucose (mmol/L)	5.72	5.27
Insulin (uU/mL)	21	14
Interleukin-6 (pg/mL)	4.5	3.1
CRP (mg/L)	3.3	1.9
Systolic BP (mm Hg)	127	124
Diastolic BP (mm Hg)	86	82
Physical activity level (minutes per week)	48	195
Total daily calorie intake (calories)	2,390	1,950
Fiber intake (g)	15	25
Saturated fat (% calories)	14	9
Ratio of omega-6:3	12	6

Abbreviations: *BMI* body mass index, *HDL* high-density lipoprotein, *CRP* C-reactive protein, *BP* blood pressure
[a]Data are from [124]. See Chap. 1 for specific dietary and other lifestyle interventions utilized in this clinical trial

In this trial, ED scores increased significantly ($p=0.008$) compared with controls by three points [124]. A total of 17 men in the intervention group reported an erectile score of 22 or higher, which is tantamount to normal function. In other words, approximately 33 % of the men with ED in this study regained normal erectile function within 2 years, and the majority of men experienced at least some improvement in sexual function and a simultaneous reduction in the risk of well-accepted CVD markers. Multivariate statistical analysis demonstrated that several changes were independently and significantly associated with a higher rate of improved erectile health on the IIEF, including a lower BMI or BMI reduction, increased physical activity/exercise, and lower CRP levels. Still, the comprehensive lifestyle intervention (specifics of this program are reviewed in Chap. 1) had one limitation, which was the lack of evaluation of psychological factors, because it is also plausible that these lifestyle changes improved mood and self-esteem, which could have been another mechanism of action for improved erectile function.

Another notable and unique randomized study by this same research group utilizing a similar intervention protocol was also published in 2004 [125]. This trial was also conducted over a 2-year period, but in participants with metabolic syndrome. A total of 180 men and women ($n=90$ in each group) demonstrated significant resolution of metabolic syndrome prevalence (over 50 % reduction), reduction in cardiovascular risk, and endothelial function improvement compared with controls. IL-6, which is associated with CRP production, was also significantly reduced in both clinical trials [124, 125]. IL-6 and hs-CRP (inflammatory markers) are gaining acceptance as potential markers of cardiac and overall health [126], and perhaps sexual function, and may provide a novel mechanism for ED reduction after nerve-sparing radical prostatectomy [127]. A recent follow-up from this research group of 209 men participating in these and other past clinical trials (mean age 45 years and BMI 31–32) continues to espouse the notion that erectile function rates can be significantly normalized in as many as 34–56 % of participants compared with controls through comprehensive lifestyle changes alone [128]. Other intensive lifestyle programs in different patient populations continue to support lifestyle interventions as a standard treatment to improve erectile health and overall health [129, 130].

The question remains that if comprehensive lifestyle changes such as a Mediterranean diet pattern have such profound impacts on men's and women's health and male sexual health, then what is the potential impact on FSD? This question needs immediate research and lags behind male sexual health research. Yet, the preliminary evidence is also potentially profound [131, 132], and the following is a basic review of what is partially involved (apart from more frequent and longer durations of exercise) in these Mediterranean lifestyle studies for ED and FSD [133, 134]:

- High intake of fruits (3–4 servings per day) and vegetables (2–3 servings per day)
- High intake of monounsaturated-to-saturated fats (ratio of 2 or more)

- Higher intake of olive oil (a monounsaturated fat, used daily)
- Daily intake of cereals (whole grain) and legumes
- Moderate intake of fish and nuts (3–5 servings/week)
- Moderate intake of wine (1–2 servings per day)
- Low intake of red and processed meat (4–5 servings per month)
- Daily intake of low-fat dairy products

In a large study, 595 women with type 2 diabetes, ages 35–70 years, were analyzed based on adherence to the Mediterranean diet and FSD using the FSFI validated questionnaire [132]. Primarily based on the threshold of 23 as the cut-off score for FSD with the FSFI, women with greater adherence to the diet had significantly ($p=0.01$) lower risk of FSD compared to women with less adherence after adjusting for confounding variables. Another 2-year randomized trial by this similar research team placed 31 women with metabolic syndrome on a Mediterranean diet compared to 28 in the control group [131]. FSFI significantly ($p=0.01$) improved in the diet group from a mean of 19.7–26.1 at the end of the trial, but were "stable" in the control arm. Two additional findings from this trial did not appear to receive attention but are noteworthy. First, no single domain of the FSFI (desire, arousal, orgasm, satisfaction, pain) was significantly reduced by the Mediterranean diet, which suggests that multiple minimal to moderate changes in diverse areas of sexual health may be cumulative in significantly reducing FSD as a whole. Second, CRP levels were significantly ($p<0.02$) reduced in the diet group, which suggests thus far in these studies that men and women may share this as a novel marker for heart disease and sexual dysfunction or improvement from this condition [124, 131].

A clinical trial of obese (mean BMI 43–45) fertile women (ages 18–49 years, mean 36 years) with FSFI-6 scores of 19 or less who were placed in only 16-week intervention programs again highlight the potential for improving FSD with comprehensive lifestyle programs [135]. Women were assigned increased physical activity and reduced caloric intake at a specialized clinical site or at home. Women assigned to the clinic oversight program had significantly higher improvement in sexual activity and FSFI-6 and significant improvements in arousal, lubrication, and satisfaction domain scores (all $p<0.01$). Significant improvements in insulin sensitivity, endothelial function and weight, BMI, fat mass, and percentage of fat mass were also found for the intensive clinic intervention group compared to the home-based lifestyle changes group. It should be kept in mind that the intensive clinic program consisted of a personalized nutrition program designed for the participant with a reduced caloric intake, protein intake of 0.8–1 g of protein per kilogram of body weight, and exercise at 60–70 % of maximum heart rate for an average of 10 h per week. This trial suggests that morbidly obese women who make profound changes in their lifestyle guided by a multidisciplinary weight loss clinic could see profound changes (average weight loss of 16 kg or over 35 pounds) or improvement in FSD. It is concerning that the home-based educational group did not experience any significant changes in any parameter. This would suggest that intensive clinic-based supervision is far superior to simple education and so-called "do it yourself" self-improvement programs. I would agree with this finding for patients who are in desperate need of more extreme changes based on their current status and past inadequate performance in the area of weight loss for overall and specific health improvements. Intense focus for FSD or even ED treatment should also be placed on subtle and simplistic changes that could prevent or improve these conditions. FSD appears to not only be prevalent, but be at a higher risk in women of a variety of ages who have one or several markers of a heart-unhealthy profile. For example, younger women with dyslipidemia are more likely to report worse scores on FSFI diverse domains compared to women of similar age and characteristics that do not have cholesterol issues [136], and this also may be true for multiple heart-healthy markers [137]. If the sexual health benefits in men and women derived from one or more lifestyle changes alone are not adequate, then it should be a clinical marker of the potential true need to add other conventional medical treatments for individuals concerned about ED and FSD.

Conclusion

It is time to reinforce simplistic general and specific advice for clinicians and patients trying to prevent ED and FSD or improve outcomes if already experiencing sexual dysfunction. Some suggestions derived from this chapter and from other sources are found in Table 5.3 [66].

Currently, the relationship between cardiovascular and erectile health is so strong that perhaps ED is a potential risk factor or

Table 5.3 Suggested comprehensive general and specific lifestyle changes with clinical evidence to be included in sexual dysfunction (ED and FSD) prevention and treatment guidelines that could be utilized with or without conventional medicines by healthcare professionals and patients[a]

Lifestyle/health parameter	General recommendation for men
Alcohol	Eliminate or reduce when dieting; otherwise, 1–2 standard drinks per day maximum. Hidden source of large calories, weight gain, and hormonal changes that negatively impact sexual function (e.g., reduced Leydig and Sertoli cell function, LH and FSH, and testosterone, and increased estradiol in men and increased testosterone in women with weight gain)
Calories (dietary)	Reduce by 100–750 cal per day according to weight-loss goals. Very low calorie-restricted diets (500 cal per day) have provided sexual health benefits in as little as 8 weeks, but compliance is always the issue
Dairy	Low-fat and low-calorie dairy generally contains lower caloric levels compared to higher fat dairy options and still provide adequate nutrition (e.g., calcium)
Carbohydrates	Reduce simple sugars and increase consumption of complex carbohydrates or "good" carbohydrates, especially fiber (see below). Simple sugars (soda, fruit juices, etc.) and simple calorie consumption increase insulin levels that can temporarily inhibit testosterone production for several hours. Testosterone blood testing should arguably be changed to a fasting blood test for more accurate results based on the impact of insulin increases on short-term testosterone production
Exercise	Approximately 30 min minimum per day on average or a goal of at least 300–500 cal expended per daily physical activity (any form of exercise is beneficial from Tai Chi, treadmill, rapid walking, treadmill, elliptical, etc.). Some effective clinical trials of women and men consisted of more than 1 h of exercise per day on average. Resistance exercise should also occur 1–2 times a week to improve metabolic rate, lean muscle mass, and testosterone levels with age
Fat (dietary)	Reduce saturated fat to less than 10 % calories and increase intake of monounsaturated and other healthy fat (e.g., omega-3)
Fiber	20–30 g per day of a combination of soluble and insoluble fiber or approximately 15 g of fiber per 1,000 kcal consumed per day
Fruits and vegetables	Several servings per day of whole fruits and vegetables (not processed)
Glucose, lipid, testosterone, and inflammatory blood marker testing	These should all be considered fasting blood tests, especially glucose, lipid, and testosterone
Meat	Lean meat, game, and grass-fed meats should be encouraged over high-saturated fat or processed meat, and moderate to minimal consumption should also be encouraged. Lean meat is one of the best sources of concentrated protein and can provide appetite satiation for some individuals
Mental health (depression/stress/anxiety)	Awareness and discussion and evaluation on a regular basis. Depression, e.g., is linked to higher rates of ED and FSD. This is one area of FSD research that has arguably as much data compared to any other lifestyle change with the exception of obesity
Nuts and seeds	Several servings a week (high in fiber, magnesium, potassium, and healthy fats)
Omega-3 fatty acids	Consume healthy fatty fish at least twice a week and increase consumption of plant omega-3 (chia, flaxseed, soy, etc.)

(continued)

Table 5.3 (continued)

Lifestyle/health parameter	General recommendation for men
Polypharmacy and/or excessive dietary supplement use	Review the list on a regular basis to determine impact on sexual health. Prescription medications and dietary supplements that attempt to mimic prescription drugs (e.g., BPH supplements) in excess have the ability to impair sexual health
Processed food	Choose unprocessed options when possible (whole fruit instead of juice, whole grain, etc.)
Protein consumption	0.8–1.0 g of protein per kg of body weight should be a normal intake; utilize low-calorie animal (casein, egg white, whey) or plant-based (hemp, pea, rice, soy, etc.) protein powders, if needed
Sleep	A total of 6–8 h on average per night and become educated on specific sleep issues (apnea, nocturia, snoring, etc.). Laboratory and home-based testing of sleep patterns are now available for the patient to determine the etiology of a sleep abnormality with a clinician
Sodium (or potassium-to-sodium ratio)	Consume less than 1,500 mg per day of sodium if highly salt sensitive and in need of aggressive blood pressure control, or 2,500 mg per day or less if salt sensitive and need minimal to moderate pressure control; otherwise, choose foods with high (≥2:1) potassium-to-sodium ratio (unsalted nuts, seeds, fruits, vegetables, etc.)
Tobacco (including cigars, smokeless, and secondhand/passive), marijuana, and other drug use	Eliminate or educate on current cessation options because 20 % or more of the population still smokes. Smoking cessation leads to 4–5 kg (10 lb) of weight gain in the first year of cessation, so clinicians and patients must aggressively address ways to reduce this often neglected negative impact of smoking cessation. Marijuana may increase the risk of sexual dysfunction in women and men
Weight and waist size	Maintain a healthy weight/waist, or a 5–10 % weight reduction over several months or years is associated with sexual and overall health improvements. Become educated on local weight-loss medical organizations and publications. Obesity shows a strong link with sexual dysfunction in men and women. Overweight has been studied to a smaller extent, but overweight and normal-weight individuals have lower risk of ED and FSD compared to obese individuals

[a]Note: Discussion with a hospital, clinic, or community nutritionist should also be encouraged, and a goal of reducing cardiovascular risk to as close to zero as possible with the primary care doctor or specialist should be discussed with each patient

marker for all-cause morbidity and mortality [138]. The evidence correlating FSD with morbidity and mortality is more anemic, but perhaps this is due to the lack of clinical data in this discipline. Perhaps with more time and research funding, the lines between ED and FSD risk factors will not be as demarcated. In the meantime, if heart-healthy changes are not emphasized in a clinical setting to patients, regardless of the data, then what is the point of all this research that has occurred? It appears that a focus only on over-the-counter, prescription, or other extrinsic interventional options is not the healthiest initial method of trying to improve sexual health in some men and women because intrinsic or personalized lifestyle changes may be the issue by itself; if not, they still provide a perfect ancillary enhancement to conventional treatment. My concern is that with all the emphasis and focus in medicine and sexual health on extrinsic solutions for patients, then what it might create is a large group of clinicians and patients who have become completely, or at least primarily, dependent on and entranced by these methods. I hope I am incorrect, but in the meantime, some past surveys and countless medical reviews, in my opinion, suggest that my perception is arguably the reality [139–141].

References

1. National Cholesterol Education Program (NCEP) Expert Panel on the Detection, Evaluation, and Treatment of High Blood Cholesterol in Adults (Adult Treatment Panel III). Third Report of the National Cholesterol Education Program (NCEP) Expert Panel on Detection, Evaluation, and Treatment of high blood cholesterol in Adults (Adult Treatment Panel III) final report. Circulation 2002;106:3143–421.
2. Brown JP, Josse RG, Scientific Advisory Council of the Osteoporosis Society of Canada. 2002 clinical practice guidelines for the diagnosis and management of osteoporosis in Canada. CMAJ. 2002;167(10 Suppl):S1–34.
3. Hatzimouratidis K, Amar E, Eardley I, Giuliano F, Hatzichristou D, Montorsi F, European Association of Urology, et al. Guidelines on male sexual dysfunction: erectile dysfunction and premature ejaculation. Eur Urol. 2010;57:804–14.
4. Pischon T, Boeing H, Hoffman K, European Prospective Investigation into Cancer and Nutrition (EPIC) Investigators. General and abdominal adiposity and risk of death in Europe. N Engl J Med. 2008;359:2105–20.
5. Moyad MA. Current methods used for defining, measuring, and treating obesity. Semin Urol Oncol. 2001;19:247–56.
6. Koster A, Leitzmann MF, Schatzkin A, Mouw T, Adams KF, van Eijik JT, et al. Waist circumference and mortality. Am J Epidemiol. 2008;167:1465–75.
7. Jacobs EJ, Newton CC, Wang Y, Patel AV, McCullough ML, Campbell PT, et al. Waist circumference and all-cause mortality in a large US cohort. Arch Intern Med. 2010;170:1293–301.
8. Flegal KM, Kit BK, Orpana H, Graubard BI. Association of all-cause mortality with overweight and obesity using standard body mass index categories: a systematic review and meta-analysis. JAMA. 2013;309:71–82.
9. Boggs DA, Rosenberg L, Cozier YC, Wise LA, Coogan PF, Ruiz-Narvaez EA, et al. General and abdominal obesity and risk of death among black women. N Engl J Med. 2011;365:901–8.
10. Pischon T, Boeing H, Weikert S, European Prospective Investigation into Cancer and Nutrition (EPIC) Investigators. Body size and risk of prostate cancer in the European prospective investigation into cancer and nutrition. Cancer Epidemiol Biomarkers Prev. 2008;17:3252–61.
11. Pischon T, Nothlings U, Boeing H. Obesity and cancer. Proc Nutr Soc. 2008;67:128–45.
12. Shaeer O, Shaeer K. The global online sexuality survey (GOSS): the United States of America in 2011. Chapter I: erectile dysfunction among English-speakers. J Sex Med. 2012;9:3018–27.
13. Bacon CG, Mittleman MA, Kawachi I, Giovannucci E, Glasser DB, Rimm EB, et al. Sexual function in men older than 50 years of age: results from the Health Professionals follow-up study. Ann Intern Med. 2003;139:161–8.
14. Riedner CE, Rhoden EL, Ribeiro EP, Fuchs SC. Central obesity is an independent predictor of erectile dysfunction in older men. J Urol. 2006;176:1519–23.
15. Esposito K, Giugliano F, Martedi E, Feola G, Marfella R, D'Armiento M, et al. High proportions of erectile dysfunction in men with the metabolic syndrome. Diabetes Care. 2005;28:1201–3.
16. Walczak MK, Lokhandwala N, Hodge MB, Guay AT. Prevalence of cardiovascular risk factors in erectile dysfunction. J Gend Specif Med. 2002;5:19–24.
17. Moore RH, Sarwer DB, Lavenberg JA, Lane IB, Perez JL, Volger S, et al. Relationship between sexual function and quality of life in obese persons seeking weight reduction. Obesity (Silver Spring). 2013 [Epub ahead of print].
18. Fung MM, Bettencourt R, Barrett-Connor E. Heart disease risk factors predict erectile dysfunction 25 years later: the Rancho Bernardo Study. J Am Coll Cardiol. 2004;43:1405–11.
19. Thompson IM, Tangen CM, Goodman PJ, Probstfield JL, Moinpour CM, Coltman CA. Erectile dysfunction and subsequent cardiovascular disease. JAMA. 2005;294:2996–3002.
20. Miner M, Esposito K, Guay A, Montorsi P, Goldstein I. Cardiometabolic risk and female sexual health: the Princeton III summary. J Sex Med. 2012;9:641–51.
21. Martelli V, Vallisela S, Moscatiello S, Matteucci C, Lantadilla C, Costantino A, et al. Prevalence of sexual dysfunction among postmenopausal women with and without metabolic syndrome. J Sex Med. 2012;9:434–41.
22. MacDonald AA, Herbison GP, Showell M, Farquhar CM. The impact of body mass index on semen parameters and reproductive hormones in human males: a systematic review with meta-analysis. Hum Reprod Update. 2010;16:293–311.
23. Ramlau-Hansen CH, Hansen M, Jensen CR, Olsen J, Bonde JP, Thulstrup AM. Semen quality and reproductive hormones according to birth weight and body mass index in childhood and adult life: two decades of follow-up. Fertil Steril. 2010;94:610–8.
24. Rohrmann S, Shiels MS, Lopez DS, Rifai N, Nelson WG, Kanarek N, et al. Body fatness and sex steroid hormone concentrations in US men: results from NHANES III. Cancer Causes Control. 2011;22:1141–51.
25. Cabler S, Agarwal A, Flint M, du Plessis SS. Obesity: modern man's fertility nemesis. Asian J Androl. 2010;12:480–9.
26. Mogri M, Dhindsa S, Quattrin T, Ghanim H, Dandona P. Testosterone concentrations in young pubertal and post-pubertal obese males. Clin Endocrinol (Oxf). 2013;78:593–9.
27. Norman RJ, Dewailly D, Legro RS, Hickey TE. Polycystic ovary syndrome. Lancet. 2007;370:685–97.
28. Samojlik E, Kirschner MA, Silber D, Schneider G, Ertel NH. Elevated production and metabolic clearance

rates of androgens in morbidly obese women. J Clin Endocrinol Metab. 1984;59:949–54.
29. Hakonsen LB, Thulstrup AM, Aggerholm AS, Olsen J, Bonde JP, Andersen CY, et al. Does weight loss improve semen quality and reproductive hormones? Results from a cohort of severely obese men. Reprod Health. 2011;8:24.
30. Ernst B, Wilms B, Thurnheer M, Schultes B. Reduced circulating androgen levels after gastric bypass surgery in severely obese women. Obes Surg. 2012;23:602–7.
31. Mehrabani HH, Salehpour S, Amiri Z, Farahani SJ, Meyer BJ, Tahbaz F. Beneficial effects of a high-protein, low-glycemic-load hypocaloric diet in overweight and obese women with polycystic ovary syndrome: a randomized controlled intervention study. J Am Coll Nutr. 2012;31:117–25.
32. Svendsen PF, Jensen FK, Hoist JJ, Haugaard SB, Nilas L, Madsbad S. The effect of a very low calorie diet on insulin sensitivity, beta cell function, insulin clearance, incretin hormone secretion, androgen levels and body composition in obese young women. Scand J Clin Lab Invest. 2012;72:410–9.
33. Khoo J, Piantadosi C, Worthley S, Wittert GA. Effects of low-energy diet on sexual function and lower urinary tract symptoms in obese men. Int J Obes (Lond). 2010;34:1396–403.
34. Govonlu S, Wooding FG. Pharmacological management of benign prostatic hypertrophy with phosphodiesterase-5 inhibitors. Consult Pharm. 2009;24: 769–71.
35. Cantrell MA, Baye J, Vouri SM. Tadalafil: a phosphodiesterase-5 inhibitor for benign prostatic hyperplasia. Pharmacotherapy. 2013;33:639–49.
36. Khoo J, Piantadosi C, Duncan R, Worthley SG, Jenkins A, Noakes M, et al. Comparing effects of a low-energy diet and a high-protein low-fat diet on sexual and endothelial function, urinary tract symptoms, and inflammation in obese diabetic men. J Sex Med. 2011;8:2868–75.
37. Schroeder R, Garrison Jr JM, Johnson MS. Treatment of adult obesity with bariatric surgery. Am Fam Physician. 2011;84:805–14.
38. Rao SR, Kini S, Tamler R. Sex hormones and bariatric surgery in men. Gend Med. 2011;8:300–11.
39. Legro RS, Dodson WC, Gnatuk CL, Estes SJ, Kunselman AR, Meadows JW, et al. Effects of gastric bypass surgery on female reproductive function. J Clin Endocrinol Metab. 2012;97:4540–8.
40. Hammoud A, Gibson M, Hunt SC, Adams TD, Carrell DT, Kolotkin RL, et al. Effect of Roux-en-Y gastric bypass surgery on the sex steroids and quality of life in obese men. J Clin Endocrinol Metab. 2009;94:1329–32.
41. Reis LO, Favaro WJ, Barreiro GC, de Oliveira LC, Chaim EA, Fregonesi A, et al. Erectile dysfunction and hormonal imbalance in morbidly obese male is reversed after gastric bypass surgery: a prospective randomized controlled trial. Int J Androl. 2010;33: 736–44.
42. Dallal RM, Chernoff A, O'Leary MP, Smith JA, Braverman JD, Quebbemann BB. Sexual function is common in the morbidly obese male and improves after gastric bypass surgery. J Am Coll Surg. 2008;207:859–65.
43. Assimakopoulos K, Karaivazoglou K, Panaylotopoulos S, Hyphantis T, Iconomou G, Kalfarentzos F. Obes Surg. 2011;21:362–6.
44. Bond DS, Wing RR, Vlthiananthan S, Sax HC, Roye GD, Ryder BA, et al. Significant resolution of female sexual dysfunction after bariatric surgery. Surg Obes Relat Dis. 2011;7:1–7.
45. Bond DS, Llthiananthan S, Leahey TM, Thomas JG, Sax HC, Pohl D, et al. Prevalence and degree of sexual dysfunction in a sample of women seeking bariatric surgery. Surg Obes Relat Dis. 2009;5: 698–704.
46. Ranasinghe WK, Wright T, Attia J, McElduff P, Doyle T, Bartholomew M, et al. Effects of bariatric surgery on urinary and sexual function. BJU Int. 2011;107:88–94.
47. Kaukua J, Pekkarinen T, Sane T, Mustajoki P. Sex hormones and sexual function in obese men losing weight. Obes Res. 2003;11:689–94.
48. Olivera CK, Herron DM, Kini SU, Vardy MD, Ascher-Walsh CJ, Garely AD, et al. Long-term quality of life and pelvic floor dysfunction after bariatric surgery. Am J Obstet Gynecol. 2012;207:431.e1–e4.
49. Kaukua J, Pekkarinen T, Sane T, Mustajoki P. Health-related quality of life in obese outpatients losing weight with very-low-energy diet and behaviour modification—2-y follow-up study. Int J Obes Relat Metab Disord. 2003;27:1233–41.
50. Corona G, Rastrelli G, Monami M, Saad F, Luconi M, Lucchese M, et al. Body weight loss reverts obesity-associated hypogonadotropic hypogonadism: a systematic review and meta-analysis. Eur J Endocrinol. 2013;168:829–43.
51. Cheng JY, Ng EM, Ko JS, Chen RY. Physical activity and erectile dysfunction: meta-analysis of population-based studies. Int J Impot Res. 2007;19:245–52.
52. Lamina S, Agbanusi E, Nwacha RC. Effects of aerobic exercise in the management of erectile dysfunction: a meta analysis study on randomized controlled trials. Ethiop J Health Sci. 2011;21:195–201.
53. Hsiao W, Shrewsberry AB, Moses KA, Johnson TV, Cai AW, Stuhldreher P, et al. Exercise is associated with better erectile function in men under 40 as evaluated by the International Index of Erectile Dysfunction. J Sex Med. 2012;9:524–30.
54. Feldman HA, Johannes CB, Derby CA, Kleinman KP, Mohr BA, Araujo AB, et al. Erectile dysfunction and coronary risk factors: prospective results from the Massachusetts Male Aging Study. Prev Med. 2000;30:328–38.
55. Bacon CG, Mittleman MA, Kawachi I, Giovannucci E, Glasser DB, Rimm EB. A prospective study of risk factors for erectile dysfunction. J Urol. 2006;176:217–21.

56. Ponholzer A, Temmi C, Mock K, Marszalek M, Obermayr R, Madersbacher S. Prevalence and risk factors for erectile dysfunction in 2869 men using a validated questionnaire. Eur Urol. 2005;47:80–5.
57. Rosen RC, Wing RR, Schneider S, Wadden TA, Foster GD, West DS, et al. Erectile dysfunction in type 2 diabetic men: relationship to exercise fitness and cardiovascular risk factors in the Look AHEAD trial. J Sex Med. 2009;6:1414–22.
58. Lamina S, Okoye CG, Dagogo TT. Therapeutic effect of an interval exercise training program in the management of erectile dysfunction in hypertensive patients. J Clin Hypertens (Greenwich). 2009;11:125–9.
59. Esposito K, Maiorino MI, Bellastella G, Giugliano F, Romano M, Giugliano D. Determinants of female sexual dysfunction in type 2 diabetes. Int J Impot Res. 2010;22:179–84.
60. Lorenz TA, Meston CM. Acute exercise improves sexual arousal in women taking antidepressants. Ann Behav Med. 2012;43:352–61.
61. Cheng JY, Ng EM. Body mass index, physical activity and erectile dysfunction: an U-shaped relationship from population-based study. Int J Obes. 2007;31:1571–8.
62. Janiszewski PM, Janssen I, Ross R. Abdominal obesity and physical inactivity are associated with erectile dysfunction independent of body mass index. J Sex Med. 2009;6:1990–8.
63. Kratzik CW, Lackner JE, Mark I, Rucklinger E, Schmidbauer J, Lunglmayr G, et al. How much physical activity is needed to maintain erectile function? Results of the Androx Vienna Municipality Study. Eur Urol. 2009;55:509–16.
64. Pohjantahti-Maaroos H, Palomaki A, Hartikainen J. Erectile dysfunction, physical activity and metabolic syndrome: differences in markers of atherosclerosis. BMC Cardiovasc Disord. 2011;22:36.
65. Maio G, Saraeb S, Marchiori A. Physical function and PDE5 inhibitors in the treatment of erectile dysfunction: results of a randomized controlled study. J Sex Med. 2010;7:2201–8.
66. Moyad MA. Male sexual health. Ann Arbor, MI: Spry; 2012.
67. Belkoff LH, McCullough A, Goldstein I, Jones L, Bowden CH, Didonato K, et al. An open-label, long-term evaluation of the safety, efficacy and tolerability of avanafil in male patients with mild to severe erectile dysfunction. Int J Clin Pract. 2013;67:333–41.
68. Campbell KL, Foster-Schubert KE, Alfano CM, Wang CC, Wang CY, Duggan CR, et al. Reduced-calorie dietary weight loss, exercise, and sex hormones in postmenopausal women: randomized controlled trial. J Clin Oncol. 2012;30:2314–26.
69. Claudino MA, Delbin MA, Franco-Penteado CF, Priviero FB, De Nucci G, Antunes E, et al. Exercise training ameliorates the impairment of endothelial and nitrergic corpus cavernosum responses in diabetic rats. Life Sci. 2011;88:272–7.
70. Claudino MA, Franco-Penteado CF, Priviero FB, Camargo EA, Teixeira SA, Muscara MN, et al. Upregulation of gp91phox subunit of NAD(P)H oxidase contributes to erectile dysfunction caused by long-term nitric oxide inhibition in rats: Reversion by regular physical training. Urology. 2010;75:961–7.
71. Zheng H, Mayhan WG, Patel KP. Exercise training improves the defective centrally mediated erectile responses in rats with type I diabetes. J Sex Med. 2011;8:3086–97.
72. Dogru MT, Basar MM, Haciislamoglu A. The difference in heart rate recovery between males with and without erectile dysfunction. Ann Noninvasive Electrocardiol. 2010;15:223–9.
73. Lee JY, Joo KL, Kim JT, Cho ST, Cho DS, Won YY, et al. Heart rate variability in men with erectile dysfunction. Int Neurourol J. 2011;15:87–91.
74. Nauman J, Janszky I, Vatten LJ, Wisloff U. Temporal changes in resting heart rate and deaths from ischemic heart disease. JAMA. 2011;306:2579–87.
75. Jensen MT, Marott JL, Jensen GB. Elevated resting heart rate is associated with greater risk of cardiovascular and all-cause mortality in current and former smokers. Int J Cardiol. 2011;151:148–54.
76. Pohjantahti-Maaroos H, Palomaki A. Comparison of metabolic syndrome subjects with and without erectile dysfunction-levels of circulating oxidized LDL and arterial elasticity. Int J Clin Pract. 2011;65:274–80.
77. Raman K, Chong M, Akhtar-Danesh GG, D'Mello M, Hasso R, Ross S, et al. Genetic markers of inflammation and their role in cardiovascular disease. Can J Cardiol. 2013;29:67–74.
78. Tan HM, Tong SF, Ho CC. Men's health: sexual dysfunction, physical, and psychological health-is there a link? J Sex Med. 2012;9:663–71.
79. Montejo A, Liorca G, Izquierdo J, Rico-Villademoros F. Incidence of sexual dysfunction associated with antidepressant agents: a prospective multicenter study of 1022 outpatients. Spanish Working Group for the study of psychotropic-related sexual dysfunction. J Clin Psychiatry. 2001;62 Suppl 3:10–21.
80. Nahas R, Sheikh O. Complementary and alternative medicine for the treatment of major depressive disorder. Can Fam Physician. 2011;57:659–63.
81. Rimer J, Dwan K, Lawlor DA, Greig CA, McMurdo M, Morley W, et al. Exercise for depression. Cochrane Database Syst Rev. 2012;7, CD004366.
82. Krogh J, Nordentoft M, Sterne JA, Lawlor DA. The effect of exercise in clinically depressed adults: systematic review and meta-analysis of randomized controlled trials. J Clin Psychiatry. 2011;72:529–38.
83. Bridle C, Spanjers K, Patel S, Atherton NM, Lamb SE. Effect of exercise on depression severity in older people: systematic review and meta-analysis of randomized controlled trials. Br J Psychiatry. 2012;201:180–5.
84. Rethorst CD, Sunderajan P, Greer TL, Grannemann BD, Nakonezny PA, Carmody TJ, et al. Does exercise improve self-reported sleep quality in non-remitted major depressive disorder? Psychol Med. 2013;43:699–709.

85. Barnes PM, Schoenborn CA. Trends in adults receiving a recommendation for exercise or other physical activity from a physician or other health professional. NCHS Data Brief. 2012;86:1–8.
86. Melnik T, Soares BG, Nasselo AG. Psychological interventions for erectile dysfunction. Cochrane Database Syst Rev. 2007;3, CD004825.
87. Londono DC, Slezak JM, Quinn VP, Van Den Eeden SK, Loo RK, Jacobsen SJ. Population-based study of erectile dysfunction and polypharmacy. BJU Int. 2012;110:254–9.
88. Serretti A, Chiesa A. Sexual side effects of pharmacological treatment of psychiatric diseases. Clin Pharmacol Ther. 2011;89:142–7.
89. Traish AM, Hassani J, Guay AT, Zitzmann M, Hansen ML. Adverse side effects of 5alpha-reductase inhibitors therapy: persistent diminished libido and erectile dysfunction and depression in a subset of patients. J Sex Med. 2011;8:872–84.
90. Gleason JM, Slezak JM, Jung H, Reynolds K, Van den Eeden SK, Haque R, et al. Regular nonsteroidal anti-inflammatory drug use and erectile dysfunction. J Urol. 2011;185:1388–93.
91. Shiri R, Koskimaki J, Hakkinen J, Tammela TL, Auvinen A, Hakama M. Effect of nonsteroidal anti-inflammatory drug use on the incidence of erectile dysfunction. J Urol. 2006;175:1812–5.
92. Wilt TJ, Macdonald R, Ishani A. B-sitosterol for the treatment of benign prostatic hyperplasia: a systematic review. BJU International. 1999;83:976–83.
93. Wilt TJ, Ishani A, MacDonald R, Stark G, Mulrow CD, Lau J. Beta-sitosterols for benign prostatic hyperplasia. Cochrane Database of Syst Rev. 2000;2, CD001043.
94. Wilt TJ, Ishani A, Stark G, MacDonald R, Lau J, Mulrow C. Saw palmetto extracts for treatment of benign prostatic hyperplasia: a systematic review. JAMA. 1998;280:1604–9.
95. Tengs TO, Osgood ND. The link between smoking and impotence: two decades of evidence. Prev Med. 2001;32:447–52.
96. Polsky JY, Aronson KJ, Heaton JP, Adams MA. Smoking and other lifestyle factors in relation to erectile dysfunction. BJU Int. 2005;96:1355–9.
97. Kupelian V, Link CL, McKinlay JB. Association between smoking, passive smoking, and erectile dysfunction: results from the Boston Area Community Health (BACH) Survey. Eur Urol. 2007;52:416–22.
98. He J, Reynolds K, Chen J, Chen CS, Wu X, Duan X, et al. Cigarette smoking and erectile dysfunction among Chinese men without clinical vascular disease. Am J Epidemiol. 2007;166:803–9.
99. Ferlay J, Shin HR, Bray F, Forman D, Mathers C, Parkin DM. GLOBOCAN 2008, Cancer Incidence and Mortality Worldwide, IARC CancerBase No. 10. Lyon, France: International Agency for Research on Cancer; 2010. Available from: http://globocan.iarc.fr.
100. Laniado-Laborin R. Smoking cessation intervention: an evidence-based approach. Postgrad Med. 2010; 122:74–82.
101. Current cigarette smoking among adults-United States, 2011. MMWR 2012;44:889–94.
102. Farley AC, Hajek P, Lycett D, Aveyard P. Interventions for preventing weight gain after smoking cessation. Cochrane Database Syst Rev. 2012;1, CD006219.
103. Aubin HJ, Farley A, Lycett D, Lahmek P, Aveyard P. Weight gain in smokers after quitting cigarettes: meta-analysis. BMJ. 2012;345:e4438.
104. Safarinejad MR. Female sexual dysfunction in a population-based study in Iran: prevalence and associated risk factors. Int J Impot Res. 2006;18: 382–95.
105. Diehl A, Silva RL, Laranjeira R. Female sexual dysfunction in patients with sub-stance-related disorders. Clinical (Sao Paulo). 2013;68:205–12.
106. Clair C, Rigotti NA, Porneala B, Fox CS, D'Agostino RB, Pencina MJ, et al. Association of smoking cessation and weight change with cardiovascular disease among adults with and without diabetes. JAMA. 2013;309:1014–21.
107. Christensen BS, Gronbaek M, Pedersen BV, Graugaard C, Frisch M. Associations of unhealthy lifestyle factors with sex inactivity and sexual dysfunctions in Denmark. J Sex Med. 2011;8:1903–16.
108. Lee AC, Ho LM, Yip AW, Fan S, Lam TH. The effect of alcohol drinking on erectile dysfunction in Chinese men. Int J Impot Res. 2010;22:272–8.
109. Cheng JY, Ng EM, Chen RY, Ko JS. Alcohol consumption and erectile dysfunction: meta-analysis of population-based studies. Int J Impot Res. 2007;19:343–52.
110. Chew KK, Bremner A, Stuckey B, Earle C, Jamrozik K. Alcohol consumption and male erectile dysfunction: an unfounded reputation for risk. J Sex Med. 2009;6:1386–94.
111. Emanuele MA, Emanuele NV. Alcohol's effects on male reproduction. Alcohol Health Res World. 1998;22:195–201.
112. George WH, Davis KC, Heiman JR, Norris J, Stoner SA, Schacht RL, et al. Women's sexual arousal: effects of high alcohol dosages and self-control instructions. Horm Behav. 2011;59:730–8.
113. Nielsen SJ, Kit BK, Fakhouri T, Ogden CL. Calories consumed from alcoholic beverages by U.S. adults, 2007–2010. NCHS Data Brief. 2012;110:1–8.
114. Axelsson J, Ingre M, Akerstedt T, Holmback U. Effects of acutely displaced sleep on testosterone. J Clin Endocrinol Metab. 2005;90:4530–5.
115. Luboshitzky R, Shen-Orr Z, Herer P. Middle-aged men secrete less testosterone at night than young healthy men. J Clin Endocrinol Metab. 2003;88: 3160–6.
116. Andersen ML, Tufik S. The effects of testosterone on sleep and sleep-disordered breathing in men: its bidirectional interaction with erectile function. Sleep Med Rev. 2008;12:365–79.
117. Leproult R, Van Cauter E. Effect of 1 week of sleep restriction on testosterone levels in young healthy men. JAMA. 2011;305:2174–5.

118. Caronia LM, Dwyer AA, Hayden D, Amati F, Pitteloud N, Hayes FJ. Abrupt decrease in serum testosterone levels after an oral glucose load in men: implications for screening for hypogonadism. Clin Endocrinol (Oxf). 2013;78:291–6.
119. Iranmanesh A, Lawson D, Veldhuis JD. Glucose ingestion lowers pulsatile LH and basal testosterone secretion in men. Am J Physiol Endocrinol Metab. 2012;302:E724–30.
120. Sartorius G, Spasevska S, Idan A, Turner L, Forbes E, Zamojska A, et al. Serum testosterone, dihydrotestosterone and estradiol concentrations in older men self-reporting very good health: the healthy man study. Clin Endocrinol. 2012;77:755–63.
121. Wang C, Catlin DH, Starcevic B, Heber D, Ambler C, Berman N, et al. Low-fat high-fiber diet decreased serum and urine androgens in men. J Clin Endocrinol Metab. 2005;90:3550–9.
122. Gann PH, Chatterton RT, Gapstur SM, Liu K, Garside D, Giovanazzi S, et al. The effects of a low-fat/high-fiber diet on sex hormone levels and menstrual cycling in premenopausal women: a 12-month randomized trial (the diet and hormone study). Cancer. 2003;98:1870–9.
123. Lee DM, Tajar A, Ravindrarajah R, Pye SR, O'Connor DB, Corona G, The European Male Aging Study Group, et al. Frailty and sexual health in older European men. J Gerontol A Biol Sci Med Sci. 2013;68:837–44.
124. Esposito K, Giugliano F, Di Palo C, Giugliano G, Marfella R, D'Andrea F, et al. Effect of lifestyle changes on erectile dysfunction in obese men: a randomized controlled trial. JAMA. 2004;291: 2978–84.
125. Esposito K, Marfella R, Ciotola M, Di Palo C, Giugliano F, Giugliano F, et al. Effect of a Mediterranean-style diet on endothelial dysfunction and markers of vascular inflammation in the metabolic syndrome: a randomized trial. JAMA. 2004;292:1440–6.
126. Gulec S. The JUPITER trial: a new approach in primary prevention. Turk Kardiyol Drn Ard. 2009;37 Suppl 4:18–26.
127. Yamashita S, Kato R, Kobayashi K, Hisasue S, Arai Y, Tsukamoto T. Inhibition of interleukin-6 attenuates erectile dysfunction in a rat model of nerve-sparing radical prostatectomy. J Sex Med. 2011;8:1957–64.
128. Esposito K, Ciotola M, Giugliano F, Maiorino MI, Autorino R, De Sio M, et al. Effects of intensive lifestyle changes on erectile dysfunction in men. J Sex Med. 2009;6:243–50.
129. Wing RR, Rosen RC, Fava JL, Bahnson J, Brancati F, Gendrano Iii IN, et al. Effects of weight loss intervention on erectile function in older men with type 2 diabetes in the Look AHEAD trial. J Sex Med. 2010;7:156–65.
130. Kolotkin RK, Binks M, Crosby RD, Ostbyte T, Mitchell JE, Hartley G. Improvements in sexual quality of life after moderate weight loss. Int J Impot Res. 2008;20:487–92.
131. Esposito K, Ciotola M, Giugliano F, Schisano B, Autorino R, Iuliano S, et al. Mediterranean diet improves sexual function in women with the metabolic syndrome. Int J Impot Res. 2007;19:486–91.
132. Giugliano F, Maiorino MI, Di Palo C, Autorino R, De Sio M, Giugliano D, et al. Adherence to Mediterranean diet and sexual function in women with type 2 diabetes. J Sex Med. 2010;7:1883–90.
133. Esposito K, Giugliano F, Maiorino MI, Giugliano D. Dietary factors, Mediterranean diet and erectile dysfunction. J Sex Med. 2010;7:2338–45.
134. Esposito K, Giugliano F, Ciotola M, De Sio M, Armiento MD, Giugliano D. Obesity and sexual dysfunction, male and female. Int J Impot Res. 2008;20:358–65.
135. Aversa A, Bruzziches R, Francomano D, Greco EA, Violl F, Lenzi A, et al. Weight loss by multidisciplinary intervention improves endothelial and sexual function. J Sex Med. 2013;10:1024–33.
136. Esposito K, Ciotola M, Malorino MI, Giugliano F, Autorino R, De Sio M, et al. Hyperlipidemia and sexual function in premenopausal women. J Sex Med. 2009;6:1696–703.
137. Veronelli A, Mauri C, Zecchini B, Peca MG, Turri O, Valitutti MT, et al. Sexual dysfunction is frequent in premenopausal women with diabetes, obesity, and hypothyroidism, and correlates with markers of increased cardiovascular risk. A preliminary report. J Sex Med. 2009;6:1561–8.
138. Dong JY, Zhang YH, Qin LQ. Erectile dysfunction and risk of cardiovascular disease: meta-analysis of prospective cohort studies. J Am Coll Cardiol. 2011;58:1378–85.
139. Montague DK, Jarow JP, Broderick GA, Dmochowski RR, Heaton JP, Lue TF, Erectile dysfunction guideline update panel, et al. Chapter 1: The management of erectile dysfunction: an AUA update. J Urol. 2005;174:230–9.
140. Tal R, Teloken P, Mulhall JP. Erectile function after radical prostatectomy: practice patterns among AUA members. J Sex Med. 2011;8:2370–6.
141. Brien JC, Trussell JC. Erectile dysfunction for primary care providers. Can J Urol. 2008;15 Suppl 1:63–70.

6 Complementary and Alternative Medicine for Erectile Dysfunction, Testosterone Replacement Therapy, and Female Sexual Dysfunction

Introduction

One area of medicine that appears to be in the highest need of better objective teaching of CAM recommendations or non-recommendations is in the area of male and female sexual dysfunction, especially erectile dysfunction (ED) [1–4]. Part of the reason for the dearth of objective education is due to the poor quality-control record of numerous ED dietary supplements and arguably the unctuous history associated with this over-the-counter category of products [5–8]. The FDA has removed more male-enhancement products from the market for contaminants compared to any other category of health products [9]. For example, some of the compounds that have been found in dietary supplements that mimic PDE-5 inhibitors are listed in Table 6.1 [10].

Still, such negative perceptions and realities should not completely cloud objectivity over the small number of products and methods that do have some scientific merit. Therefore, the purpose of this chapter is to review the male and female products that do and do not have clinical data to espouse their use. The reader might be pleasantly surprised that a few CAM options are beginning to garner enough data to recommend their use in a clinical setting. After much thought, placing ED and FSD options in the same chapter appeared to make the most sense because some of the CAM products with the most efficacy in ED are showing efficacy for FSD and vice versa. In order to gain comprehensive education in the area of male and female sexual function and CAM again they are placed and discussed together. On the heels of the constant interest in and controversies of ED supplements is the overlapping subject of the testosterone replacement treatment (TRT) supplements, which are also included in this chapter.

In my experience, it is important to keep in mind that TRT CAM products, especially some commercialized dietary supplements, usually offer several methods or theories whereby their product increases testosterone:

1. Increase testosterone by acting as an aromatase inhibitor (block the conversion of testosterone to estrogen). For example, this has been proposed as the mechanism of action of the herbal fenugreek by some commercial entities, but this has not been proven. Although this makes sense, I am concerned about this method because estradiol is needed for proper male skeletal health (see section "Miscellaneous").
2. Increase testosterone by acting as a 5-alpha-reductase inhibitor (block the conversion of testosterone to dihydrotestosterone or DHT). For example, this has been proposed as the mechanism of action of saw palmetto and other BPH supplements by some commercial entities but has not been proven (see Chaps. 2 and 3). Although this makes sense, I am also concerned about this method because of the potential adverse effects of prescription 5-alpha-reductase inhibitors.
3. Increase testosterone by functioning as a precursor to testosterone—for example, DHEA.

M.A. Moyad, *Complementary & Alternative Medicine for Prostate and Urologic Health*,
DOI 10.1007/978-1-4614-8492-9_6, © Springer Science+Business Media New York 2014

Table 6.1 A list of potential drug-like contaminants that could be utilized to adulterate herbal medicines touted for sexual health

Acetildenafil (Hongdenafil)
Aminotadalafil
Carbodenafil
Dimethylsildenafil
Gendenafil
Homosildenafil
Hydroxyacetildenafil
Hydroxyhomosildenafil
Hydroxythiohomosildenafil
Imidazosagatriazinone
N-Desmethylacetildenafil
Nor-acetildenafil (desmethylacetildenafil)
Norneosildenafil
Piperiacetildenafil
Pseudovardenafil
Sildenafil citrate
Sildenafil coupled
Tadalafil
Thiodimethylsildenafil
Thiohomosildenafil
Thiosildenafil
Udenafil
Vardenafil
Xanthoanthrafil (benzamidenafil)

The problem with this method is the somewhat similar issue with prescription testosterone pill in that HDL decreases are common and DHEA is unpredictable in terms of response and can raise estrogen levels only or more than testosterone (see section "DHEA").

4. Increase testosterone by stimulating the Leydig cells in the testicles or by LH increase, for example—in other words, simply stimulating the cells that produce testosterone either directly or indirectly. This would represent the ideal supplement for TRT in terms of efficacy, safety, and reliability, in my opinion. For example, this has been proposed as one of the mechanisms of action for tongkat ali (*Eurycoma longifolia*) but has not been proven (see section "tongkat ali"). The problem is that no such CAM product exists that can adequately perform this function, but some may have an ability to partially operate by this mechanism now and in the future.

Now that the controversies and some of the background on ED, FSD, and TRT have been addressed, it is important to review multiple CAM options that can be discussed with patients. Similar to conventional medicine, I believe that the underlying theme is that some of these products are overhyped and some deserve more attention based on their research and/or low cost, but most of all, there needs to be more objectivity when addressing these options.

Acupuncture

This method has inconsistent data in terms of efficacy in ED. One meta-analysis found minimal data to support the use of this technique based on methodology issues of past clinical trials [11]. Still, it would seem plausible that acupuncture does have a potential role for some forms of ED such as one with a psychogenic etiology [12–14]. Preliminary studies have suggested a high placebo response rate but an even higher response with acupuncture treatment for psychogenic ED. Acupuncture does not have adequate research in the area of FSD to make a recommendation.

Androstenedione and/or DHEA (Better, Worse, the Same, or an Ancillary to Prescription Testosterone Replacement Therapy?)

On January 20, 2005 it became illegal to sell androstenedione dietary supplements in the United States [15, 16]. Androstenedione was considered a "prohormone" supplement that some men used in an attempt to build muscle. It was utilized by several notable US professional athletes before being banned, and it created much controversy. It was a potentially dangerous supplement because it had been associated with a reduction in "good cholesterol" or HDL and it had potentially other health consequences such as significantly increasing estrogen (estrone and estradiol) in healthy young men (ages 26–32 years) taking 100 mg or 300 mg per day for 7 days and significantly increasing testosterone levels at 300 mg per day (from 526 to 872 ng/dL on average in one study) [17]. Other studies of young men demonstrated just increases in estrogen with these dosages [18], which is why it would not been surprising that some individual reports of ED from these supplements can also occur arguably because of the suppression of the pituitary and gonadal axis [19]. The individual variability in the response is also what is striking about androstenedione (or DHEA) in men and women, except for the estrogen increases in young and older primarily eugonadal men. Men ages 35–65 years taking 200 mg of androstenedione had significant increases in estrogen but not testosterone over 12 weeks [20]. In postmenopausal women, a significant increase in estrone occurred, but the individual variability in the response was always notable, which is again part of the problem [21]. Regardless of the population, studied variability or unpredictability of the physiologic response should be mentioned to patients. It has also been my experience that men and women without overt hormone deficiencies have variable results and men experience dramatic increases in estrogen and potentially a small increase in testosterone the more testosterone deficient the male [22].

Therefore, there were so many concerns with these supplements that eventually the FDA and the US government decided to remove almost all of them, including androstenedione, from the market [15]. Other so-called "prohormone" supplements like DHEA were not banned but are still being allowed for sale. Now, if DHEA is similar to androstenedione in that it has similar effects, then why is this supplement still allowed to be for sale over the counter? This is part of the strange circumstances surrounding some dietary supplements and the inconsistency in the policies that are applied. DHEA supplements enjoy a unique exemption under federal law, because of a bill approved by Congress in late 2004. How did DHEA survive when other similar to identical supplements did not? Sports officials were in favor of an overall ban on steroids and related products, including DHEA. DHEA has been banned by the Olympics, the World Anti-Doping Agency, the National Collegiate Athletics Association, the National Football League, the National Basketball Association, and minor league baseball. The 2005 law that impacts prohormone supplements, passed without objection, also gave the Drug Enforcement Administration more authority to ban new or novel steroids, with one exemption: DHEA. The term "anabolic steroid" is defined now as any drug or hormonal substance chemically and pharmacologically related to testosterone (other than estrogens, progestins, corticosteroids, and DHEA). In my opinion, since such a large percentage of Congressional men and women use dietary supplements and some perceived DHEA as unique, the proposal to ban all over-the-counter prohormone supplements in the USA would have not passed Congress if DHEA were included in the proposal. Now, with this pertinent history, what about any new data to support DHEA for men's health or sexual health?

Population studies such as the Massachusetts Male Aging Study have suggested a higher risk of ED with lower blood levels of DHEA-S [23]. Yet, what gets missed in referencing these studies is that there were also inverse associations of HDL with ED and a higher risk of ED in those with heart disease, hypertension, smoking, and diabetes, for example, which is a more tangible and productive conversation. It should be kept in mind that DHEA levels decrease substantially with aging, and this has been utilized in deceptive advertising in my opinion to encourage men and women to purchase this supplement. Other studies suggest that a lower level of DHEA and an increase risk of ED is only a weak association [24]. DHEA is produced primarily by the adrenal cortex and in smaller amounts by the testes and the ovaries, and then it is quickly sulfated by sulfotransferases into DHEA-S, which is more stable with a longer half-life and its concentrations stay stable most of the day [25]. DHEA is arguably the most abundant steroid in the human body (more than testosterone); thus, for this and many other reasons there will always be sufficient physiologic facts to give it some advertising cache. Yet, it does not appear to have a role for androgen-deficient or androgen-insufficient men because it is not predictable.

So, does DHEA appear to be of benefit in men with ED and low DHEA levels? Small studies of men utilizing 50 mg for 6 months (DHEA-S level<1.5 μmol/L) showed some improvements in function in those with hypertension and ED or those without organic etiology, but not in those with diabetes or neurologic issues [26, 27]. These men were all generally tested with prostaglandin E1 first to ensure that they were capable of having a full erection with pharmacologic intervention.

The problem with DHEA is a lack of large studies with good methodology and no really novel findings with DHEA and ED or in the area of male sexual health. DHEA-S levels are also not easy to acutely or chronically predict with lifestyle interventions; for example, in some studies there are minimal or large changes in this hormonal marker for men and women after large reduction in weight [28–30]. Perhaps this is due to the fact that DHEA levels need to be monitored over many years. Obesity appears to attenuate the association or correlation between higher DHEA and lower morbidity [31].

The problem with DHEA in women is that longer randomized trials in postmenopausal women (26+ weeks) have not shown results better than placebo on sexual desire, for example, at 50 mg per day [32]. Also, more women experienced acne and increased hair growth in the DHEA arm. Overall the results are so mixed that reviews of past data tend to discourage the use of oral DHEA for sexual health improvements in women with FSD [33]. The good news is that overall the safety of 50 mg of DHEA tends to be excellent in 1-year studies, but I still am concerned about reductions in HDL over time with this and higher dosages [34]. Although, some of the criticism with DHEA studies is that the dosages utilized are not high enough for efficacy. Older studies of higher DHEA dosages (300 mg and more) in small groups of postmenopausal women have suggested a benefit over placebo that could have an impact on mental and physical sexual health and arousal within 60 min of visual sexual stimuli [35]. Yet, these are acute dosage studies and the positives and negatives of several days/months of high-dose DHEA ingestion have not received adequate attention. For example, a DHEA supplementation study (1,600 mg/day for 28 days) was published that showed profound reductions in HDL and significant increases in testosterone in postmenopausal women (no changes in estrogen) [36].

DHEA is not a promising or predictable option for those that need TRT or postmenopausal FSD, but perhaps those with adrenal or androgen insufficiency might benefit? Replacement with DHEA in those with androgen or especially "adrenal insufficiency" (e.g., adrenal adenectomy, autoimmune, or secondary from pituitary issues) appears practical and has some preliminary older data in women [37, 38], but the decision of whether or not it has consistent benefits is still very subjective. For example, a retrospective review (non-placebo) of over 100 women with androgen insufficiency and sexual dysfunction ingesting 50 mg of DHEA on average for 4 months reported a significant reduction in sexual distress and increases in desire, arousal, lubrication, satisfaction, and orgasm [38]. Women in this study (mean age of 43 years) had testosterone and DHEA-S levels that were in the lower range of normal. Increased facial hair (11 %), weight gain (7 %), acne (5 %), temporary breast tenderness, loss of head hair, and skin rash (1 % each) were the most commonly reported side effects. Thus, there is fairly general agreement that women with androgen or especially adrenal insufficiency are the best potential candidates for DHEA, especially if there is a need to increase mood and/or libido [39]. This is not tantamount to a solid recommendation. Small studies against placebo of women with adrenal insufficiency for 4 months suggest some benefit of DHEA supplementation of 50 mg per day on general sexual health [40]. Still, these data in patients with adrenal insufficiency are controversial, and there is always concern about long-term toxicity in these individuals [41]. Additionally, there have been several studies showing no impact on sexual health, which is arguably why one of the only meta-analyses performed on randomized trials for DHEA and quality of life in women with adrenal insufficiency did not recommend it [42]. This is a classic example of a mixed-data situation where the decision to add small amounts of DHEA for women who are androgen- or adrenal-insufficient should be left to the patient and clinician.

What about DHEA for specific and general antiaging health purposes? In one of the longest-duration clinical trials in the history of DHEA [43], the supplement was given for 2 years at a dose of 75 mg per day in men and 50 mg per day in women, and these researchers decided to look at the impact of this hormone on the body, physical performance, insulin, and other factors compared to a placebo. There were a total of 87 men (29 received DHEA, 27 received testosterone, and 31 received placebo) in this study and 57 women (27 received DHEA and 30 received placebo), and the average age of the participants ranged from 66 to 70 years. Men and women in this study were just slightly overweight, with a body mass index (BMI) of 26–27. Women who had low levels of DHEA (median value of 0.4 mcg/mL or 1.1 mmol/L), and men with low levels of DHEA (median value of 0.7 mcg/mL or 1.9 mmol/L) had their levels increased by approximately 3.5 mcg/mL or 9.5 mmol/L after taking DHEA. This is a 500 % increase in blood levels of this hormone in some of the patients. This current study showed that quality of life did not change on DHEA, but perhaps a larger study would have provided more clarity in this area. There were no changes in oxygen intake (a measure of metabolism change), muscle strength, or insulin. The DHEA group experienced an unhealthy drop in HDL or "good" cholesterol, which was a significant five-point reduction in women and an almost significant three-point reduction in men during the study (US units). No such HDL drop occurred in the testosterone-receiving group of men during the study. Men receiving testosterone had a slight reduction in fat tissue, and bone mineral density increased at the hip area in men on DHEA and testosterone. In women, DHEA increased bone mineral density only in the area of the wrist, but not at other sites. So, again this study leaves open the possibility of testing higher doses of DHEA and testosterone, but safety will ultimately also be an issue. Higher doses of DHEA need to be studied, but in the meantime, reversing the signs of aging with hormones has little to no evidence and may do harm.

Why not just give TRT to the men who truly require or qualify for testosterone or smaller amounts (10 % or less) to women deficient in androgen? This seems to make more sense as opposed to playing a guessing game with a dietary supplement for general antiaging purposes that also seems to possess safety and quality-control issues [15, 16, 44]. This is also a concern because just because someone purchases DHEA does not necessarily guarantee that DHEA is found in the bottle at the reported concentrations [41]. Finally, other areas of men's health, such as muscle strength and physical function, have shown minimal impact with this supplement from short and long-term studies [45]. Other long-term (2 years) studies of women's health suggest that a significant improvement in spinal bone mineral density (BMD) with 50 mg per day of DHEA in women (ages 65–75) also receiving 650 IU per day of vitamin D and 700 mg per day of calcium versus vitamin D and calcium alone suggests that this may be an area worth pursuing [46].

What does the future hold for DHEA? Vaginally administered DHEA (e.g., Prasterone, 0.25–1 % DHEA) appears to provide sexual health benefits (desire, arousal, lubrication, orgasm, and reduced dryness) for women with vaginal atrophy and estrogen deficiency in menopause [33, 47], but I would not consider this a CAM. It is applied intravaginally with an applicator at bedtime. Vaginal DHEA requires daily application, whereas other steroids (estradiol or estriol) require dosing two to three times a week and safety has been well established with vaginal estrogen [48]. So, how popular this will be in the future is a matter of opinion.

L-Arginine or L-Arginine Aspartate + Pycnogenol

Nitric oxide (NO) is produced from L-arginine by nitric oxide synthase (NOS) [22]; thus, the idea of utilizing L-arginine supplements to enhance the treatment of ED appears logical and is an option for some patients. In fact, L-arginine, with its ability to increase NO and lower blood pressure, makes it a potential preventive or treatment option in other areas of medicine such as hypertension and preeclampsia [49–51].

Still, over the years of clinical research there appear to be multiple questionable areas with

L-arginine supplements that needed to be answered, in my opinion. These are:

1. Safety
2. Metabolism
3. Efficacy by itself
4. L-arginine aspartate + pycnogenol (the best current arginine option)
5. Why not just citrulline?

Safety

One of the best studies completed on L-arginine (not L-arginine aspartate) by itself on heart/vascular health for individuals with a history of having a myocardial infarction found a higher rate of health problems and possibly mortality in the L-arginine group compared to placebo, and this study, conducted at Johns Hopkins, was terminated based on these early results [52]. The clinical trial was known as the "VINTAGE MI," and researchers attempted to eventually have the participants ingest up to 9 g of L-arginine per day. Another well-known clinical trial, but for those with peripheral artery disease (PAD), known as the "Nitric Oxide in Peripheral Artery Insufficiency (NO-PAIN)" study found that 3 g a day of L-arginine for 6 months compared to placebo not only did not improve NO production, but the improvement in patients was actually significantly better in the placebo group [53]. This suggests that in some individuals L-arginine might not be a good option, including those with a history of a myocardial infarction or PAD until more clarity or research adequately resolves the issue, because other studies have found some benefits or at least no immediate safety issues in similar patient populations [54, 55].

Metabolism

Three serious problems with L-arginine supplementation in terms of metabolism include:

1. The potential for extensive first-pass liver metabolism (arginase enzyme) that occurs when ingesting this compound [56–58].
2. The additional intestinal enzymes (gut arginases) that also exist in the GI tract to further potentially deactivate this agent [56–58].
3. The presence of an endogenous inhibitor of NOS that is known as ADMA (asymmetrical dimethylarginine) [59, 60].

Thus, large dosages of L-arginine will usually needed to achieve some success in general medicine and in the area of ED and FSD, and this can be daunting for the patient. For example, 3–6 g of L-arginine would require 6–12 large pills or capsules per day.

Perhaps this is one reason large intakes of dietary arginine or supplemental arginine have not been proven beneficial in other areas of medicine such as athletic performance [61, 62]. More research is needed in less trained and elderly individuals because past studies do focus on highly trained athletes, which are arguably less likely to benefit from these products because they are already in peak physical condition. Still, either a better substitute or form of L-arginine or an ancillary agent to enhance the efficacy at lower dosages appears to be needed.

Efficacy by Itself

Low dosages of L-arginine alone (1,500 mg/day) do not appear to work better compared to placebo [63] for ED. Other studies of high dosages of L-arginine (5 g/day, $n=50$) over 6 weeks appear to work mildly to moderately better than placebo in terms of subjective (not objective) outcomes, especially for those with organic ED that may produce or secrete low amounts of nitrite and nitrate (metabolites of nitric oxide that are fairly stable) from urinary measurements [64]. Urinary nitric oxide metabolites appear to double when taking 5 g per day. One area that needed better research was whether L-arginine efficacy could be enhanced when combining it with other agents, as has been preliminarily demonstrated, for example, with yohimbine [65, 66]. L-arginine glutamate at 6 g a day with 6 mg of yohimbine hydrochloride 1–2 h before sexual activity appears to improve the efficacy of yohimbine alone, and these preliminary data exist in ED and for arousal improvement in FSD.

L-Arginine Aspartate + Pycnogenol (Prelox and Others)

An impressive amount of clinical data has been garnered for the use of L-arginine aspartate at a lower dosage (2,800–3,000 mg) when used with pycnogenol (80 mg) [67–69]. The most commonly tested supplement in this form is Prelox (Horphag Research Ltd., London, UK). Perhaps this solves part of the metabolism problem when utilizing L-arginine by itself.

A randomized, double-blind, placebo-controlled crossover study of 50 participants with moderate ED (IIEF score of 11–17) and a mean age of 37 years was conducted [68]. The total daily dose of Prelox was 3,000 mg of L-arginine aspartate and 80 mg of pycnogenol. This total dosage was divided into four tablets, two taken between 7 and 9 A.M. and two between 7 and 9 P.M. with 200 mL of water. IIEF scores from 11 to 17 at baseline approximately doubled to 26–30 ($p > 0.001$) after 1 month. The earliest improvement was 1 day, and the latest response was after 9 days (mean 4.9 days). IIEF domains, including orgasmic function, sexual desire, intercourse satisfaction, overall satisfaction, and percent sexual response, also approximately doubled ($p > 0.001$). Systolic and diastolic blood pressure also dropped significantly ($p < 0.001$), and side effects were similar to placebo.

It should be kept in mind that men with severe cardiovascular disease or hypertension were excluded from this study.

The clinical trial that has established Prelox as a definite CAM option for men with mild to moderate ED, in my opinion, and arguably one of the three best CAM options for ED was a 6-month randomized, double-blind trial, placebo-controlled parallel-arm study ($n = 124$, mean age 44 years) [69]. Men in this trial had IIEF scores at baseline of 11–17, and diabetics and those with severe hypertension were excluded. Again, two tablets were utilized in the morning and evening, and each table contained 700 mg L-arginine aspartate and 20 mg of pycnogenol (total daily dose was 2,800 mg L-arginine aspartate and 80 mg pycnogenol). The erectile domain of the IIEF (questions 1–5 and 15) improved from a baseline of 15–25 after 3 months and 27 after 6 months compared to placebo, where an increase of 15–19 was observed ($p < 0.05$). These results are in the same range of prescription PDE-5 inhibitors. There was an insignificant drop in blood pressure in the Prelox group from a systolic of 139–131 and a diastolic from 86 to 82 (6-point drop in the placebo arm). Total testosterone also increased significantly ($p < 0.05$) from 15.9 to 18.9 nmol/L in the Prelox group (16.9–17.3 nmol/L with placebo). It is plausible that testosterone increased from increased sexual activity and/or another mechanism, and this should be followed in patients to answer this question because it would be a tremendous ancillary benefit for some men if this was the case. Increases in the domain of orgasmic function, sexual desire, intercourse satisfaction, and overall satisfaction were all significantly improved over placebo ($p < 0.05$) with Prelox. A total of 13 men were lost to follow-up in this trial, so 111 men completed the trial. The question is whether or not the data were analyzed based on intention-to-treat principle (this does not appear to be the case), which is important because all significant values reached the minimum of $p < 0.05$. Regardless, there is adequate efficacy with Prelox, and it should be offered as an option for healthy men with mild to moderate ED and no significant comorbidity and no hepatic or renal abnormalities. The number of pills needed per day (four) could be problematic in the long term along with cost, and whether or not those with cardiovascular disease should utilize it is questionable, but the overall efficacy is still notable and again makes it one of the best CAM options available based on the scientific evidence for men with mild to moderate ED. Interestingly, a female version of Perlox is also receiving some clinical trials with some early promising results [70].

In the area of FSD, another combination proprietary product (ArginMax, GNC, Inc.,

Pittsburgh, PA, USA) utilizing multiple compounds including L-arginine appears to have garnered enough data to potentially recommend it to some patients. Two previous placebo-controlled studies published of this combination dietary supplement (L-arginine, *Panax ginseng*, *Ginkgo biloba*, damiana leaf, multiple vitamins and minerals, etc.) helped to improve arousal, desire, orgasm, sexual frequency, clitoral sensation, and increased sexual function scores [71, 72]. These preliminary studies ($n=77$ and $n=108$, ages 22–73 years) are suggesting that pre-, peri-, and postmenopausal women with FSD could benefit. Pre- and perimenopausal appeared to derive more diverse benefits, whereas desire was primarily increased in postmenopausal women. The more recent clinical study showed a benefit within 4 weeks. This supplement does not appear to have estrogenic enhancement properties, which means that it could be appropriate option for women with breast cancer or those that do not want to use hormone replacement therapy. It could also be argued that the benefits of ArginMax could also have occurred from other well-known herbals such as *P. ginseng* because the concentrations of the active ingredients (ginsenosides) were high (30 %; see section "*P. ginseng*"). Whether or not L-arginine or *P. ginseng* or other supplements alone could be just as effective as this combination approach has not been tested.

Why Not Just Citrulline?

Perhaps the solution to the L-arginine metabolism and/or questionable safety problem and the need for higher dosages lies in L-citrulline, an amino acid derived from watermelon rind [22, 73, 74]. L-citrulline is produced by L-arginine in the formation of nitric oxide and can be recycled back to produce more L-arginine. In other words, the first-pass metabolism issues do not occur with L-citrulline supplements compared to L-arginine supplements and lower dosages for efficacy appear to be needed. This will be discussed in more detail in the "L-citrulline" section.

L-Carnitine

L-carnitine is an amino acid that transports fatty acids from the cytosol to the mitochondria for energy production in each cell of the body [75]. Humans can produce carnitine de novo in the liver from lysine and methionine (25 %), but dietary intake is the primary source of carnitine (75 %). Foods high in carnitine include dairy and meat and a plant-based diet is in general a poor source of carnitine. Excretion of carnitine occurs from the kidneys, but reabsorption is also efficient, so that vegans are still able to maintain close to normal blood levels of this amino acid despite only 10 % of less the consumption of carnitine compared to omnivores.

There are several minimally different forms of L-carnitine available for purchase that have been used in clinical trials, including L-carnitine, acetyl-L-carnitine (ALC), and propionyl-L-carnitine (PLC). These other types of L-carnitine have been tested because L-carnitine itself tends to be unstable. Yet, these other forms of L-carnitine do not necessarily have better data in other areas of urology such as male subfertility, especially when compared to each other at higher dosages such 3,000 mg per day [76], and are more costly for the patient. Still, the potential minimal to moderate impact of L-carnitine on male subfertility has become better known because of multiple clinical trials in this area of medicine [77–82] (see fertility chapter 4).

There are a few serious potential issues with utilizing L-carnitine for ED and FSD. Most of the efficacy data stems from its use in combination products, such as L-arginine and niacin with or without a PDE-5 inhibitor, and the small number of participants in some studies [83–86].

In my opinion, one clinical trial of carnitine from Italy clearly stands out among the rest and should be discussed [87]. This was a trial of 120 men with symptoms of androgen reduction and a free testosterone lower than 6 pg/mL. Participants were randomized to one of three groups: testosterone undecanoate 160 mg/day, propionyl-L-carnitine 2,000 mg/day + acetyl-L-carnitine

2,000 mg per day, or placebo for 6 months (mean age 66 years). Carnitine and testosterone significantly improved the mean IIEF score. The only real issue with this trial is the 4,000 mg per day of total carnitine needed for efficacy, which can be costly and the number of pills needed per day can be as high as eight because most carnitine large tablets or pills are 500 mg each. Additionally, oral testosterone is not standard of care in many areas where other delivery systems appear to be more efficacious and safer [22]. Still, it was notable in this trial that the duration was 6 months and IIEF-15 erectile function, orgasm, sexual desire, and general well-being domain scores significantly increased at 3 months ($p < 0.01$). Erectile function and orgasm increased significantly at 6 months ($p < 0.01$), but sexual desire and general well-being did not. Sexual intercourse satisfaction had significantly increased at 6 months ($p < 0.01$), but not at the 3-month evaluation period. Nocturnal penile tumescence (NPT) also increased significantly with this supplement at 3 months. Carnitine was more efficacious compared to placebo but in terms of NPT, IIEF, and improving mood, it was more effective than oral testosterone. The authors noted that propionyl-L-carnitine was registered in Italy for intermittent claudication, which suggests an improvement in circulation with carnitine, and increases in peak systolic and diastolic velocity in this trial suggest a benefit. Improvement in mood were also noted, but not testosterone levels, so whether or not this could be an option for men needing symptomatic improvement that do not qualify for prescription TRT is controversial at this time because other trials with this supplement have not been published specifically in this area. Still, it is worthy of mentioning it to patients with a strong need for symptomatic changes because of low testosterone without actually wanting or qualifying for TRT. Still, L-carnitine is a controversial supplement in terms of true efficacy and heart health [22], so it would be nice to have another clinical trial support or refute the original 4,000-mg positive trial in men with low levels of free testosterone. L-carnitine has received little to no attention in the area of FSD.

L-Citrulline

Penile erection is initiated by the relaxation of smooth muscle in the corpus cavernosum and its arterioles [88, 89]. During sexual stimulation, NO is released from nerve endings of parasympathetic nonadrenergic, noncholinergic neurons, and endothelial cells in the corpus cavernosum. NO causes a molecular cascade that results in the relaxation of smooth-muscle cells in the corpus cavernosum. NO accomplishes this by activating the enzyme guanylate cyclase, resulting in increased synthesis of cyclic guanosine monophosphate (cGMP) in these cells. The available cGMP in turn triggers the smooth-muscle relaxation, which permits increased blood flow into the penis and an erection. Citrulline could function as a better precursor to arginine and NO production compared to arginine itself [89].

As mentioned earlier in the section of this chapter on "L-arginine", oral L-arginine is extensively metabolized by arginase in the gut wall and liver [56–58] and is converted to ornithine and proline or used as a substrate in the liver for ureagenesis. Therefore, trials of L-arginine in the treatment of ED have found that large doses are necessary to have an effect. Another problem with L-arginine has been the questionable safety in some studies [52, 53] and the possibility that ADMA (endogenous inhibitor of nitric oxide production) levels can increase in time on L-arginine [59, 60, 90], which may be another reason that larger dosages of arginine might be needed over time to overcome this negative-feedback mechanism (tachyphylaxis effects).

The major source of L-arginine within the endothelial cell is from L-citrulline, and both L-arginine and L-citrulline raise vascular NO levels [73]. Yet, it appears that in some individuals L-citrulline may be at least twice as efficient at increasing NO levels compared to L-arginine, which could solve some of the dosage and other issues mentioned with L-arginine. In a double-blind, randomized, placebo-controlled crossover study, 20 (mean age 57 years) healthy volunteers received six different dosing regimens of placebo, citrulline, and arginine. L-citrulline was significantly more effective at increasing L-arginine plasma levels compared to L-arginine itself ($p<0.01$). At a dosage of only 1.5 g per day of oral L-citrulline, L-arginine blood levels were raised to a similar degree as 3.2 g per day of oral L-arginine. L-citrulline raised the ratio of L-arginine to ADMA, and the arginine/ADMA ratio is again thought to determine substrate availability of arginine to the endothelium. The correlation observed in this study between increases in the arginine/ADMA ratio and forearm flow-mediated vasodilatation indicated a dose–response relationship with NO production. The highest dose of L-citrulline (3 g twice a day or 6 g total) was the most effective at raising NO levels compared to L-arginine ($p<0.01$). Urinary nitrate (a marker of NO) and cGMP (another potential indicator of systemic NO production and bioactivity) were significantly ($p=0.01$, $p=0.04$) increased over arginine. Neither blood urea nitrogen (BUN) nor serum creatinine was changed, and there were no safety issues over placebo.

It is interesting that the 1.5 g of L-citrulline used as one dosage in the previously mentioned study was the same daily dosage found to be effective in 1-month crossover trial of men with mild to moderate ED [74]. A total of 24 men (mean age is 56.5 years ±9.8 years) took 1.5 g of L-citrulline a day or placebo for 1 month. An improvement in erection hardness score (a validated ED instrument) was found after 1 month in the L-citrulline group compared to placebo ($p<0.01$). No adverse events occurred over placebo, and 37.5 % of participants had hypertension, 21 % had high cholesterol, 12.5 % had BPH, and 12.5 % had diabetes. This is preliminary but potentially exciting research, suggesting that L-citrulline could be one of the best CAM options for ED and should also be researched as ancillary supplementation to conventional ED options. L-citrulline should also be tested in women with FSD.

Still, the question of short- and long-term safety with L-citrulline needs to be addressed. High dosages of L-citrulline have been utilized in some short-term clinical trials with good safety. For example, a total of ten healthy volunteers were given 0.18 g/kg body weight of oral L-citrulline at one time [91]. The average age was 24 years, and BMI was 22.5. This dosage equates to a 70-kg man receiving 12.6 g of L-citrulline. Plasma and urine were evaluated every 3 h from 11 A.M. to 8 P.M. Significant increases in plasma (fivefold or 490 %), urine, and red blood cell citrulline (p of at least 0.001) occurred and doubling of the plasma arginine level without changes in blood urea or urinary urea excretion. The authors concluded that oral citrulline could be used to enhance systemic citrulline and arginine availability, because citrulline is bioavailable and very little citrulline is lost in urine. This may also explain the safety of L-citrulline, because these authors note that past research suggested that "citrulline may be a better candidate than arginine for supplementation, because extensive uptake and metabolism of arginine by the liver may cause excessive ureagenesis." Citrulline was efficiently absorbed in the gut and reabsorbed by the kidney. In addition, the authors concluded that this study is one of the first to suggest that oral citrulline can be used to increase arginine availability without affecting urea excretion and may enhance nitrogen balance. It does appear that adequate renal function is needed for maximum citrulline conversion into arginine, and this should be kept in mind.

Another 1-day study of eight fasting, healthy males undergoing four separate (2, 5, 10, and 15 g) oral loading doses of citrulline in random order was published [92]. Blood was drawn ten times over an 8-h period for measurement of biomarkers, and urine samples were collected at baseline and after 24 h. No adverse events occurred at any dosage. Even at the highest dosages, there was very little urine excretion of citrulline. Plasma insulin and growth hormone were not impacted. Citrulline increased in the plasma at higher dosages, while plasma arginine levels increased less than expected. This may be due to saturation of the renal conversion of citrulline into arginine. Citrulline administration had no impact on total nitrogen or calcium excretion, and no effect on hematologic or other biochemical markers or blood pressure. No side effects were observed, and again this study confirmed that acutely citrulline bypasses splanchnic extract. Still, a limitation that one could derive (not mentioned) from this and other studies is that in individuals without adequate kidney function, there could be inadequate conversion of citrulline into arginine because again this is where the primary reaction appears to occur. Additionally, this study suggested that the 15-g daily dose of citrulline is when saturation occurs, so that 10 g a day should be the maximum amount used in clinical practice. It is also interesting that another form of L-citrulline, citrulline malate, has a good safety record and has been given in large dosages (e.g., 8 g) to reduce muscle fatigue [93], but this form of citrulline has not gone through an ample number of nitric oxide generating studies nor a single ED study compared to just the free form of L-citrulline [74]. It is also of interest that citrulline from synthetic or watermelon extract supplements have not been known to cause acute side effects and is another source of citrulline and arginine, but blood pressure reductions could occur, especially in prehypertensive and hypertensive patients, and this has to be noted to anyone before starting citrulline supplementation [94].

Several 1-week studies of L-citrulline have supported the potential for short-term use in healthy individuals with adequate safety. For example, a double-blind, randomized, placebo-controlled parallel-group trial of 15 healthy male subjects (mean of 58 years old) were given 5.6 g of L-citrulline per day or placebo for 7 days and a variety of measurement were conducted including arterial stiffness [95]. No differences in blood pressure were found, and the serum nitrogen oxide (NOx, the sum of nitrite plus nitrate) and NO metabolic products were significantly increased only in the L-citrulline group ($p<0.05$). This study also suggested that L-citrulline could improve arterial stiffness, independent of blood pressure and without short-term adverse effects. Another 1-week study of a mean of 11.7 g of citrulline per day or placebo in young adults with a mean age of 22 years was conducted [96]. There was no impact on insulin or IGF-1 concentrations and no impact on nitrogen balance. Arginine is known to be a stimulus of insulin secretion, which could be another favorable reason to use citrulline in some individuals over arginine. No side effects were observed. Additionally, no side effects were noted in a citrulline compared to placebo cross-over study of 6 g a day for 4 weeks each [97] or an 8-week study of 3 g of citrulline malate or 8 g of L-arginine per day for those with heart failure [98]. Some experts now believe that citrulline is the ideal amino acid to deliver arginine to endothelial and immune cells and appears to have the ability to prevent abnormally excessive uncontrolled NO production, thus having a better potential safety profile compared to L-arginine [99]. Still, other interesting questions remain unanswered but look encouraging at this time, such as can citrulline really also act in other favorable ways in the body such as an accelerator of injury repair or protein synthesis [100, 101]? And, since NO production inhibits platelet aggregation as demonstrated from L-arginine infusion studies [102], it should be expected that L-citrulline can do the same but needs more research. More short- and long-term studies are needed in the area of ED, FSD, and potentially with TRT to determine the best potential use of this interesting amino acid from watermelon. Since citrulline has the potential to be heart healthy, this also makes it a potential ideal candidate in the area of ED and hopefully FSD in the future [22].

Maca (*Lepidium meyenii*)

L. meyenii or "maca" is an Andean plant that is a part of the Brassica family and has been used for centuries in the Andes to enhance fertility and sexual health in humans and animals [103, 104]. Maca may also slightly improve sexual function from a series of recent and past preliminary clinical trials in men, and it does not appear to alter testosterone levels [105, 106]. The data points toward good preliminary safety and a potential enhancement in fertility that should receive attention in the future as much as its potential impact on ED.

The potential issues with maca are threefold: this product has not been tested beyond preliminary studies with small numbers of individuals, high dosages are required in some studies to observe an impact (2,400–3,000 mg), and there is a question of what to look for when standardizing the ingredients of maca. This is also the case in FSD, where maca appeared to significantly increase libido in nine women with SSRI-induced FSD when taking 3 g per day compared to seven individuals taking 1.5 g per day, but there was no placebo arm [107]. However, one older clinical trial appeared to find an improvement in libido at 1,500 mg per day after 8 and 12 weeks that was as good as 3,000 mg [105]. A past systematic review also agrees that although interesting it is difficult to comment with more certainty whether or not this product can be a stand-alone or ancillary option for ED or FSD [108]. My biggest concern is standardization of maca during a clinical trial because it appears that dried maca roots need to be standardized to a specific amount of the "macamide" and "macaene" (polyunsaturated fatty acids and their amides) amount from a lipidic extract of this herb because these are the proposed potential active ingredients, and macamides, for example, are a unique class of secondary metabolites not found in another plant species [109, 110]. Therefore, they would be useful markers of not only efficacy but also quality control. It appears that a product with at least 0.6 % macamides and macaenes should be the minimum quality-control marker of standardization [111]. Maca also contains diverse amino acids, including almost 100 mg of arginine per gram of maca [112]. It is concerning that a large study to determine if maca really improves sexual desire and other parameters of sexual health in men and women has not been conducted based on the preliminary results with this herbal product.

Niacin (Vitamin B_3)

Niacin used to be a logical choice to study as a potential ED treatment, in my opinion, because of its past success of improving heart-healthy parameters (increase HDL, reduce triglycerides, lower LDL, etc.) [113]. However, niacin is immersed in ongoing controversy because of its recent lack of efficacy beyond intense statin therapy and because the newer prescription form of niacin has not performed any better and there may be toxicity concerns [114, 115]. It is for these and other reasons that I believe the future of this supplement and drug in medicine is very questionable. It is also difficult to purchase and tolerate niacin as a dietary supplement, even in dosages of 100 mg (immediate release niacin) because of the cutaneous flushing that can occur, liver toxicity, exacerbation of gout, hyperglycemia, peptic ulcer disease, and perhaps other issues such as increasing the risk of dry eye [116, 117]. Prescription niacin (extended release) may be easier to tolerate even at higher dosages of 500–2,000 mg, and fewer pills are needed, but similar side effects of over-the-counter niacin and new concerns of a lack of efficacy in heart disease only fuel the ongoing controversy of using this drug or supplement. Yet, for those that believe that niacin still has a future in cardiovascular or sexual medicine, there was one notable trial in men with ED using the prescription form (Niaspan) that deserves some attention [118]. This was a single-center prospective randomized, placebo-controlled parallel-group trial of 160 men (mean age 58 years) with ED and dyslipidemia. Men were randomized to receive 1,500 mg of oral niacin daily or placebo for 12 weeks.

No significant differences overall were found between groups. However, when men were stratified and analyzed based on ED severity, men with mild ED also showed no improvement, but men with moderate and severe ED (50 % or more of men) on niacin showed a significant improvement on IIEF-3 and -4 (maintenance of erection questions) compared to baseline values. A significant improvement for niacin compared to baseline values was also found for IIEF-3 in men not on statins. Flushing (36 vs. 3 %) and itchiness (33 vs. 9 %) were significantly greater side effects with niacin compared to placebo. A total of 12 patients from the niacin group and six from the placebo group dropped out of the study. Using niacin in combination dietary supplements for ED does have some minimal clinical research [83, 84]. Still, the near future will determine the fate of prescription niacin in cardiovascular medicine, which should determine the fate of niacin as a dietary supplement; for reasons already outlined, I am not optimistic, but I hope I am incorrect.

P. ginseng and Ginsenosides (Korean Red Ginseng and Others)

Ginseng actually refers to the root of several species in the genus *Panax*, of which *P. ginseng* is one of the most widely utilized species and is native to Asian countries such as China and Korea [119–122]. *P. ginseng* has a medical history stretching over thousands of years. The word is derived from the Greek words *pan*, meaning all, and *axos*, meaning cure. The species name is derived from the Chinese word *rensheng*, which means "human," because ginseng roots have some resemblance to the human body. In China and Korea, ginseng roots are usually harvested after 3–6 years. In Korea, fresh ginseng is less than 4 years old, white ginseng is 4–6 years old and dried after peeling, and red ginseng is harvested when it is 6 years old and then steamed and dried (red ginseng is not skinned before it is steamed). These different processes appear to increase the concentration and number of active ingredients (ginsenosides) in ginseng, especially Korean red ginseng.

Ginsenosides, which are also known as ginseng saponins or glycosylated steroidal saponins, are unique to the *Panax* species and are the primary active ingredients in ginseng [119–122]. More than 30 different ginsenosides have been isolated from the root of *P. ginseng*, and although ginseng contains other miscellaneous compounds, the individual and collective ginsenosides appear to be the generally agreed upon active ingredients whose clinical effects are supported by basic science [119–126].

Ginsenosides have multiple mechanisms of action, and each ginsenoside may have tissue-specific impacts [123–126]. The backbone of each ginsenoside is similar and consists of a common four-ring steroid-like structure that includes multiple carbon atoms with attached sugar moieties. Each ginsenoside has a different type, position, and number of sugar moieties attached by a glycosidic bond at C-3 and C-6. Each type of ginsenoside also has at least three side chains at the C-3, C-6, or C-20 position. These side chains are free or are attached to monomers, dimers, or trimers of sugars. It is these sugar compounds that may provide the cellular-specific or receptor effects of each ginsenoside. The ginseng species, age, part of the plant, harvest season, preservation, and extraction method can all impact the compounds found in ginseng and even alter somewhat the ginsenoside content.

Over several decades, the content of ginsenoside standardized extracts utilized in clinical trials has varied, from approximately 4 % ginsenosides in the 1990s to 4–7 % ginsenosides in the mid-2000s, and higher standardized extracts are offered today (e.g., >8 %) [127, 128]. The ginsenoside content should be considered when comparing different efficacy doses from clinical trials. When the ginsenoside concentration is isolated, it appears to elicit the same or better results than the sum of the total ginseng components [128], which again supports the accepted general philosophy that ginsenosides are the active medical components of *P. ginseng* [119–128]. In other words, the more concentrated the specific ginsenosides, the greater the potential impact and the lower the dosage needed for that impact. Yet, as ginseng becomes more concentrated, in my opinion, the overall cost can become quite high for the consumer and adverse effects have less research at these concentrations, so patients need to be aware of this issue.

One of the more influential evidence-based endorsements for ginseng and male sexual function was a clinical evidence guideline of conventional and alternative medicines [129]. The authors used *P. ginseng* data from six randomized trials conducted over a period of approximately 15 years that included a total of 349 men. The investigators found that ginseng significantly ($p<0.00001$) improved erectile function compared with placebo over 4–12 weeks. Approximately 58 % of men experienced an improvement in some aspect of sexual function compared with 20 % of men who received the placebo. No other dietary or truly CAM supplement was recommended. Ginseng was found to have "moderate-quality evidence" and the investigators concluded that ginseng is "likely to be beneficial" in men with erectile dysfunction of any etiology (organic and psychogenic causes).

The final clinical evidence-based guideline provided in this review stated "Ginseng is a traditional Asian remedy with rare adverse effects in the recommended dose of 0.5–2.0 g daily." What was not mentioned in this review and any others to date to my knowledge, and should be kept in mind, is that these dosages recommended were for the older, less concentrated form of ginseng (4–7 % ginsenosides).

In this same systematic review [129], the authors mentioned that they still needed to evaluate a more concentrated ginsenoside randomized trial by Park and colleagues that was published in Korean in the Korean Journal of Urology [130] but that the article was being translated. Interestingly, I had this study by Park and colleagues translated into English, and it arguably provides some of the best preliminary clinical data to date for a dietary supplement compared with placebo over 8 weeks for men with ED. This was a multicenter, randomized, double-blind, placebo-controlled study of 69 participants that used a highly concentrated ginsenoside product (800 mg/day) [130]. The primary endpoint was the response to the erectile function domain of the International Index of Erectile Function (IIEF) questionnaire at baseline and 8 weeks. The other domains of the IIEF were secondary endpoints, and safety was monitored. Every single sexual health domain from the IIEF-15 was significantly improved by Korean ginseng compared with placebo: erectile function (primary endpoint), sexual desire, orgasmic function, intercourse satisfaction, and overall satisfaction. Additionally, every question on the IIEF (15 out of 15) was improved significantly in this specific clinical trial. The sexual desire domain, frequency, and degree of sexual desire were all also significantly increased ($p<0.001$). In other words, both the primary and the secondary endpoints significantly favored ginseng over placebo.

Additionally, there were no significant differences in adverse events reported for ginseng compared with placebo [130]. The results of this trial will strengthen the clinical evidence for *P. ginseng* and the evidence that highly concentrated ginsenosides are the active or effective ingredients in ginseng. The product used was from a Korean Ginseng Company (BT Gin) that I have had discussions with in terms of their unique ability to concentrate ginsenosides, and they are conducting multiple clinical trials in other areas of medicine, including as cardiovascular health product. Still, the current and future cost of this and other products need to be discussed, because again they can be quite high depending on the source and time of year.

Another prominent review of systematic reviews of alternative medicines for sexual function [131] arrived at a similar conclusion as the previous review [129]. The qualitative methods utilized from past clinical trials were evaluated by two independent experts, and the only dietary supplement that received a cautiously positive conclusion with no safety issues was *P. ginseng*. Another older systematic review of all randomized data from *P. ginseng* trials up to that time period also deserves to be mentioned [132]. This meta-analysis emphasized the significant ($p<0.00001$) effect of ginseng on erectile function. Subgroup analyses also found a significant ($p=0.001$) impact of ginseng on the psychogenic etiology of sexual dysfunction. The authors stated that adverse events or side effects were "scarce and those that were reported were mild." No significant side effects compared with placebo were reported. According to this review, the methodology of future trials must be improved, but still numerous randomized trials met the inclusion criteria set by these investigators.

Thus, the three most recent comprehensive reviews of conventional or alternative medicine in the treatment of sexual dysfunction all arrived at a similar conclusion, which is that ginseng is a potential option for men at diverse dosages and ginsenoside concentrations [129, 131, 132]. The onset of action or efficacy of ginseng could arguably occur within days to months [130, 132]. The time period is variable and requires further elucidation, but at least 4–8 weeks should be attempted on a *P. ginseng* supplement before deciding upon efficacy. The onset of action will not be as rapid on average as PDE-5 inhibitors, but the impact on libido, lower cost in some cases, and safety afford ginseng its own set of advantages for certain patients. In addition, the potential for combining ginseng with conventional ED treatments should be explored.

Interestingly, a more natural (wild form) and older *P. ginseng* known as "tissue-cultured mountain ginseng extract" that was approved by the Korean Food and Drug Administration in 2003 also has preliminary clinical data as a treatment for ED [133]. This form of ginseng has a structure similar to that of *P. ginseng*, and collectively these trials included over 100 participants with fairly adequate overall methodology [133, 134], especially the most recent clinical trial [133]. Significantly greater improvements were observed over placebo in terms of erectile function, intercourse satisfaction, overall satisfaction, and total IIEF score [133]. This form of ginseng apparently contains higher concentrations of ginsenoside Rb [135] but could arguably be potentially less efficacious owing to its lack of ginsenoside standardization, scarcity, and costs. This mountain ginseng extract was still shown to be clinically effective and should be considered in future meta-analysis or systematic reviews in terms of the overall quality and quantity of the evidence and safety analysis for *P. ginseng*.

Both *P. ginseng* and *P. quinquefolius* (American ginseng) have been shown in the past in laboratory studies to positively impact male sexual behavior [136, 137]. Since 1995, however, favorable clinical trial results in men with ED of diverse etiologies have been published only for *P. ginseng*. Yet, it is unfortunate that research has not continued for American ginseng in the area of ED or FSD. In terms of *P. ginseng*, the laboratory data for ginsenosides suggest multiple mechanisms of action. In cultured bovine endothelial cells, ginsenosides were shown to stimulate the conversion of [14C]L-arginine to [14C]L-citrulline and to promote vasorelaxation [138]. More specific studies in rabbit corpus cavernosum tissue continue to support the potential of increasing endogenous NO concentrations via the addition of ginsenosides [139]. Other basic laboratory investigations and reviews support this thought and mechanism whereby the stimulation of NO synthase may produce higher quantities of NO and peripheral neurophysiologic enhancement may also occur [140–143]. Other laboratory investigations of a primary ginsenoside (Rg1) from *P. ginseng* showed significantly increased mounting and pelvic thrusting frequency and intromission numbers with male mice [144]. Ginseng components also increased testosterone (not observed in clinical trials), cyclic GMP accumulation, and NO release. Thus, the potential to isolate and concentrate one particular ginsenoside for nutraceutical or pharmaceutical investigation will hopefully be of interest in the near future because at least seven or more ginsenosides appear to have some mechanism of action in *P. ginseng*.

A past human interventional mechanistic study of 12 males demonstrated that a single oral administration of *P. ginseng* water extract (500 mg/50 kg) significantly ($p<0.05$) increased NO levels for about a 2-h period 45 min after ingestion [145]. Ginseng increased NO in exhaled breath and reduced blood pressure and heart rate. The correlation between NO levels and heart rate was significant ($p<0.01$). The active components of ginseng may enhance the release of NO from endothelial cells, and ginseng components may act synergistically with other vasoactive substances and specific nerves in the corpus cavernosum. Via this central mechanism of action, these endothelial and neurogenic impacts of ginseng in causing relaxation of the corpus cavernosum may also be responsible for the aphrodisiac effect of *P. ginseng*. For example, the central and not just peripheral mechanism of action with ginseng deserves more research. Ginsenosides compete with agonists for binding to GABA-A and GABA-B receptors [146, 147], which could also explain a central mechanism of action impacting desire or arousal. Anxiolytic effects have also been demonstrated in mice and maze models. Ginseng and ginsenosides have been shown to positively impact striatal dopaminergic activity and dopamine receptors [148]. Ginseng may exert a direct effect on the hypothalamus or pituitary to also suppress prolactin secretion, but I believe these hormonal changes are minor at best because past clinical trials measuring hormonal changes in men did not find significant or consistent increases in prolactin or testosterone [149]. The neurotransmitter or centrally acting effects of ginsenosides require further investigation, because animal models continue to demonstrate central or neurotransmitter effects [150, 151].

Heart-healthy changes could occur with ginseng, which theoretically could explain the improvement in sexual function. A randomized, controlled, double-blind, crossover trial of 17 healthy, fasted individuals examined the effects of *P. ginseng* on arterial stiffness [128]. On separate occasions, 3 g of placebo, *P. ginseng* root, or a bioequivalent dose of *P. ginseng* root ginsenoside or polysaccharide fractions was used. Blood pressure and arterial health as measured by the augmentation index were recorded 1, 2, and 3 h after treatment. Three grams of ginseng significantly lowered the radial augmentation index by 4.6 % compared with placebo ($p = 0.05$), and the ginsenoside fraction reduced it by 4.8 %; no significant effect was found with the polysaccharide fraction. No significant difference in blood pressure was found, but this was one of the first recent investigations to demonstrate a potential improvement in arterial stiffness. The researchers concluded, "…it appears that ginsenosides may be the principal pharmacologically active component of the root, rather than the polysaccharide fraction." The potential improvement in multiple potential cardiovascular parameters, including glucose, lipids, and blood pressure, should also be of interest [152, 153].

For this reason and others, it should also be further tested in postmenopausal women with FSD. For example, a *P. ginseng* double-blind randomized parallel trial of 72 postmenopausal women over 12 weeks found a significant benefit for relieving menopausal symptoms and significant reductions in low-density lipoprotein and carotid intima-media thickness compared with placebo without significant changes in estradiol [154].

The antifatigue effect or improved energy levels with ginseng should also be considered another potential mechanism of action, whereby ED or FSD could theoretically be improved. A large ($n = 290$) Mayo Clinic trial of American ginseng found sufficient improvements in cancer-related fatigue over placebo to warrant further clinical study [155]. Interestingly, no side effects over placebo were found in the low (750 mg) or higher (1,000 or 2,000 mg) ginseng dose group. The mental or physical energy-enhancing effects of ginseng are of interest in both sexes [156, 157] and again could theoretically explain some of the sexual health improvements. It is interesting that 4–8 weeks were needed to improve energy levels over placebo.

In our opinion, one ancillary mechanism of action that appears most fascinating as of yet may be the neurologic improvement or protection via ginsenosides from degenerative or abnormal conditions in the central or peripheral nervous system [158–163]. Ginsenosides have demonstrated some anti-inflammatory, antioxidant, anti-apoptotic, neuronal growth factor enhancement, and other mechanisms of action. Therefore, the potential of ginsenosides to improve sexual function with prescription agents after prostate cancer treatment (e.g., surgery or radiation) should be investigated. An intervention that generates some excitement in the area of neuronal protection and regeneration outside of sexual health should be of interest within sexual health. High doses of ginseng have already been utilized in patients with neuronal degenerative diseases with at least a hint of some clinical efficacy, which should increase the interest in diverse neurological research with ginseng extracts [164, 165]. Ginseng's potential impact on cognition is preliminary but notable from past clinical trials [166], and quality-of-life improvements in an aging population are also of interest [167].

Laboratory studies have consistently found no overt safety or toxicity issues of concern with unadulterated ginseng. *P. ginseng* was nominated by the US National Institutes of Health to the US National Toxicology Program for assessment of its carcinogenic potential because it is one of the most popular and widely used herbs in the world [168, 169]. Researchers examined chronic toxicity, tumorigenicity, and safety in multiple studies in male and female mice (B6C3F1) and rats (Fischer 344). Studies included a 2-week, repeated-dose toxicity study (0, 125, 250, 500, 1,000, or 2,000 mg/kg) for 5 days per week for 16 days. Another study was a 3-month ingestion study (0, 1,000, 2,000, 3,000, 4,000, or 5,000 mg/kg) in which *P. ginseng* was ingested 5 days per week for 14 weeks. In yet another study, male and female rats and mice were given 0, 1,250, 2,500, or 5,000 mg/kg 5 days per week for 104 weeks. Ginseng was also tested in two independent bacterial mutagenicity assays. No significant safety issues were found in animals in the 2-week, 3-month, or 2-year gavage studies. The results of the US National Toxicology Program acute and chronic toxicity and tumorigenic bioassays found *P. ginseng* to be neither toxic nor tumorigenic even when administered at doses of 5,000 mg/kg. Interestingly, the incidence of mammary gland fibroadenoma was significantly decreased in female rats administered 5,000 mg/ kg.

Past laboratory studies investigating the impact of *P. ginseng* on sexual function also noted no safety issues of concern. For example, in the most recent investigation, the researchers reported no animal (mouse) mortality even with doses up to 20 g/kg for 10 days [144]. In another ancillary study by this same group and noted in the same publication, no signs of toxicity were observed in beagle dogs that were treated with a primary ginsenoside (Rg1) at a dose of 500 mg/ kg by mouth daily for 5 months.

The consistency of safety data from human studies is also notable and is derived from a variety of sources. One analysis included a systematic review from five electronic databases and all articles with original data on adverse events and drug interactions with *P. ginseng* [170]. Information was also requested from 12 manufacturers of preparations of ginseng, the spontaneous reporting of the World Health Organization, and national drug safety bodies. No language restrictions were imposed. The incidence of side effects of ginseng was found to be similar to that of placebo. More serious side effects were reported in isolated case reports and through spontaneous reporting and not in randomized trials. The authors concluded, "Collectively, these data suggest that *P. ginseng* monopreparations are rarely associated with adverse events or drug interactions. The ones that are documented are usually mild and transient. Combined preparations are more often associated with such events but causal attribution is usually not possible." An update to this manuscript reached a similar conclusion and stated that the potential for drug-ginseng interactions is "low" and the concern over other medications is primarily based on isolated case reports [171].

A rare but still surprising concern with some herbal preparations, in my opinion, is the chance for them to be inappropriately and falsely labeled with an acute safety issue on the basis of isolated case reports or uncontrolled investigation without an examination of the of the majority of the objective laboratory and clinical evidence. One perpetuated example is a 1979 observational series in a notable medical journal that associated the self-reported utilization of ginseng products with hypertension in 14 individuals after 3 months of use [172]. Despite no control group, and other basic methodology quality-control issues, including a lack of correction for other confounders, such as high intakes of caffeine and potentially other stimulants, this investigation was used by multiple authors as cause and effect or evidence [173–175]. These hypertensive effects have not been replicated since 1979 in a controlled setting. Randomized trials of hypertensive and non-hypertensive individuals have demonstrated no impact or a partial reduction in blood pressure with *Panax* or American ginseng and isolated ginsenosides, regardless of dose utilized and time period (up to 3 months) [176–181].

Regardless, long-term studies (several years) are needed to confirm this consistent finding in the acute setting. In my experience, other compounds found with ginseng commercial products such as caffeine or caffeine mimics I believe have the ability to exacerbate the stimulant effects of ginseng itself or be the sole cause of blood pressure or heart rate increases in rare patients. It is for this reason that a patient with controlled or uncontrolled hypertension should receive some objective education on the past history of ginseng in combination with adulterants that could theoretically change blood pressure values. Again, the data suggest no change in blood pressure with ginseng itself, but when stimulants are added to any supplement, the potential always exists.

Potential interactions with warfarin or hemostatic issues have also been suggested on the basis of case reports [170, 171, 182], but controlled studies have not been able to substantiate any consistent impact of ginseng on warfarin anticoagulation or hemostasis in general (prothrombin time, partial thromboplastin time, and international normalized ratio [INR]) [181, 183–187]. Still, this needs to be further elucidated based on studies of other types of ginseng that could have some impact on platelet activity, and this could explain some cardiovascular benefits. And, since ginseng may improve NO levels [188, 189], and NO is known, as mentioned earlier in the chapter, to inhibit platelet aggregation, it is plausible there could be a blood-thinning-type effect.

More long-term randomized studies are always needed. One 2-year study in patients with diabetes did not demonstrate concerns [190], and a lengthy observational study may provide some assurance [191]. The observational study analyzed ginseng intake and mortality over an 18.8-year follow-up period in a cohort of 6,282 subjects aged 55 years or older. The analyses were adjusted for age, education, occupation, drinking, self-reported chronic disease, body mass index, and blood pressure. All-cause mortality for male regular users of ginseng was significantly improved compared with that for nonusers of ginseng (HR = 0.90), but this association was not observed for women (HR = 1.03). Cancer-specific mortality was also improved in female ginseng users compared with nonusers (HR = 0.80). Mortality from cardiovascular diseases was not associated with ginseng intake. The 18.8-year progressive cohort study showed that ginseng intake favorably impacted all-cause mortality in older males but not in women. The test for trends demonstrated that male all-cause mortality improved significantly with increasing frequency of ginseng intake regardless of adjustment for variables. Overall, it should be kept in mind that almost 50 years of Medline publications have failed to note a serious toxic event or even a case study on the topic of ginseng alone and coagulation issues [192], but again there could be some individual variability with these issues.

Past human studies of ginseng and sexual health have reported gastrointestinal side effects [129–132] (e.g., stomach upset), but these were not reported at a rate significantly higher than the rate for placebo. Ingesting ginseng with a meal seems more appropriate because of potential gastrointestinal issues with most dietary supplement interventions or placebo, and there are no reports that ginseng is less or more efficacious in this scenario. More rigorous monitoring of ginseng safety in clinical trials should be conducted to provide some clarity on adverse events. The dose of ginseng and ginsenoside concentration should always be noted in clinical trials, and again reviews on this topic have been lacking. Ginsenoside concentrations should be required for publication in any clinical trial of ginseng.

P. ginseng has arguably the longest and perhaps one of the most impressive CAM records to date for use in men with mild to moderate ED. Approximately ten randomized trials have suggested that *P. ginseng* and its ginsenosides have potential efficacy in diverse areas of male sexual health [129–134]. Still, this is not meant to suggest that it is the most effective ED CAM option because others (arginine combinations and citrulline) have their own advantages and disadvantages and methodologic quality of future clinical trials needs to be improved. The isolation of the more active ginsenosides also needs more research, and in my experience, quality control is a real problem with many ginseng products. Also, I have to reiterate that the price issues need to be resolved, because at the time of this writing, Korean red ginseng and Chinese ginseng with more concentrated ginsenosides were no longer of low cost.

What about FSD? There is some interesting preliminary basic science and clinical trial data that suggest that *P. ginseng* (Korean red ginseng) could significantly improve some domains of FSD [193–196]. A crossover trial ($n = 28$ completed the study) of postmenopausal women at a dosage of 3 g per day (approximately 8 % ginsenoside concentration) for 8 weeks demonstrated a significant improvement in arousal, but not other domains, utilizing the FSFI questionnaire [196]. Mean estradiol levels did not change, and side effects were similar to placebo. Two women experienced vaginal bleeding during the trial on ginseng, and one of these participants had a significant increase in estradiol (less than 10–27 pg/mL). There is no current suggestion that ginseng can improve sexual health or FSD in premenopausal women.

Tongkat Ali (*E. longifolia*, Also Known as or Nicknamed "Malaysian Ginseng," but It Is Not in the Ginseng Family)

This CAM or dietary supplement was well reviewed in the chapter on male fertility. It is derived from a plant or a common shrub found along the slopes of hilly areas in the Malaysian rainforest [197]. It has preliminary human data that show it might improve various aspects of male health, including sex drive, erectile function, testosterone, and improved sperm quality and quantity at only 200–300 mg a day [198–204].

The product that has the most research and only one with real clinical data is the standardized water-soluble extract (Physta) of *E. longifolia* root from the company Biotropics Malaysia Berhad, Kuala Lumpur, Malaysia [198, 202–204]. The company has also financially supported most of these studies. Their proprietary standardized water-soluble extract from the root of the plant and other tongkat ali studies show that this root has multiple diverse ingredients such as:

- Tannins
- High-molecular-weight polysaccharides
- Glycoproteins mucopolysaccharides
- Quassinoid alkaloids
- Amino acid isoleucine
- Calcium, magnesium, and potassium

It is theorized to also benefit in the area of male health because it may have a prohormone effect or DHEA mimic, or it could be directly stimulating Leydig cells or reducing testicular oxidative stress, or perhaps it is acting more like a diverse multivitamin for men [198, 202–204]. The mechanism of action or standardization of this herbal product has not been pinpointed. Yet a product that increases testosterone and improves or maintains fertility would also be suggested to have a direct or indirect Leydig cell stimulatory function (e.g., similar to clomiphene citrate or human chorionic gonadotropin in the pharmaceutical world). Still, again, there is no consensus as to specifically how it is working at the current time, and the supplement known as "Physta" is a water-soluble extract of tongkat ali that is proprietary, so specifically what compounds from the plant are reliably found in the CAM product, and at what concentrations is not known as this time. It could be that this product is no better than a really low-cost source or another supplement of tongkat ali, but the problem is that other brands or just generic tongkat ali does not have adequate clinical trials in these similar areas of men's health or quality-control testing for common and uncommon contaminants (for lead, arsenic, etc.). Tongkat ali does have preliminary clinical evidence to recommend its use in men with mild to moderate ED or low testosterone but its long-term safety and efficacy is not known. Few herbal supplements have even received adequate laboratory and clinical testing in this area with quality-control and standardization measures. Thus, it could be utilized for a trial period if other less costly products appear not to be efficacious.

There are at least two clinical trials in the area of male sexual health that the reader should be familiar with in order to discuss the preliminary results with patients [203, 204]. A total of 109 men (ages 30–55 years, mean age 43; 33 % in the tongkat group and 44 % in the placebo group were smokers) received either 300 mg of the water extract of tongkat (also known as "Physta") or placebo [204]. The group receiving Physta after 12 weeks had significant improvement in the erectile function domain of the IIEF compared to placebo ($p<0.001$) and also significant improvements in libido, sperm motility, and semen volume. Men with a BMI of 25 or more even had a significant reduction in fat mass ($p=0.008$). Men in this study had no or mild ED. Side effects were similar to placebo. There were no significant increases in testosterone over placebo, but the mean testosterone was in the normal range. The sperm parameter improvements reflect the results of an earlier clinical study with this supplement [202]. The second clinical trial (open label) involved only men taking Physta at 200 mg per day who had low testosterone ("late-onset hypogonadism") [203]. There was no placebo group in this study, and the mean age was 51 years of age (range 28–70 years). Aging Male Symptoms (AMS score) were in the "mild complaints" range and significantly improved to "no complaints" after 1 month ($p<0.001$). These changes were significantly correlated with an increase in total testosterone levels. A total of 90 % of participants had complaints from the AMS, and this was reduced to 29 % with the supplements, and at baseline 35 % of men had normal testosterone and after 1 month 90 % had normal testosterone values. A closer look at these data showed that a median testosterone of 5.60 nmol (161 ng/dL) increased to 7.60 nmol (219 ng/dL) after 1 month. In other words, most of the testosterone increases were mild (less than 100 ng/dL); it should be kept in mind that they were not in the range of what could be observed with pharmaceutical testosterone replacement.

If these data can be replicated in a placebo-controlled trial, it would be an interesting and mild testosterone-increasing dietary supplement, since currently I do not believe there is an effective CAM option for TRT that has been proven safe on the market. And if men with mild to moderate ED could improve with this herbal, this would represent a unique dual action not consistently observed before with any dietary supplement. I have been in contact with this company from Malaysia and what I am impressed most by is the large number of clinical trials that have been initiated with this product. Tongkat ali has not been adequately tested in the area of FSD, but it seems that some of the properties or proposed mechanisms of action of this herbal (e.g., adrenal- or testosterone-enhancing/metabolism-like effects) could provide some potential benefit in the area of FSD. Again, I am enthusiastic about this product, but future clinical trials will determine if this herbal really is effective or will go the same unreliable, inconsistent, and at times unsafe route of DHEA and androstenedione supplements. Currently, no safety issues have been published with this product, which is a preliminary step in the right direction.

Tribulus terrestris

This is an herbal product that has been suggested by some commercial entities to have DHEA or prohormone type effects (for ED and TRT). It has been around for decades, but there is simply no positive or adequate evidence to support its use for ED, TR, or FSD. Human studies have failed to demonstrate that this herb acts like "DHEA" to increase testosterone or just increases testosterone by an independent mechanism, which is what it is advertised to do in many places [22]. For example, in a small clinical trial, Australian elite male rugby players ($n=22$) were placed on *Tribulus* or placebo for 5 weeks, and no alterations in testosterone or muscle mass occurred [205]. Another small trial of healthy men ages 20–36 years of age with body weights ranging from 60 to 125 kg ($n=14$) was published [206]. Participants consumed 10 or 20 mg/kg body weight of *Tribulus* (divided into three daily intakes) for 4 weeks. No significant changes in any parameter occurred in the *Tribulus* group, and this included testosterone, androstenedione, or LH. The authors concluded that this supplement does not contain any indirect or direct testosterone-enhancing properties. In my experience, I would agree. In fact, the only adequate clinical trial where a dose of *Tribulus* (750 mg or more) appears to increase testosterone is when it is combined with 150 mg of DHEA and 300 mg of androstenedione [207–210]. Drops of 5.0 mg/dL in HDL or "good cholesterol" were observed, which have to be somewhat concerning [208] but again were probably due to the DHEA and androstenedione components. Preliminary clinical trials have failed to demonstrate an impact of *Tribulus* on body composition or exercise performance and no impact on hormone levels. Ideally, it would have been best to study this supplement in men with low testosterone to finally clarify any potential effect of this product, but I do not believe that positive results would occur based on my experience. Additionally, it is difficult to determine how *Tribulus* could show any success as a treatment for FSD when it has really not been proven to have a mechanism of action and has not shown efficacy in the area of ED or TRT.

Yohimbine Hydrochloride (Not Really a Dietary Supplement or CAM)

Yohimbine comes from the West African yohimbe tree and can be found as a supplement and a prescription drug (Yocon, etc.) [22, 211]. Whether or not it even works is controversial, but what is not controversial is that it is a "alpha-2-adrenoreceptor antagonist," and some of the side effects include headache, sweating, nausea, dizziness, nervousness/agitation, tremors, sleeplessness, antidiuresis, and elevated blood pressure and heart rate [212]. It cannot be used by individuals with kidney disease, those on antidepressants or other mood-altering drugs, and in some individuals with specific cardiovascular, neurological, and psychological issues.

Many media and other credible sources appear to suggest yohimbine is an alternative medicine or over-the-counter dietary supplement, but this is really not the case based on its clinical trial efficacy. Since it is usually characterized as an "alternative medicine" by some individuals and reviews [213], some may assume this is a dietary supplement, and there are many companies that sell "yohimbe" or tout that they sell "yohimbine HCL." The positive data with the drug or compound derived from this tree, yohimbine hydrochloride, came from European and other studies at a total of 5–10 mg per day (divided doses) [213]. The real problem here is that yohimbine HCL is a prescription drug, but many dietary supplements that mimic this drug have serious quality-control problems and are dangerous (like the drug) [211, 212]. Again, yohimbine HCL is the active ingredient found in the bark of a West African tree, but many dietary supplements really sell "yohimbe," which in many cases has little to no or variable quantities of the active ingredient "yohimbine HCL" in it. Again, if there is an interest in yohimbine HCL in the area of ED or FSD, I believe the prescription drug should be utilized because of quality-control issues and because the successful clinical trials utilized this version.

Zinc

Recent and past evidence has demonstrated that the excess/megadoses of zinc (80 or 100 mg or more per day), especially with individual supplements, has the potential to encourage the growth of prostate conditions from BPH to cancer [214, 215] and to increase the risk of hospitalization for urologic conditions from urinary tract infections and BPH to kidney stones [216, 217]. In fact, in one of the largest population studies of zinc supplements in medicine (Harvard study), researchers found a significantly higher risk of advanced prostate cancer in men consuming large intakes of these supplements [215]. Some countries such as Canada now have restrictions on dosages of zinc supplements that can be sold over the counter without evidence to back up efficacy and safety for a specific condition [218]. In other words, this supplement does little to nothing for sexual health.

The problem with zinc currently is that the recommended dietary intake is only 11 mg [219], and again megadoses of zinc supplements are replete with issues, especially in urology [214]. Some major phase III clinical trials (AREDS 2) are now testing lower zinc dosages compared to the older effective higher dosage based on this history of adverse events [220]. Dosages as low as 22 mg per day of zinc gluconate, for example, could reduce plasma copper and iron levels [221].

Therefore, when examining the larger picture of high-dose zinc supplements in general medicine, it would be difficult to research or recommend these doses in the area of ED, FSD or TRT. In fact, in individuals with a normal zinc intake and status, dosages as high as 30 mg per day of zinc have caused no changes in testosterone levels [222]. The preliminary older data that suggested that zinc could be a form of TRT was from those with overt zinc deficiency, including those on hemodialysis [223], or those with sickle-cell anemia, for example [224]. Another issue that needs to be resolved is whether or not zinc status is inversely associated with weight increase such that the majority of obese and morbidly obese individuals have a high prevalence of zinc deficiency. Preliminary research suggests this is indeed the case [225, 226]. And since testosterone deficiency is correlated and occurs with weight gain, it may be easier to associate zinc intake with testosterone increases compared to the more real impact of confounding variables such as weight. Thus, the amount of zinc (approximately 10–20 mg) found in multivitamins is ample, and whether or not increasing doses improve testosterone production in hypogonadal men has not been definitely tested. I am skeptical as to whether or not it can provide a consistent tangible benefit unless an individual is deficient in zinc.

Miscellaneous

Fenugreek (*Trigonella foenum-graecum*)

Fenugreek has been promoted by numerous commercial entities as an option for testosterone replacement or a testosterone-increasing supplement via an aromatase inhibitor mechanism of action (blocks the conversion of testosterone to estrogen) [22]. Human studies have failed to demonstrate that this herb/spice supplement increases testosterone consistently. In fact, fenugreek has been used as a spice and is utilized in Indian Ayurvedic and in Chinese Medicine as a stimulus for lactation for breastfeeding women [22, 227]. This supplement has a partial notorious history for being touted as a breast-enlarging supplement for women without human research to support this claim. Yet allergic reactions to the powder and mild gastrointestinal upset are not uncommon side effects, and increased bleeding can occur beyond what is expected in those on aspirin or anti-inflammatory drugs [227].

In terms of fenugreek as a TRT supplement, in one clinical study, fenugreek (standardized to 70 % trigimannose) actually significantly reduced levels of free testosterone [228]. Men had a 40 ng/ml free testosterone at baseline, reduced to 33 ng/ml at 4 weeks, and then to 36 ng/ml at 8 weeks ($p=0.02$) when taking 500 mg per day. DHT levels were reduced in the fenugreek group. Other studies demonstrate that fenugreek either causes no change or slightly increases testosterone in men with an already normal testosterone at baseline [229, 230]. In other words, it is an unpredictable supplement in the area of TRT. One clinical trial of fenugreek of 500 mg per day (standardized for grecunin) over 8 weeks showed average increases of 6.6 % and 12.3 % for total testosterone and bioavailable testosterone [229]. Even if fenugreek operates as an aromatase inhibitor, as explained earlier in this chapter, I do not recognize this as a positive mechanism of action because it could cause bone loss in healthy men based on some past clinical trials of prescription drugs that have this same mechanism of action.

One ancillary health advantage of fenugreek is that the natural seeds can be purchased at health food stores and used in most diet plans (soups, yogurt, oatmeal, etc.) and they may slightly lower blood sugar and cholesterol because they are a good source of fiber (1 tablespoon = 3 g of fiber) [22, 231]. A role for fenugreek as a treatment for FSD is highly unlikely.

Horny Goat Weed (*Epimedium* Species)

Very little clinical data exist for this herbal compound, but laboratory studies suggest that several ingredients in it have a somewhat similar structure to natural PDE-5 inhibitor [232, 233]. A compound called "icariin" is arguably the active ingredient found in this herbal product. It is for this reason that there is enthusiasm for clinical research because it may also exhibit some neurotrophic and NO effects in addition to its PDE-5 inhibiting properties [233, 234]. What role this product could have in FSD has not been researched and is not known. It is my hope that this compound gets into a good clinical trial soon based on the isolation of some of these interesting natural compounds.

Lubricants (Zestra for FSD)

Zestra is a female massage oil with some minimal clinical data to suggest it can increase warmth and sensitivity and increase the probability of arousal when applied to the clitoris, labia, and vaginal opening [235]. This is an over-the-counter massage oil that is composed of borage seed oil, evening primrose oil, angelica root extract, and coleus extract. Interestingly, borage seed and evening primrose contain high concentrations of gamma-linolenic acid (GLA) that can be metabolized into dihomo-gamma-linolenic acid (DGLA), and into prostaglandin E1 or E2, which may increase nerve conduction, protection, and blood flow in other medical situations, but the impact could be subtle in some cases [236–238]. A small preliminary study of 20 women with sexual arousal disorder and some with normal sexual functioning had significant improvements in the level of arousal, desire, genital sensation, ability to achieve orgasm, and overall sexual pleasure [235]. Mild genital burning in three participants was reported that resolved in 5–30 min and was the only reported adverse effect of Zestra.

The problem with the study of CAM and lubricants in general for sexual health is that there is minimal research published in this category. There is little doubt that in studies of water- or silicon-based lubricants, the effectiveness can be clinically significant, especially for women experiencing dyspareunia [239, 240]. Yet it is remarkable that more studies of lubricants to potentially improve other aspects of FSD or even ED have not been attempted or published. Lubricants are not only commonly used and popular but in general they are associated with greater sexual pleasure and satisfaction during solo and partnered sexual activity [239, 241]. Hopefully, research on ingredients that have the potential to improve arousal or another aspect of FSD and ED such as L-arginine or L-citrulline will receive more research.

SAM-e for SSRI-Induced Sexual Dysfunction

S-adenosyl methionine (SAM-e) is a naturally occurring compound that functions as a methyl donor in human metabolism; it may have an individual treatment role for major depressive disorder (MDD) or an ancillary role to enhance conventional treatment [22, 242–246]. A Harvard Medical School clinical study of 73 serotonin reuptake inhibitor non-responders with MDD over 6 weeks found a benefit in those receiving 800 mg twice daily of SAM-e compared to placebo [243]. A significantly higher response and remission rate occurred with SAM-e over placebo. Side effects were similar to placebo. Still, gastrointestinal side effects and headaches have occurred in other studies [244], and SAM-e is not a low-cost CAM in general.

Preliminary research also suggests that in those with MDD, this dietary supplement may have a positive effect on male arousal and ED, such that scores improved in these areas compared to placebo [247]. SSSRIs and other antidepressant medications could have a profound impact on male and female sexual function [248]. I am hopeful that research on SAM-e to support its minimal or even positive effect on sexual function (ED or FSD) in those with MDD continues. It is also of interest that SAM-e has been used as a prescription drug, given as an IV or an injectable in numerous European countries since the 1970s, and its ability to reduce osteoarthritic pain is also notable, well published, and on par with NSAIDs but with less toxicity at dosages of up to 600 mg per day [249, 250].

Conclusion

What is the minimal threshold for any CAM or dietary supplement to receive any form of endorsement in clinical guidelines or by clinicians on a regular basis in the area of ED, TRT, or FSD? It appears that the threshold is rather high, arguably for many reasons, including the fact that the history of CAM products in this area of medicine are the most notorious and infamous in terms of quality-control issues, safety, and the addition of drug adulterants. And this terrible trend of cheating, especially in the category of medicine, is unlikely to be greatly reversed in the near future, especially in countries such as the United States [251]. This is a shame, because although this chapter covered numerous noneffective products, the reader should be encouraged because of the number of potentially safe and effective CAM options listed in this chapter. In fact, a complete listing of all CAM products that may or may not have evidence can be found in Table 6.2.

On the other hand, I am bothered and perplexed by the idea of why only effective prescription pills with an average cost that is 20–40 times that of several CAM products, with a definitive number of minor and serious toxicity and compliance issues, should be the only acceptable ingestible option for patients? This has seemed very odd and counterintuitive and counterproductive for patients for a considerable amount of

Table 6.2 A summary of the CAM options for male and female sexual health that have and do not have clinical evidence

CAM	ED and/or TRT	FSD
Acupuncture	For psychogenic ED, it appears to be an option. It may provide a mental health benefit. Otherwise, there is weak or no evidence in the area of ED or TRT	No adequate clinical research to allow for any type of recommendation
Ashwagandha	No adequate clinical research or safety studies to allow for any type of recommendation	No adequate clinical research or safety studies to allow for any type of recommendation
Avena sativa	No adequate clinical research or safety studies to allow for any type of recommendation	No adequate clinical research or safety studies to allow for any type of recommendation
Catuaba	No adequate clinical research or safety studies to allow for any type of recommendation	No adequate clinical research or safety studies to allow for any type of recommendation
Coenzyme Q10	No adequate clinical research to allow for any type of recommendation. Preliminary evidence for some potential efficacy in Peyronie's disease (300 mg/day). Appears to interfere with blood-thinning medication	No adequate clinical research to allow for any type of recommendation
Cordyceps	No adequate clinical research or safety studies to allow for any type of recommendation	No adequate clinical research or safety studies to allow for any type of recommendation
Damiana	No adequate clinical research or safety studies to allow for any type of recommendation	No adequate clinical research or safety studies to allow for any type of recommendation
DHEA (or androstenedione)	Adrenal insufficiency patients may potentially benefit. Not a reliable or dependable TRT option and can increase estrogen levels in men and reduce HDL cholesterol. Unpredictable and wide variations in individual results. Quality control is also a large problem	Androgen and especially adrenal insufficiency (low DHEA or testosterone patients) may slightly benefit. Increased facial hair, weight gain, acne, and temporary breast tenderness and rarely loss of head hair and skin rash on dosages as low as 50 mg/day. Can also reduce HDL cholesterol. Quality control is a problem. Vaginal DHEA may be the most promising future option for DHEA, but daily application will be a potential compliance issue
Eleuthero	No adequate clinical research or safety studies to allow for any type of recommendation	No adequate clinical research or safety studies to allow for any type of recommendation
Fenugreek (*Trigonella foenum-graecum*)	No adequate clinical data to support the use of fenugreek in ED or even TRT where it is most heavily marketed. Studies show decreases or slight increases in testosterone in men with normal testosterone levels at baseline. And, if it really acts as a weak aromatase inhibitor as some commercial entities suggest, then it may not be bone-healthy for men. Some risk of allergies and blood thinning from ingredients in fenugreek. Using just the seeds (not the dietary supplement) on food may be healthy because they are high in fiber	Found in some breast enlargement supplements for women but does not have evidence. Minimal evidence in the area of improving lactation but no evidence in the area of FSD. Some risk of allergies and blood thinning from ingredients in fenugreek. Using just the seeds (not the dietary supplement) on food may be healthy because they are high in fiber
Folic acid	Clinical evidence is weak and using high doses of folic acid in elderly men is concerning and controversial enough for concern from a prostate cancer incidence or progression standpoint	Clinical evidence is weak and using high doses of folic acid in elderly women is concerning and controversial enough from a cancer incidence and progression standpoint. This issue needs to be resolved in women

(continued)

Table 6.2 (continued)

CAM	ED and/or TRT	FSD
Ginkgo biloba	Weak clinical evidence and has the potential to potentiate the effects of blood-thinning medications. Most interesting data was for SSRI-induced sexual dysfunction benefits, but the research has not matured and there is little confidence that it works much beyond a placebo. Studies outside of urology have failed recently to reduce the risk of cognitive impairment, for example, which raises more doubts over efficacy	Weak clinical evidence and has the potential to potentiate the effects of blood-thinning medication. Most interesting data was for SSRI-induced sexual dysfunction but the research has not matured, and there is little confidence that it works much beyond a placebo. Studies outside of urology have failed recently to reduce the risk of cognitive impairment, which raises more doubts over efficacy in other areas of medicine
Horny goat weed (*Epimedium sagittatum*)	Laboratory studies suggest that a compound in this herb ("icariin") may mimic or have a PDE-5 inhibitor effect. Needs human clinical trials and should receive clinical trials based on such positive laboratory data	No adequate research. Although "icariin" should be tested in FSD
L-Arginine or L-arginine aspartate and pycnogenol	Precursor to nitric oxide (NO). High dosage (3–6 g per day) is needed alone to observe a benefit in some individuals. Lower doses of L-arginine aspartate (2,800 mg/day) might provide a substantial benefit when combined with 80 mg of Pycnogenol ("Prelox" and others). "Prelox" has adequate clinical data and should be recommended for ED, but cost and number of pills could be issues for some patients. Blood pressure reductions can occur with L-arginine, and some safety issues have been raised in those with a recent cardiac events or peripheral artery disease (PAD). Otherwise, good safety overall	Precursor to nitric oxide (NO). High dosage (3–6 g/day) is needed to observe a benefit in some individuals. Clinical trials with the female version of "Prelox" are now being tested. Lubricants with L-arginine should be tested. Blood pressure reductions can occur with L-arginine and some safety issues have been raised in those with a recent cardiac event or peripheral artery disease (PAD). Otherwise, good safety overall. ArginMax® is a CAM supplement with preliminary clinical trials to support its use for FSD in some pre-, peri-, and postmenopausal women. It has a combination of ingredients, including L-arginine and concentrated ginsenoside *P. ginseng*. Desire was improved in postmenopausal women and in pre- and perimenopausal women multiple diverse benefits were preliminarily observed
L-Carnitine	2,000 mg of acetyl- and propionyl-L-carnitine (4,000 mg/day) may have improved symptoms of low free testosterone without increasing testosterone levels from an older clinical trial. Otherwise, dosages this high are problematic because of the number of pills needed and the cost involved. This amino acid appears to be most effective in studies when combined with CAM that has evidence (such as arginine), which is why there is skepticism on its ability to be effective by itself. There are also some heart health controversies with this compound that need to be resolved	No adequate clinical research or safety studies to allow for any type of recommendation. There are also some heart-healthy controversies with this compound that need to be resolved

(continued)

Table 6.2 (continued)

CAM	ED and/or TRT	FSD
L-Citrulline	One of the most promising CAM products for mild to moderate ED. May also be able to be combined in some patients with conventional ED options. It appears to be twice as effective as L-arginine in raising nitric oxide (NO) blood levels so lower dosages are needed. A small 1-month clinical trial of 1,500 mg/day of citrulline was effective in significantly improving erection hardness scores compared to placebo. Citrulline could arguably lower blood pressure in some patients (mixed results) and adequate kidney function is needed for maximum conversion (citrulline back to arginine to NO in the blood stream) effectiveness. Cost could be an issue	No adequate clinical research or safety studies for FSD to allow for any type of recommendation. Still, it appears to be one of the more promising CAM products because it appears to be able to work twice as effectively as L-arginine in producing nitric oxide in healthy individuals with adequate kidney function. Citrulline could arguably lower blood pressure in some patients (mixed results) and adequate kidney function is needed for maximum conversion effectiveness. Cost could be an issue
L-Theanine	No adequate clinical research studies to allow for any type of recommendation. However, this amino acid found in green tea has a good history of safety in the area of stress and anxiety reduction as a stand-alone CAM option. Thus, for some types of psychogenic ED it could be theoretical option at 100–200 mg per day	No adequate clinical research studies to allow for any type of recommendation. However, this amino acid found in green tea has a good history of safety in the area of stress and anxiety reduction as a stand-alone CAM option. It could be used in future CAM and FSD research in combination with other ingredients
Lubricants (water, silicon based and others)	Lubricants are not only commonly used and popular but in general they are associated with greater sexual pleasure and satisfaction during solo and partnered sexual activity. Lubricants with nitric oxide enhancing ingredients such as arginine and citrulline or even ginseng should receive more research. There is little doubt that CAM lubricant research in the area of male or female sexual health is one of the least studied areas of CAM in urology, and this is unfortunate because there is an adequate room for advances or improvement	Lubricants are not only commonly used and popular but in general they are associated with greater sexual pleasure and satisfaction during solo and partnered sexual activity. Zestra (borage seed oil, evening primrose oil, angelica root extract, and coleus extract) is a female massage oil with some minimal clinical data to suggest it can increase warmth and sensitivity and increase the probability of arousal when applied to the clitoris, labia, and vaginal opening. A small preliminary study of 20 women with sexual arousal disorder and some with normal sexual functioning had significant improvements in the level of arousal, desire, genital sensation, ability to achieve orgasm, and overall sexual pleasure. Mild temporary burning sensation can occur in a minority of individuals
Maca (*L. meyenii*)	Mixed results in the area of ED and does not appear to change testosterone levels. Safety has been good but quality control based on a percentage of "macamides" or other active ingredients should be reported. Dosages of 1,500–3,000 mg have been reported to have some mixed success on libido and erectile function. Should also be studied more in men with SSRI-induced sexual dysfunction	Mixed results in the area of FSD and does not appear to change hormone levels. Safety has been good but quality control based on a percentage of "macamides" or other active ingredients should be reported. Dosages of 3,000 mg (primarily in a small group of women) have been reported to have some mixed preliminary success in those with sexual dysfunction from SSRI medication
Menopausal or premenopausal ingredients that mimic hormone effects	Not applicable	Multiple commercial ingredients that have preliminary evidence for pre-, peri-, and postmenopausal symptoms (black cohosh, red clover, Vitex agnus-castus, etc.) have minimal data in the area of FSD so use with caution. Quality-of-life improvements may occur that do or do not translate to the area of FSD

(continued)

Table 6.2 (continued)

CAM	ED and/or TRT	FSD
Muira puama ("potency wood")	No adequate clinical research or safety studies to allow for any type of recommendation	No adequate clinical research or safety studies to allow for any type of recommendation
Omega-3 fatty acids	No adequate clinical research or studies to allow for any type of recommendation. Omega-3 still has some blood-thinning ability in some patients. FDA-approved to reduced "triglycerides," thus, in some patients could reduce theoretically heart disease risk and may slightly improve erectile function. Mixed data on improving mood	No adequate clinical research or studies to allow for any type of recommendation. Omega-3 still has some blood-thinning ability in some patients. Mixed data on improving mood
P. ginseng (Korean red ginseng and others)	Consistently improves libido for ED and improves erectile function at dosages of 1,600–3,000 mg/day at 8 % or less ginsenoside concentration. Regardless, methodology has been questioned on some of the ten randomized trials that have shown positive effects on ED. A dose of 800 mg at an unusually high ginsenoside concentration showed profound efficacy in ED over placebo. More concentrated and more specific ginsenosides appear far more effective. No changes in testosterone have been noted with this supplement. The biggest current issue is cost because *P. ginseng* prices (especially Korean red ginseng) have increased dramatically over the years. The libido increasing effects may make this suitable to be combined with a PDE-5 inhibitor for some patients. Controversy exists over whether or not it is safe with blood thinners and patients with hypertension	Not currently for premenopausal FSD. May improve arousal for postmenopausal FSD (approximately 8 % ginsenoside concentration at 3,000 mg/day), and some controversial data suggest it may reduce some menopausal symptoms in general. No changes in hormone levels have been noted with this supplement. More concentrated and more specific ginsenosides appear far more effective and should be tested for FSD. The biggest current issues is cost, because *P. ginseng* prices (especially Korean red ginseng) have increased dramatically over the years. Controversy exists over whether or not it is safe with blood thinners and patients with hypertension
Pycnogenol	A French maritime pine bark extract (80 mg daily) and when combined with L-arginine aspartate (2,800 mg daily) has good efficacy for men with mild to moderate ED (Prelox and other products). Pycnogenol by itself have minimal supportive evidence in the area of ED and this CAM option can be costly	Needs studies in FSD in combination with L-arginine aspartate and some of these studies are now being funded. Some preliminary evidence for pycnogenol exists to reduce generally accepted menopausal symptoms
Rhodiola rosea	Cannot be recommended now, but it does have preliminary evidence for stress and anxiety reduction so it should be tested for psychogenic ED	Cannot be recommended now, but it does have preliminary evidence for stress and anxiety reduction. It could be combined with other CAM ingredients in a future clinical trial
SAM-e (S-adenosyl methionine)	Antidepressant (800 mg twice a day) effects of this CAM option are well known and supported by adequate clinical trials and has even been used in those with a non-adequate response to serotonin-enhancing prescription antidepressants. Preliminary evidences from some of these trials suggest no sexual side effects of this antidepressant and a potential for sexual health improvement, so perhaps it can be utilized in patients with sexual dysfunction from prescription antidepressant agents. This needs more research but it is arguably already an option	Antidepressant effects of this CAM option are well known and supported by adequate clinical trials. Preliminary evidence from some of these trials suggest no sexual side effects of this antidepressant so perhaps it can be utilized in patients with sexual dysfunction from prescription antidepressant agents. This needs more research, but it is arguably already an option and has been used along with prescription serotonin-enhancing medications in some clinical trials

(continued)

Table 6.2 (continued)

CAM	ED and/or TRT	FSD
Saw palmetto and other BPH supplements (beta-sitosterol, pygeum, stinging nettle, etc.)	Proposed to increase testosterone by blocking 5-alpha-reductase, but this has not been demonstrated in an adequate clinical trial(s) and in BPH trials these ingredients actually report causing or contributing to ED in a small number of participants that use these CAM options. No research supports their use for ED or TRT	No research supports their used for FSD
Tongkat ali (*E. longifolia*, "Malaysian ginseng")	One standardized form of tongkat ali from Malaysia ("Physta") from one manufacturer (Biotropics Malaysia Berhad, Kuala Lumpur, Malaysia) appears to have the majority of the evidence at 200–300 mg/day to preliminarily and mildly improve testosterone levels in men with low testosterone and also to improve erectile function. This is preliminary, but multiple ongoing clinical trials are currently in process	Needs to be tested in the area of FSD based on the preliminary positive results in male sexual health
Tribulus terrestris	A common ingredient in ED and TRT CAM commercial products but has minimal to no research suggesting it can actually improve either condition. It is suggested to have a DHEA-like compound in it, but this has not be proven	It is suggested to have a DHEA-like compound in it, but it has failed to provide benefit in this fashion in male or female sexual health
Yohimbine HCL (yohimbe)	All of the best clinical research for ED was with the prescription version and not the CAM option. Prescription versions contain "yohimbine HCL," but CAM options primarily contain "yohimbe," which has variable and inconsistent levels of "yohimbine HCL." Side effects can be severe, and I do not recommend any CAM option with yohimbine HCL or yohimbe	Minimal research for FSD on improving arousal with arginine. I would encourage the prescription option over the CAM option if needed in rare cases. Yohimbe bark extract is sold over the counter but it generally contains minimal or variable levels of the active ingredient. Side effects can be severe, and I do not recommend any CAM option with yohimbine HCL
Zinc	Some minimal clinical evidence that in men with rare cases of overt plasma zinc deficiency (anemia, dialysis, etc.), it may help to slightly improve testosterone levels. The risk of urologic toxicity (BPH, prostate cancer, stones, UTI, etc.) with high dosages (80 mg or higher or elemental zinc) of zinc intake has enough data to simply not recommend their use	No evidence in FSD. In addition, there are multiple safety issues with ingesting high-dose zinc: from creating copper deficiency to increasing the risk of multiple potential urologic toxicities including UTI and stones

time. And what about researching the possibility of combining prescriptive and over-the-counter agents for synergistic benefits (e.g., function and libido)? It is clear that for some time, some physicians recognize that in certain cases of male or female sexual issues, CAM options exist where the benefit outweighs the risk [69, 252]. How can medicine move from a conventional-only option to one that is truly evidence based, especially in the areas of ED, FSD, and TRT? It will not be easy, but it is my hope that this chapter at least places the options and the current state of research in the right perspective, which is why I am more excited now compared to any other time in my career about utilizing some form of CAM in urology for male or female sexual health.

References

1. Hatzimouratidis K, Amar E, Eardley I, Giuliano F, Hatzichristou D, Montorsi F, European Association of Urology, et al. Guidelines on male sexual dysfunction: erectile dysfunction and premature ejaculation. Eur Urol. 2010;57:804–14.
2. Montague DK, Jarow JP, Broderick GA, Dmochowski RR, Heaton JP, Lue TF, Erectile Dysfunction Guideline Update Panel, et al. Chapter 1: The management of erectile dysfunction: an AUA update. J Urol. 2005;174:230–9.

3. Montorsi F, Adaikan G, Becher E, Giuliano F, Khoury S, Lue TF, et al. Summary of the recommendations on sexual dysfunctions in men. J Sex Med. 2010;7:3572–88.
4. Porst H, Burnett A, Brock G, Ghanem H, Giuliano F, Glina S, ISSM Standards Committee for Sexual Medicine, et al. SOP conservative (medical and mechanical) treatment of erectile dysfunction. J Sex Med. 2013;10:130–71.
5. Hasegawa T, Saijo M, Ishii T, Nagata T, Haishima Y, Kawahara N, et al. Structural elucidation of a tadalafil analogue found in a dietary supplement. Shokuhin Eiseigaku Zasshi. 2008;49:311–5.
6. Venhuis BJ, Zomer G, Hamzink M, Meiring HD, Aubin Y, de Kaste D. The identification of a nitrosated prodrug of the PDE-5 inhibitor aildenafil in a dietary supplement: a Viagra with a pop. J Pharm Biomed Anal. 2011;54:735–41.
7. No authors listed. Two dietary supplements contain undeclared ingredient. FDA Consum. 2005;39:6.
8. Lee HM, Lee BJ. A novel approach to simultaneous screening and confirmation of regulated pharmaceutical dietary supplements by LC/MS/MS with an information-dependent acquisition method. Food Addit Contam Part A Chem Anal Control Expo Risk Assess. 2011;28:396–407.
9. http://www.fda.gov. Accessed on 9 Feb 2013.
10. ChromaDex®, Boulder, CO. http://www.chromadex.com. Report accessed on 28 Sep 2010.
11. Lee MS, Shin BC, Ernst E. Acupuncture for treating erectile dysfunction: a systematic review. BJU Int. 2009;104:366–70.
12. Engelhardt PF, Daha LK, Zlis T, Simak R, Konig K, Pfluger H. Acupuncture in the treatment of psychogenic erectile dysfunction: first results of a prospective randomized placebo-controlled study. Int J Impot Res. 2003;15:343–6.
13. Yaman LS, Kllic S, Sarica K, Bayar M, Saygin B. The place of acupuncture in the management of psychogenic impotence. Eur Urol. 1994;26:52–5.
14. Aydin S, Ercan M, Caskurlu T, Tasci AI, Karaman I, Odabas O, et al. Acupuncture and hypnotic suggestions in the treatment of non-organic male sexual dysfunction. Scand J Urol Nephrol. 1997;31:271–4.
15. Kornblut Anne E, Duff W. How one pill escaped place on steroid list. The New York Times, Sunday, April 17, 2005, page 1 and page 20.
16. Brown GA, Vukovich M, King DS. Testosterone prohormone supplements. Med Sci Sports Exerc. 2006;38:1451–61.
17. Leder BZ, Longcope C, Catlin DH, Ahrens B, Schoenfeld DA, Finkelstein JS. Oral androstenedione administration and serum testosterone concentrations in young men. JAMA. 2000;283:779–82.
18. King DS, Sharp RL, Vukovich MD, Brown GA, Reifenrath TA, Uhl NL, et al. Effect of oral androstenedione on serum testosterone and adaptations to resistance training in young men: a randomized controlled trial. JAMA. 1999;281:2020–8.
19. Ritter RH, Cryar AK, Hermans MR. Oral androstenedione-induced impotence and severe oligospermia. Fertil Steril. 2005;84:217.
20. Broeder CE, Quindry J, Brittingham K, Panton L, Thomson J, Appakondu S, et al. The Andro Project: physiological and hormonal influences of androstenedione in men 35 to 65 years old participating in a high-intensity resistance training program. Arch Intern Med. 2000;160:3093–104.
21. Leder BZ, Leblanc KM, Longcope C, Lee H, Catlin DH, Finkelstein JS. Effects of oral androstenedione administration on serum testosterone and estradiol levels in post-menopausal women. J Clin Endocrinol Metab. 2002;87:5449–54.
22. Moyad MA. Dr. Moyad's guide to male sexual health: what works and what's worthless? Ann Arbor, MI: Spry; 2012.
23. Feldman HA, Goldstein I, Hatzichristou DG, Krane RJ, McKinlay JB. Impotence and its medical and psychological correlates results of the Massachusetts Male Aging Study. J Urol. 1994;151:54–61.
24. Reiter WJ, Pycha A, Schatzi G, Klingler HC, Mark I, Auterith A, et al. Serum dehydroepiandrosterone sulfate concentrations in men with erectile dysfunction. Urology. 2000;55:755–8.
25. Traish AM, Kang P, Saad F, Guay AT. Dehydroepiandrosterone (DHEA)-a precursor steroid or an active hormone in human physiology. J Sex Med. 2011;8:2960–82.
26. Reiter WJ, Schatzi G, Mark I, Zeiner A, Pycha A, Marberger M. Dehydroepiandrosterone in the treatment of erectile dysfunction in patients with different organic etiologies. Urol Res. 2001;29:278–81.
27. Reiter WJ, Pycha A, Schatzi G, Pokorny A, Gruber DM, Huber JC, et al. DHEA in the treatment of erectile dysfunction: a prospective, double-blind, randomized, placebo-controlled study. Urology. 1999;53:590–4.
28. Hellbronn LK, de Jonge L, Frisard MI, DeLany JP, Larson-Meyer DE, Rood J, Pennington CALERIE Team, et al. Effect of 6-month calorie restriction on biomarkers of longevity, metabolic adaptation, and oxidative stress in overweight individuals: a randomized controlled trial. JAMA. 2006;295:1539–48.
29. Niskanen L, Laaksonen DE, Punnonen K, Mustajoki P, Kaukua J, Rissanen A. Changes in sex hormone-binding globulin and testosterone during weight loss and weight maintenance in abdominally obese men with the metabolic syndrome. Diabetes Obes Metab. 2004;6:208–15.
30. Ernst B, Wilms B, Thurnheer M, Schultes B. Reduced circulating androgen levels after gastric bypass surgery in severely obese women. Obes Surg. 2013;23:602–7.
31. Voznesensky M, Walsh S, Dauser D, Brindisi J, Kenny AM. The association between dehydroepiandrosterone and frailty in older men and women. Age Ageing. 2009;38:401–6.
32. Panjari M, Bell RJ, Jane F, Wolfe R, Adams J, Morrow C, et al. A randomized trial of oral DHEA

treatment for sexual function, well-being, and menopausal symptoms in post-menopausal women with low libido. J Sex Med. 2009;6:2579–90.
33. Panjari M, Davis SR. DHEA for post-menopausal women: a review of the evidence. Maturitas. 2010;66:172–9.
34. Panjari M, Bell RJ, Jane F, Adams J, Morrow C, Davis SR. The safety of 52 weeks of oral DHEA therapy for post-menopausal women. Maturitas. 2009;63:240–5.
35. Hackbert L, Helman JR. Acute dehydroepiandrosterone (DHEA) effects on sexual arousal in postmenopausal women. J Women's Health Gend Based Med. 2002;11:155–62.
36. Mortola JF, Yen SS. The effects of oral dehydroepiandrosterone on endocrine-metabolic parameters in post-menopausal women. J Clin Endocrinol Metab. 1990;71:696–704.
37. Panjari M, Davis SR. DHEA therapy for women: effect on sexual function and wellbeing. Hum Reprod Update. 2007;13:239–48.
38. Munarriz R, Talakoub L, Flaherty E, Giola M, Hoag L, Kim NN, et al. Androgen replacement therapy with dehydroepiandrosterone for androgen insufficiency and female sexual dysfunction: androgen and questionnaire results. J Sex Marital Ther. 2002;28 Suppl 1:165–73.
39. Davis SR, Panjari M, Stanczyk FZ. Clinical review: DHEA replacement for post-menopausal women. J Clin Endocrinol Metab. 2011;96:1642–53.
40. Arlt W, Callies F, van Villjmen JC, Koehler I, Reincke M, Bidlingmaier M, et al. Dehydroepiandrosterone replacement in women with adrenal insufficiency. N Engl J Med. 1999;341:1013–20.
41. Allollo B, Arlt W, Hahner S. DHEA: why, when, and how much-DHEA replacement in adrenal insufficiency. Ann Endocrinol (Paris). 2007;68:268–73.
42. Alkatib AA, Cosma M, Elamin MB, Erickson D, Swigio BA, Erwin PJ, et al. A systematic and meta-analysis of randomized placebo-controlled trials of DHEA treatment effects of quality of life in women with adrenal insufficiency. J Clin Endocrinol Metab. 2009;94:3676–81.
43. Nair KS, Rizza RA, O'Brien P, Dhatariya K, Short KR, Nehra A, et al. DHEA in elderly women and DHEA or testosterone in elderly men. N Engl J Med. 2006;355:1647–59.
44. Parasrampuria J, Schwartz K, Petesch R. Quality control of dehydroepiandrosterone dietary supplement products. JAMA. 1998;280:1565.
45. Baker WL, Karan S, Kenny AM. Effect of dehydroepiandrosterone on muscle strength and physical function in older adults: a systematic review. J Am Geriatr Soc. 2011;59:997–1002.
46. Weiss EP, Shah K, Fontana L, Lambert CP, Holloszy JO, Villareal DT. Dehydroepiandrosterone replacement in older adults: 1- and 2-y effects on bone. Am J Clin Nutr. 2009;89:1459–67.
47. Labrie F, Archer D, Bouchard C, Fortier M, Cusan L, Gomez JL, et al. Effect of intravaginal dehydroepiandrosterone (Prasterone) on libido and sexual dysfunction in post-menopausal women. Menopause. 2009;16:923–31.
48. Panjari M, Davis SR. Vaginal DHEA to treat menopause related atrophy: a review of the evidence. Maturitas. 2011;70:22–5.
49. Dong J-Y, Qin L-Q, Zhang Z, Zhao Y, Wang J, Arigoni F, et al. Effect of oral L-arginine supplementation on blood pressure: a meta-analysis of randomized, double-blind, placebo-controlled trials. Am Heart J. 2011;162:959–65.
50. Vadillo-Ortega F, Perichart-Perera O, Espino S, Avila-Vergara MA, Ibarra I, Ahued R, et al. Effect of supplementation during pregnancy with L-arginine and antioxidant vitamins in medical food on pre-eclampsia in high risk population: randomized controlled trial. BMJ. 2011;342:d2901.
51. Gui S, Jia J, Niu X, Bai Y, Zou H, Deng J, et al. Arginine supplementation for improving maternal and neonatal outcomes in hypertensive disorder of pregnancy: a systematic review. J Renin Angiotensin Aldosterone Syst 2013 [Epub ahead of print].
52. Schulman SP, Becker LC, Kass DA, Champion HC, Terrin ML, Forman S, et al. L-arginine therapy in acute myocardial infarction: the Vascular Interaction with Age in Myocardial Infarction (VINTAGE MI) randomized clinical trial. JAMA. 2006;295:58–64.
53. Wilson AM, Harada R, Nair N, Balasubramanlan N, Cooke JP. L-arginine supplementation in peripheral arterial disease: no benefit and possible harm. Circulation. 2007;116:188–95.
54. Bednarz B, Jaxa-Chamiec T, Maciewjewski P, Szpajer M, Janik K, Gniot J, et al. Efficacy and safety of oral L-arginine in acute myocardial infarction. Results of multicenter, randomized, placebo-controlled ARAMI pilot trial. Kardiol Pol. 2005;62:421–6.
55. Oka RK, Szuba A, Giacomini JC, Cooke JP. A pilot study of L-arginine supplementation on functional capacity in peripheral artery disease. Vasc Med. 2005;10:265–74.
56. Morris Jr SM. Enzymes of arginine metabolism. J Nutr. 2004;134(10 Suppl):2743S–7.
57. Morris Jr SM. Arginases and arginine deficiency syndromes. Curr Opin Clin Nutr Metab Care. 2012;15:64–70.
58. Castillo L, deRojas TC, Chapman TE, Vogt J, Burke JF, Tannenbaum SR, et al. Splanchnic metabolism of dietary arginine in relation to nitric oxide synthesis in normal adult man. Proc Natl Acad Sci USA. 1993;90:193–7.
59. Boger RH. Asymmetric dimethylarginine, an endogenous inhibitor of nitric oxide synthase, explains the L-arginine paradox and acts as novel cardiovascular risk factor. J Nutr. 2004;134:2842S–7.
60. Paroni R, Barassi A, Ciociola F, Dozio E, Finati E, Fermo I, et al. Asymmetric dimethylarginine (ADMA), symmetric dimethylarginine (SDMA) and arginine in patients with arteriogenic and non-arteriogenic erectile dysfunction. Int J Androl. 2012;35:660–7.

61. Bescos R, Gonzalez-Haro C, Pujol P, Drobnic F, Alonso E, Santolaria ML, et al. Effects of dietary L-arginine intake on cardiorespiratory and metabolic adaptation in athletes. Int J Sport Nutr Exerc Metab. 2009;19:355–65.
62. Bescos R, Sureda A, Tur JA, Pons A. The effect of nitric-oxide-related supplements on human performance. Sports Med. 2012;42:99–117.
63. Klotz T, Mathers MJ, Braun M, Bloch W, Engelmann U. Effectiveness of oral L-arginine in first-line treatment of erectile dysfunction in a controlled crossover study. Urol Int. 1999;63:220–3.
64. Chen J, Wollman Y, Chernichovsky T, Iaina A, Sofer M, Matzkin H. Effect of oral administration of high-dose nitric oxide donor L-arginine in men with organic erectile dysfunction: results of a double-blind, randomized, placebo-controlled study. BJU Int. 1999;83(3):269–73.
65. Lebret T, Herve JM, Gorny P, Worcel M, Botto H. Efficacy and safety of a novel combination of L-arginine glutamate and yohimbine hydrochloride: a new oral therapy for erectile dysfunction. Eur Urol. 2002;41:608–13.
66. Meston CM, Worcel M. The effects of yohimbine plus L-arginine glutamate on sexual arousal in postmenopausal women with sexual arousal disorder. Arch Sex Behav. 2002;31:323–32.
67. Stanislavov R, Nikolova V. Treatment of erectile dysfunction with Pycnogenol and L-arginine. J Sex Marital Ther. 2003;29:207–13.
68. Stanislavov R, Nikolova V, Rohdewald P. Improvement of erectile function with Prelox: a randomized, double-blind, placebo-controlled, crossover trial. Int J Impot Res. 2008;20:173–80.
69. Ledda A, Belcaro G, Cesarone MR, Dugall M, Schonlau F. Investigation of a complex plant extract for mild to moderate erectile dysfunction in a randomized, double-blind, placebo-controlled parallel-arm study. BJU Int. 2010;106:1030–3.
70. Bottari A, Belcaro G, Ledda A, Cesarone MR, Vinciguerra G, Di Renzo A, et al. Lady Prelox® improves sexual function in post-menopausal women. Panminerva Med. 2012;54(1 Suppl 4):3–9.
71. Ito TY, Trant AS, Polan ML. A double-blind placebo-controlled study of ArginMax, a nutritional supplement for enhancement of female sexual function. J Sex Marital Ther. 2001;27:541–9.
72. Ito TY, Polan ML, Whipple B, Trant AS. The enhancement of female sexual function with ArginMax, a nutritional supplement, among women differing in menopausal status. J Sex Marital Ther. 2006;32:369–78.
73. Schwedhelm E, Maas R, Freese R, Jung D, Lukacs Z, Jambrecina A, et al. Pharmacokinetic and pharmacodynamic properties of oral L-citrulline and L-arginine: impact on nitric oxide metabolism. Br J Clin Pharmacol. 2008;65:51–9.
74. Cormio L, De Siati M, Lorusso F, Selvaggio O, Mirabella L, Sanguedolce F, et al. Oral L-citrulline supplementation improves erection hardness in men with mild erectile dysfunction. Urology. 2011;77: 119–22.
75. No authors listed. Acetyl-L-carnitine. Monograph. Altern Med Rev. 2010;15:76–83.
76. Balercia G, Regoli F, Armeni T, Koverech A, Mantero F, Boscaro M. Placebo-controlled double-blind randomized trial on the use of L-carnitine, L-acetylcarnitine, or combined L-carnitine and L-acetylcarnitine in men with idiopathic asthenozoospermia. Fertil Steril. 2005;84:662–71.
77. Lenzi A, Sgro P, Salacone P, Paoli D, Gillio B, Lombardo F, et al. A placebo-controlled double-blind randomized trial of the use of combination l-carnitine and l-acetyl-carnitine treatment in men with asthenozoospermia. Fertil Steril. 2004;81:1578–84.
78. Lenzi A, Lombardo F, Sgro P, Salacone P, Caponecchia L, Dondero F, et al. Use of carnitine therapy in selected cases of male factor infertility: a double-blind crossover trial. Fertil Steril. 2003;79:292–300.
79. Li Z, Chen GW, Shang XJ, Bal WJ, Han YF, Chen B, et al. A controlled randomized trial of the use of combined L-carnitine and acetyl-L-carnitine treatment in men with oligoasthenozoospermia. Zhonghua Nan Ke Xue. 2005;11:761–4.
80. Cavallini G, Ferraretti AP, Gianaroli L, Biagiotti G, Vitali G. Cinnoxicam and L-carnitine/acetyl-L-carnitine treatment for idiopathic and varicocele-associated oligoasthenospermia. J Androl. 2004;25: 761–70.
81. Moncada ML, Vivari E, Cimino C, Calogero AE, Monglol A, D' Agata R. Effect of acetylcarnitine treatment in oligoashtenospermic patients. Acta Eur Fertil. 1992;23:221–4.
82. Costa M, Canale D, Filicori M, D'lddio S, Lenzi A. L-carnitine in idiopathic asthenozoospermia: a multicenter study. Italian Study Group on Carnitine and Male Infertility. Andrologia. 1994;26:155–9.
83. Gianfrilli D, Lauretta R, Di Dato C, Graziadio C, Pozza C, De Larichaudy J, et al. Propionyl-L-carnitine, L-arginine, and niacin in sexual medicine: a nutraceutical approach to erectile dysfunction. Andrologia. 2012;44 Suppl 1:600–4.
84. Gentille V, Antonini G, Antonella Bertozzi M, Dinelli N, Rizzo C, Ashraf V, et al. Effect of propionyl-L-carnitine, L-arginine and nicotinic acid on the efficacy of vardenafil in the treatment of erectile dysfunction in diabetes. Curr Med Res Opin. 2009;25:2223–8.
85. Morano S, Mandosi E, Fallarino M, Gatti A, Tiberti C, Sensi M, et al. Antioxidant treatment associated with sildenafil reduces monocyte activation and markers of endothelial damage in patients with diabetic erectile dysfunction: a double-blind, placebo-controlled study. Eur Urol. 2007;52:1768–74.
86. Cavallini G, Modenini F, Vitali G, Koverech A. Acetyl-L-carnitine plus propionyl L-carnitine improve efficacy of sildenafil in treatment of erectile dysfunction after bilateral nerve-sparing radical retropubic prostatectomy. Urology. 2005;66:1080–5.

87. Cavallini G, Caracciolo S, Vitali G, Modenini F, Biagiotti G. Carnitine versus androgen administration in the treatment of sexual dysfunction, depressed mood, and fatigue associated with male aging. Urology. 2004;63:641–6.
88. McVary KT. Erectile dysfunction. N Engl J Med. 2007;357:2472–81.
89. Luiking YC, Engelen MP, Deutz NP. Regulation of nitric oxide production in health and disease. Curr Opin Clin Nutr Metab Care. 2010;13:97–104.
90. Jabecka A, Ast J, Bogdaski P, Drozdowski M, Pawlak-Lemaska K, Cielewicz AR, et al. Eur Rev Med Pharmacol Sci. 2012;16:1665–74.
91. Rouge C, Des Robert C, Robins A, Le Bacquer O, Volteau C, De La Cochetiere MF, et al. Manipulation of citrulline availability in humans. Am J Physiol Gastrointest Liver Physiol. 2007;293:G1061–7.
92. Moinard C, Nicolis I, Neveux N, Darquy S, Benazeth S, Cynober L. Dose-ranging effects of citrulline administration on plasma amino acids and hormonal patterns in healthy subjects: the Citrudose pharmacokinetic study. Br J Nutr. 2008;99:855–62.
93. Perez-Guisado J, Jakeman PM. Citrulline malate enhances athletic anaerobic performance and relieves muscle soreness. J Strength Cond Res. 2010;24:1215–22.
94. Figueroa A, Sanchez-Gonzalez MA, Wong A, Arjmandi BH. Watermelon extract supplementation reduces ankle blood pressure and carotid augmentation index in obese adults with prehypertension or hypertension. Am J Hypertens. 2012;25:640–3.
95. Ochiai M, Hayashi T, Morita M, Ina K, Maeda M, Watanabe F, et al. Short-term effects of L-citrulline supplementation on arterial stiffness in middle-aged men. Int J Cardiol. 2012;155:257–61.
96. Thibault R, Flet L, Vavasseur F, Lemerie M, Ferchaud-Roucher V, Picot D. Oral citrulline does not affect whole body protein metabolism in healthy human volunteers: results of a prospective, randomized, double-blind, cross-over study. Clin Nutr. 2011;30:807–11.
97. Figueroa A, Trivino JA, Sanchez-Gonzalez MA, Vicil F. Oral L-citrulline supplementation attenuates blood pressure response to cold pressor test in young men. Am J Hypertens. 2010;23:12–6.
98. Orozco-Gutierrez JJ, Castillo-Martinez L, Orea-Tejeda A, Vazquez-Diaz O, Valdespino-Trejo A, Narvaez-David R, et al. Effect of L-arginine oral supplementation on blood pressure and right ventricular function in heart failure patients with preserved ejection fraction. Cardiol J. 2010;17:612–8.
99. Cynober L, Moinard C, De Bandt JP. The 2009 ESPEN Sir David Cuthbertson. Citrulline: a new major signaling molecule or just another player in the pharmaconutrition game? Clin Nutr. 2010;29: 545–51.
100. Osowska S, Duchemann T, Walrand S, Pallard A, Boirie Y, Cynober L, et al. Citrulline modulates muscle protein metabolism in old malnourished rats. Am J Physiol Endocrinol Metab. 2006;291:E582–6.
101. Cynober L, de Bandt J-P, Moinard C. Leucine and citrulline: two major regulators of protein turnover. World Rev Nutr Diet. 2013;105:97–105.
102. Marietta M, Facchinetti F, Neri I, Piccinini F, Volpe A, Torelli G. L-arginine infusion decreases platelet aggregation through an intraplatelet nitric oxide release. Thromb Res. 1997;88:229–35.
103. Lentz AC, Carson III CC, Marson L. Does the new herbal supplement "Maca" enhance erectile function or female sexual function. Sem Prev Alt Med. 2006;2:85–90.
104. Gonzales GF, Gonzales C, Gonzales-Castaneda C. Lepidium meyenii (Maca): a plant from the highlands of Peru-from tradition to science. Forsch Komplementmed. 2009;16:373–80.
105. Gonzales GF, Cordova A, Vega K, Chung A, Villena A, Gonez C, et al. Effect of Lepidium meyenii (Maca) on sexual desire and its absent relationship with serum testosterone levels in adult healthy men. Andrologia. 2002;34:367–72.
106. Zenico T, Cicero AF, Valmorri L, Mercuriali M, Bercovich E. Subjective effects of Lepidium meyenii (Maca) extract on well-being and sexual performances in patients with mild erectile dysfunction: a randomized, double-blind clinical trial. Andrologia. 2009;41:95–9.
107. Dording CM, Fisher L, Papakostas G, Farabaugh A, Sonawalla S, Fava M, et al. A double-blind, randomized, pilot dose-finding study of maca root (L. meyenii) for the management of SSRI-induced sexual dysfunction. CNS Neurosci Ther. 2008;14:182–91.
108. Shin BC, Lee MS, Yang EJ, Lim HS, Ernst E. Maca (L. meyenii) for improving sexual function: a systematic review. BMC Complement Altern Med. 2010;10:44.
109. Zheng BL, He K, Kim CH, Rogers L, Shao Y, Huang ZY, et al. Effect of a lipidic extract from Lepidium meyenii on sexual behavior in mice and rats. Urology. 2000;55:598–602.
110. McCollom MM, Villinski JR, McPhail KL, Craker LE, Gafner S. Analysis of macamides in samples of Maca (Lepidium meyenii) by HPLC-UV-MS/MS. Phytochem Anal. 2005;16:463–9.
111. Ganzera M, Zhao J, Muhammad I, Khan IA. Chemical profiling and standardization of Lepidium meyenii (Maca) by reversed phase high performance liquid chromatography. Chem Pharm Bull(Tokyo). 2002;50:988–91.
112. Gonzales GF. Ethnobiology and ethnopharmacology of Lepidium meyenii (Maca), a plant from the Peruvian Highlands. Evid Based Complement Alternat Med. 2012;2012:193496.
113. MacKay D, Hathcock J, Guarneri E. Niacin: chemical forms, bioavailability, and health effects. Nutr Rev. 2012;70:357–66.
114. AIM-HIGH Investigators, Boden WE, Probstfield JL, Anderson T, Chaltman BR, Desvignes-Nickens P, Koprowicz K, et al. Niacin in patients with low HDL cholesterol levels receiving intensive statin therapy. N Engl J Med. 2011;365:2255–67.

115. HPS2-THRIVE Collaborative Group. HPS2-THRIVE randomized placebo-controlled trial in 25,673 high-risk patients of ER niacin/laropiprant: trial design, pre-specified muscle and liver outcomes, and reasons for stopping study treatment. Eur Heart J. 2013;34:1279–91.
116. Kei A, Elisaf MS. Nicotinic acid: clinical considerations. Expert Opin Drug Saf. 2012;11:551–64.
117. Askeroglu U, Alleyne B, Guyuron B. Pharmaceutical and herbal products that may contribute to dry eyes. Plast Reconstr Surg. 2013;131:159–67.
118. Ng C-F, Lee C-P, Ho AL, Lee VW. Effect of niacin on erectile function in men suffering erectile dysfunction and dyslipidemia. J Sex Med. 2011;8: 2883–93.
119. Choi KT. Botanical characteristics, pharmacological effects and medicinal components of Korean Panax ginseng C A Meyer. Acta Pharmacol Sin. 2008;29:1109–18.
120. Yue PY, Mak NK, Cheng YK, Leung KW, Ng TB, Fan DT, et al. Pharmacogenomics and the Yin/Yang actions of ginseng: anti-tumor, angiomodulating and steroid-like activities of ginsenosides. Chin Med. 2007;2:6.
121. Lee DC, Lau AS. Effects of Panax ginseng on tumor necrosis factor-alpha-mediated inflammation: a mini-review. Molecules. 2011;16:2802–16.
122. Chu SF, Zhang JT. New achievements in ginseng research and its future prospects. Chin J Integr Med. 2009;15:403–8.
123. Kiefer D, Pantuso T. Panax ginseng. Am Fam Physician. 2003;68:1539–42.
124. Christensen LP. Ginsenosides chemistry, biosynthesis, analysis, and potential health effects. Adv Food Nutr Res. 2009;55:1–99.
125. Attele AS, Wu JA, Yuan CS. Ginseng pharmacology: multiple constituents and multiple actions. Biochem Pharmacol. 1999;58:1685–93.
126. Jia L, Zhao Y. Current evaluation of the millennium phytomedicine-ginseng (I): etymology, pharmacognosy, phytochemistry, market and regulations. Curr Med Chem. 2009;16:2475–84.
127. Bucci LR. Selected herbals and human exercise performance. Am J Clin Nutr. 2000;72(suppl):624S–34.
128. Jovanovski E, Jenkins A, Dias AG, Peeva V, Sievenpiper J, Arnason JT, et al. Effects of Korean red ginseng (Panax ginseng C.A. Mayer) and its isolated ginsenosides and polysaccharides on arterial stiffness in healthy individuals. Am J Hypertens. 2010;23:469–72.
129. Khera M, Goldstein I. Erectile Dysfunction. Clin Evid (Online) 2011 29 June 2011.
130. Ham WS, Kim WT, Lee JS, Ju HJ, Kang SJ, Oh JH, et al. Efficacy and safety of red ginseng extract powder in patients with erectile dysfunction: multicenter, randomized, double-blind, placebo-controlled study. Kor J Urol. 2009;50(2):159–64.
131. Ernst E, Posadzki P, Soo LM. Complementary and alternative medicine (CAM) for sexual dysfunction and erectile dysfunction in older men and women: an overview of systematic reviews. Maturitas. 2011;70: 37–41.
132. Jang DJ, Soo Lee M, Shin B-C, Lee Y-C, Ernst E. Red ginseng for treating erectile dysfunction: a systematic review. Br J Clin Pharmacol. 2008;66: 444–50.
133. Kim TH, Jeon SH, Hahn E-J, Paek K-Y, Park JK, Youn NY, et al. Effects of tissue-cultured mountain ginseng (Panax ginseng CA Meyer) extract on male patients with erectile dysfunction. Asian J Androl. 2009;11:356–61.
134. Kim HS, Woo SH, Jo S, Hahn E-J, Youn NY, Lee HL. Double-blind, placebo-controlled, multi-center study for therapeutic effects of Mountain Panax Ginseng C.A. Meyer extract in men with erectile dysfunction: a preliminary report. Kor J Androl. 2006;24(2):84–8.
135. Kim SJ, Murthy HN, Hahn EJ, Lee HL, Paek KY. Parameters affecting the extraction of ginsenosides from the adventitious roots of ginseng (Panax ginseng C.A. Meyer). Sep Purif Technol. 2007;56:401–6.
136. Murphy LL, Cadena RS, Chavez D, Ferraro JS. Effect of American ginseng (Panax quinquefolium) on male copulatory behaviour in the rat. Physiol Behav. 1998;64:445–50.
137. Kim C, Choi H, Kim CC, Kim JK, Kim MS. Influence of ginseng on mating behavior of male rats. Am J Chin Med (Gard City NY). 1976;4:163–8.
138. Kim H, Chen X, Gillis CN. Ginsenosides protect pulmonary vascular endothelium against free radical-induced injury. Biochem Biophys Res Commun. 1992;189:670–6.
139. Chen X, Lee TJ. Ginsenosides-induced nitric oxide-mediated relaxation of the rabbit corpus cavernosum. Br J Pharmacol. 1995;115:15–8.
140. Chen X. Cardiovascular protection by ginsenosides and their nitric oxide releasing action. Clin Exp Pharmacol Physiol. 1996;23:728–32.
141. Choi YD, Xin ZC, Choi HK. Effect of Korean red ginseng on the rabbit corpus cavernosal smooth muscle. Int J Impot Res. 1998;10:37–43.
142. Choi YD, Rha KH, Choi HK. In vitro and in vivo experimental effect of Korean red ginseng on erection. J Urol. 1999;162:1508–11.
143. Kim HJ, Woo DS, Lee G, Kim JJ. The relaxation effects of ginseng saponin in rabbit corporal smooth muscle: is it a nitric oxide donor? Br J Urol. 1998;82:744–8.
144. Wang X, Chu S, Qian T, Chen J, Zhang J. Ginsenoside Rg1 improves male copulatory behavior via nitric oxide/cyclic guanosine monophosphate pathway. J Sex Med. 2010;7(2 Pt 1):743–50.
145. Han K, Shin IC, Choi KJ, Yun YP, Hong JT, Oh KW. Korea red ginseng water extract increases nitric oxide concentrations in exhaled breath. Nitric Oxide. 2005;12:159–62.
146. Kimura T, Saunders PA, Kim HS, Rheu HM, Oh KW, Ho IK. Interactions of ginsenosides with ligand-bindings of GABA(A) and GABA(B) receptors. Gen Pharmacol. 1994;25:193–9.

147. Park JH, Cha HY, Seo JJ, Hong JT, Han K, Oh KW. Anxiolytic-like effects of ginseng in the elevated plus-maze model: comparison of red ginseng and sun ginseng. Prog Neuropsychopharmacol Biol Psychiatry. 2005;29:895–900.
148. Watanabe H, Ohta H, Imamura L, Asakura W, Matoba Y, Matsumoto K. Effect of Panax ginseng on age-related changes in the spontaneous motor activity and dopaminergic nervous system in the rat. Jpn J Pharmacol. 1991;55:51–6.
149. de Andrade E, de Mesquita AA, Claro Jde A, de Andrade PM, Ortiz V, Paranhos M, et al. Study of the efficacy of Korean red ginseng in the treatment of erectile dysfunction. Asian J Androl. 2007;9:241–4.
150. Dang H, Chen Y, Liu X, Wang Q, Wang L, Jia W, et al. Antidepressant effects of ginseng total saponins in the forced swimming test and chronic mild stress models of depression. Prog Neuropsychopharmacol Biol Psychiatry. 2009;33:1417–24.
151. Lee B, Kim H, Shim I, Lee H, Hahm DH. Wild ginseng attenuates anxiety- and depression-like behaviors during morphine withdrawal. J Microbiol Biotechnol. 2011;21:1088–96.
152. Buettner C, Yeh GY, Phillips RS, Mittleman MA, Kaptchuk TJ. Systematic review of the effects of ginseng on cardiovascular risk factors. Ann Pharmacother. 2006;40:83–95.
153. Karmazyn M, Moey M, Gan XT. Therapeutic potential of ginseng in the management of cardiovascular disorders. Drugs. 2011;71:1989–2008.
154. Kim SY, Seo SK, Choi YM, Jeon YE, Lim KJ, Choi YS, et al. Effects of red ginseng supplementation on menopausal symptoms and cardiovascular risk factors in postmenopausal women: a double-blind randomized controlled trial. Menopause. 2012;19:461–6.
155. Barton DL, Soori GS, Bauer BA, Sloan JA, Johnson PA, Figueras C, et al. Pilot study of Panax quinquefolius (American ginseng) to improve cancer-related fatigue: a randomized, double-blind, dose-finding evaluation: NCCTG trial N03CA. Support Care Cancer. 2010;18:179–87.
156. Tode T, Kikuchi Y, Hirata J, Kita T, Nakata H, Nagata I. Effect of Korean red ginseng on psychological functions in patients with severe climacteric syndromes. Int J Gynaecol Obstet. 1999;67:169–74.
157. Reay JL, Kennedy DO, Scholey AB. Effects of Panax ginseng, consumed with and without glucose, on blood glucose levels and cognitive performance during sustained "mentally demanding" tasks. J Psychopharmacol. 2006;20:771–81.
158. Rausch WD, Liu S, Gille G, Radad K. Neuroprotective effects of ginsenosides. Acta Neurobiol Exp (Wars). 2006;66:369–75.
159. Ma J, Li W, Tian R, Lei W. Ginsenoside Rg1 promotes peripheral nerve generation in rat model of nerve crush injury. Neurosci Lett. 2010;478:66–71.
160. Zheng GQ, Cheng W, Wang Y, Wang XM, Zhao SZ, Zhou Y, et al. Ginseng total saponins enhance neurogenesis after focal cerebral ischemia. J Ethnopharmacol. 2011;133:724–8.
161. Fang F, Chen X, Huang T, Lue LF, Luddy JS, Yan SS, et al. Multi-faced neuroprotective effects of ginsenoside Rg1 in an Alzheimer mouse model. Biochim Biophys Acta. 1822;2012:286–92.
162. Liang W, Ge S, Yang L, Yang M, Ye Z, Yan M, et al. Ginsenosides Rb1 and Rg1 promote proliferation and expression of neurotrophic factors in primary Schwann cell cultures. Brain Res. 2010;1357:19–25.
163. Lopez MV, Cuadrado MP, Ruiz-Poveda OM, Del Fresno AM, Accame ME. Neuroprotective effect of individual ginsenosides on astrocytes primary culture. Biochim Biophys Acta. 2007;1770:1308–16.
164. Lee ST, Chu K, Sim JY, Heo JH, Kim M. Panax ginseng enhances cognitive performance in Alzheimer disease. Alzheimer Dis Assoc Disord. 2008;22:222–6.
165. Heo JH, Lee ST, Chu K, Oh MJ, Park HJ, Shim JY, et al. An open-label trial of Korean red ginseng as an adjuvant treatment for cognitive impairment in patients with Alzheimer's disease. Eur J Neurol. 2008;15:865–8.
166. Geng J, Dong J, Ni H, Lee MS, Wu T, Jiang K, et al. Ginseng for cognition. Cochrane Database Syst Rev. 2010; CD007769.
167. Colman CI, Hebert JH, Reddy P. The effects of Panax ginseng on quality of life. J Clin Pharm Ther. 2003;28:5–15.
168. Chan PC, Peckham JC, Malarkey DE, Kissling GE, Travlos GS, Fu PP. Two-year toxicity and carcinogenicity studies of Panax ginseng in Fischer 344 rats and B6C3F1 mice. Am J Chin Med. 2011;39:779–88.
169. National Toxicology Program. Toxicology and carcinogenesis studies of ginseng (CAS No. 50647-08-0) in F344/N rats and B6C3F1 mice (gavage Studies). Natl Toxicol Program Tech Rep Ser 2011;567:1–149.
170. Coon JT, Ernst E. Panax ginseng: a systematic review of adverse effects and drug interactions. Drug Saf. 2002;25:323–44.
171. Izzo AA, Ernst E. Interactions between herbal medicines and prescribed drugs. An updated systematic review. Drugs. 2009;69:1777–98.
172. Siegel RK. Ginseng abuse syndrome. Problems with the panacea. JAMA. 1979;241:1614–5.
173. Baldwin CA, Anderson LA, Phillipson JA. What pharmacists should know about ginseng. Pharm J. 1986;237:583–6.
174. Miller LG. Herbal medicinals: selected clinical considerations focusing on known or potential drug-herb interactions. Arch Intern Med. 1998;158:2200–11.
175. Klepser TB, Klepser ME. Unsafe and potentially safe herbal therapies. Am J Health Syst Pharm. 1999;56:125–41.
176. Stavro PM, Woo M, Heim TF, Leiter LA, Vuksan V. North American ginseng exerts a neutral effect on blood pressure in individuals with hypertension. Hypertension. 2005;46:406–11.
177. Stavro PM, Woo M, Leiter LA, Heim TF, Sievenpiper JL, Vuksan V. Long-term intake of North American ginseng has no effect on 24-hour blood pressure and renal function. Hypertension. 2006;47:791–6.

178. Caron MF, Hotsko AL, Robertson S, Mandybur L, Kluger J, White CM. Electrocardiographic and hemodynamic effects of panax ginseng. Ann Pharmacother. 2002;36:758–63.
179. Han JH, Choe SC, Kim HS, Sohn DW, Nam KY, Oh BH, et al. Effect of red ginseng on blood pressure in patients with essential hypertension and white coat hypertension. Am J Chin Med. 1998;26: 199–209.
180. Rhee MY, Kim YS, Bae JH, Nah DY, Kim YK, Lee MM, et al. Effect of Korean ginseng on arterial stiffness in subjects with hypertension. J Altern Complement Med. 2011;17:45–9.
181. Vuksan V, Sung MK, Sievenpiper JL, Stavro PM, Jenkins AL, Di Buono M, et al. Korean red ginseng (Panax ginseng) improves glucose and insulin regulation in well-controlled, type 2 diabetes: results of a randomized, double-blind, placebo-controlled study of efficacy and safety. Nutr Metab Cardiovasc Dis. 2008;18:46–56.
182. Ang-Lee MK, Moss J, Yuan CS. Herbal medicines and perioperative care. JAMA. 2001;286:208–16.
183. Jiang X, Williams KM, Liauw WS, Ammit AJ, Roufogalis BD, Duke CC, et al. Effect of St John's wort and ginseng on the pharmacokinetics and pharmacodynamics of warfarin in healthy subjects. Br J Clin Pharmacol. 2004;57:592–9.
184. Shao J, Jia L. Potential serious interactions between nutraceutical ginseng and warfarin in patients with ischemic stroke. Trends Pharmacol Sci. 2013;34: 85–6.
185. Jiang X, Blair EY, McLachlan AJ. Investigation of the effects of herbal medicines on warfarin response in healthy subjects: a population pharmacokinetic-pharmacodynamic modeling approach. J Clin Pharmacol. 2006;46:1370–8.
186. Lee YH, Lee BK, Choi YJ, Yoon IK, Chang BC, Gwak HS. Interaction between warfarin and Korean red ginseng in patients with cardiac valve replacement. Int J Cardiol. 2010;145:275–6.
187. Lee S-H, Ahn Y-M, Ahn S-Y, Doo H-K, Lee B-C. Interaction between warfarin and Panax ginseng in ischemic stroke patients. J Altern Complement Med. 2008;14:715–21.
188. Yuan CS, Wei G, Dey L, Karrison T, Nahlik L, Maleckar S, et al. Brief communication: American ginseng reduces warfarin's effect in healthy patients: a randomized, controlled trial. Ann Intern Med. 2004;141:23–7.
189. Yu JY, Jin YR, Lee JJ, Chung JH, Noh JY, You SH, et al. Antiplatelet and antithrombotic activities of Korean red ginseng. Arch Pharm Res. 2006;29: 898–903.
190. Tetsutani T, Yamamura M, Yamaguchi T, Onoyama O, Kono M. Can red ginseng control blood glucose in diabetic patients. Ginseng Rev. 2000;28:44–7.
191. Sang-Wook Y, Sull JW, Hong JS, Linton JA, Ohrr H. Association between ginseng intake and mortality: Kangwha cohort study. J Altern Complement Med. 2009;15:921–8.
192. Vaes LP, Chyka PA. Interactions of warfarin with garlic, ginger, ginkgo, or ginseng: nature of the evidence. Ann Pharmacother. 2000;34:1478–82.
193. Kim S-O, Kim MK, Lee H-S, Park JK, Park K. The effect of Korean red ginseng extract on the relaxation response in isolated rabbit vaginal tissue and its mechanism. J Sex Med. 2008;5:2079–84.
194. Lee H-S, Lee MN, Hwang IS, Kim SO, Ahn K, Park K. Effect of Korean red ginseng on vaginal blood flow and structure in hypercholesterolemic female rats. Kor J Androl. 2005;23:159–64.
195. Kim S-O, Kim MK, Chae MJ, Kim HY, Park JK, Park K. Effect of Korean red ginseng on the relaxation of clitoral corpus cavernosum in rabbit. Kor J Androl. 2006;24:29–34.
196. Oh K-J, Chae M-J, Lee H-S, Hong H-D, Park K. Effects of Korean red ginseng on sexual arousal in menopausal women: placebo-controlled, double-blind crossover clinical study. J Sex Med. 2010;7: 1469–77.
197. Chua LS, Abdul-Rahman N, Rosidi B, Lee CT. Plant proteins, minerals and trace elements of Eurycoma longifolia (Tongkat ali). Nat Prod Res. 2013;27:314–8.
198. Low BS, Das PK, Chan KL. Standardized quassinoid-rich Eurycoma longifolia extract improved spermatogenesis and fertility in male rats via the hypothalamic-pituitary-gonadal axis. J Ethnopharmacol. 2013;13(145):706–14.
199. Erasmus N, Solomon MC, Fortuin KA, Henkel RR. Effect of Eurycoma longifolia Jack (Tongkat ali) extract on human spermatozoa in vitro. Andrologia. 2012;44:308–14.
200. Wahab NA, Mokhtar NM, Halim WN, Das S. The effect of eurycoma longifolia Jack on spermatogenesis in estrogen-treated rats. Clinics (Sao Paulo). 2010;65:93–8.
201. Chan KL, Low BS, The CH, Das PK. The effect of Eurycoma longifolia on sperm quality of male rats. Nat Prod Commun. 2009;4:1331–6.
202. Tambi MI, Imran MK. Eurycoma longifolia Jack in managing idiopathic male infertility. Asian J Androl. 2010;12:376–80.
203. Tambi MI, Imran MK, Henkel RR. Standardized water-soluble extract of Eurycoma longifolia, Tongkat ali, as testosterone booster for managing men with late-onset hypogonadism. Andrologia. 2012;44 Suppl 1:226–30.
204. Ismall SB, Wan Mohammad WM, George A, Nik Hussain NH, Musthapa Kamal ZM, Liske E. Randomized clinical trial on the use of PHYSTA freeze-dried water extract on Eurycoma longifolia for the improvement of quality of life and sexual well-being in men. Evid Based Complement Alternat Med. 2012;2012:429268.
205. Rogerson S, Riches CJ, Jennings C, Weatherby RP, Meir RA, Marshall-Gradisnik SM. The effect of five weeks of Tribulus terrestris supplementation on muscle strength and body composition during preseason training in elite rugby league players. J Strength Cond Res. 2007;21:348–53.

206. Neychev VK, Mitev VI. The aphrodisiac herb Tribulus terrestris does not influence the androgen production in young men. J Ethnopharmacol. 2005;101:319–23.
207. Kohut ML, Thompson JR, Campbell J, Brown GA, Vukovich MD, Jackson DA, et al. Ingestion of a dietary supplement containing dehydroepiandrosterone (DHEA) and androstenedione has minimal effect on immune function in middle-aged men. J Am Coll Nutr. 2003;22:363–71.
208. Brown GA, Vukovich MD, Martini ER, Kohut ML, Franke WD, Jackson DA, et al. Effects of androstenedione-herbal supplementation on serum sex hormone concentrations in 30- to 59-year-old men. Int J Vitam Nutr Res. 2001;71:293–301.
209. Brown GA, Vukovich MD, Reifenrath TA, Uhl NL, Parsons KA, Sharp RL, et al. Effects of anabolic precursors on serum testosterone concentrations and adaptations to resistance training in young men. Int J Sport Nutr Exerc Metab. 2000;10:340–59.
210. Antonio J, Uelmen J, Rodriguez R, Earnest C. The effects of Tribulus terrestris on body composition and exercise performance in resistance-trained males. Int J Sport Nutr Exerc Metab. 2000;10:208–15.
211. Moyad MA, Barada JH, Lue TF, Mulhall JP, Goldstein I, Fawzy A, Sexual Medicine Society (SMS) Nutraceutical Committee. Prevention and treatment of erectile dysfunction using lifestyle changes and dietary supplements: what works and what is worthless, part II. Urol Clin N Am. 2004;31:259–73.
212. Yohimbe. http://www.nlm.nih.gov/medlineplus/druginfo/natural/759.html. Accessed on 23 April 2013.
213. Ernst E, Pittler MH. Yohimbine for erectile dysfunction: a systematic review and meta-analysis of randomized clinical trials. J Urol. 1998;159:433–6.
214. Moyad MA. Zinc for prostate disease and other conditions: a little evidence, a lot of hype, and a significant potential problem. Urol Nurs. 2004;24: 49–52.
215. Leitzmann MF, Stampfer MJ, Wu K, Colditz GA, Willett WC, Giovannucci EL. Zinc supplement use and risk of prostate cancer. J Natl Cancer Inst. 2003;96:1004–7.
216. Age-Related Eye Disease Study Research Group. A randomized, placebo-controlled, clinical trial of high-dose supplementation with vitamins C and E, beta-carotene, and zinc for age-related macular degeneration and vision loss: AREDS Report Number 8. Arch Ophthalmol. 2001;119:1417–36.
217. Johnson AR, Munoz A, Gottlieb JL, Jarrard DF. High dose zinc increases hospital admissions due to genitourinary complications. J Urol. 2007;177:639–43.
218. Health Canada Website. Multi-vitamin/Mineral Supplements. http://www.hc-sc.gc.ca/dhp-mps/prodnatur/applications/licen-prod/monograph/multi_vitmin_suppl-eng.php. Accessed on 20 Apr 2013.
219. Food and Nutrition Board, National Academy of Sciences. Dietary reference intakes for vitamin A, vitamin K, arsenic, boron, chromium, copper, iodine, iron, manganese, molybdenum, nickel, silicon, vanadium, and zinc. Washington, DC: National Academy Press; 2001. p. 177–204. 351–98.
220. AREDS2 Research Group, Chew EY, Clemons T, SanGiovanni JP, Danis R, Domalpally A, McBee W, et al. The Age-Related Eye Disease Study 2 (AREDS2): study design and baseline characteristics (AREDS2 report number 1). Ophthalmology. 2012;119:2282–9.
221. de Oliveira Kde J, Donangelo CM, de Oliveira Jr AV, da Silveira CL, Koury JC. Effect of zinc supplementation on the antioxidant, copper, and iron status of physically active adolescents. Cell Biochem Funct. 2009;27:162–6.
222. Koehler K, Parr MK, Geyer H, Mester J, Schanzer W. Serum testosterone and urinary excretion of steroid hormone metabolites after administration of a high-dose zinc supplement. Eur J Clin Nutr. 2009;63:65–70.
223. Mahajan SK, Abbasi AA, Prasas AS, Rabbani P, Briggs WA, McDonald FD. Effect of oral zinc therapy on gonadal function in hemodialysis patients. A double-blind study. Ann Intern Med. 1982;97:357–61.
224. Prasad AS, Abbasi AA, Rabbani P, DuMouchelle E. Effect of zinc supplementation on serum testosterone level in adult male sickle cell anemia subjects. Am J Hematol. 1981;10:119–27.
225. de Luis DA, Pacheco D, Izaola O, Terroba MC, Cuellar L, Cabezas G. Micronutrient status in morbidly obese women before bariatric surgery. Surg Obes Relat Dis. 2013;9:323–7.
226. Sanchez C, Lopez-Jurado M, Planells E, Liopis J, Aranda P. Assessment of iron and zinc intake and related biochemical parameters in an adult Mediterranean population from southern Spain: influence of lifestyle factors. J Nutr Biochem. 2009;20:125–31.
227. Tiran D. The use of fenugreek for breast feeding women. Complement Ther Nurs Midwifery. 2003;9: 155–6.
228. Poole C, Bushey B, Foster C, Campbell B, Willoughby D, Kreider R, et al. The effects of a commercially available botanical supplement on strength, body composition, power output, and hormonal profiles in resistance-trained males. J Int Soc Sports Nutr. 2010;7:34.
229. Steels E, Rao A, Vietta L. Physiological aspects of male libido enhanced by standardized Trigonella foenum-graecum extract and mineral formulation. Phytother Res. 2011;25:1294–300.
230. Wilborn C, Taylor L, Poole C, Foster C, Willoughby D, Kreider R. Effects of a purported aromatase and 5alpha-reductase inhibitor on hormone profiles in college-age men. Int J Sport Nutr Exerc Metab. 2010;20:457–65.
231. Hannan JM, All L, Rokeya B, Khaleque J, Akhter M, Flatt PR, Abdel-Wahab YH. Soluble dietary fibre fraction of Trigonella foenum-graecum (fenugreek) seed improves glucose homeostasis in animal models of type 1 and type 2 diabetes by delaying carbohydrate digestion and absorption, and enhancing insulin action. Br J Nutr. 2007;97:514–21.

232. Dell'Agli M, Galli GV, Dal Cero E, Belluti F, Matera R, Zironi E, et al. Potent inhibition of human phosphodiesterase-5 by icariin derivatives. J Nat Prod. 2008;71:1513–7.
233. Shindel AW, Xin ZC, Lin G, Fandel TM, Huang YC, Banie L, et al. Erectogenic and neurotrophic effects of icariin, a purified extract of horny goat weed (Epimedium spp.) in vitro and in vivo. J Sex Med. 2010;7(4 Pt 1):1518–28.
234. Liu WJ, Xin ZC, Xin H, Yuan YM, Tian L, Guo YL. Effects of icariin on erectile function and expression of nitric oxide synthase isoforms in castrated rats. Asian J Androl. 2005;7:381–8.
235. Alexander J, Crosby M, Ferguson D, Singh G, Steidle C, Weimiller M. Randomized, placebo-controlled, double-blind, crossover design trial of the efficacy and safety of Zestra for women in women with and without female sexual arousal disorder. J Sex Marital Ther. 2003;29 Suppl 1:33–44.
236. Pitel S, Raccah D, Gerbi A, Pieroni G, Vague P, Coste TC. At low doses, a gamma-linolenic acid-lipoic acid conjugate is more effective than docosahexaenoic acid-enriched phospholipids in preventing neuropathy in diabetic rats. J Nutr. 2007;137: 368–72.
237. Hornych A, Oravec S, Girault F, Forette B, Horrobin DF. The effect of gamma-linolenic acid on plasma and membrane lipids and renal prostaglandin synthesis in older subjects. Bratisl Lek Listy. 2002;103: 101–7.
238. Belch JJ, Shaw B, O'Dowd A, Saniabadi A, Leiberman P, Sturrock RD, et al. Evening primrose oil (Efamol) in the treatment of Raynaud's phenomenon: a double blind study. Thromb Haemost. 1985;54:490–4.
239. Herbenick D, Reece M, Hensel D, Sanders S, Jozkowski K, Fortenberry JD. Association of lubricant use with women's sexual pleasure, sexual satisfaction, and genital symptoms: a prospective daily diary study. J Sex Med. 2011;8:202–12.
240. Sutton KS, Boyer SC, Goldfinger C, Ezer P, Pukall CF. To lube or not to lube: experiences and perceptions of lubricant use in women with and without dyspareunia. J Sex Med. 2012;9:240–50.
241. Herbenick D, Reece M, Sanders SA, Dodge B, Ghassemi A, Fortenberry JD. Women's vibrator use in sexual partnerships: results from a nationally representative survey in the United States. J Sex Marital Ther. 2010;36:49–65.
242. Papakostas GI. Evidence for S-adenosyl-L-methionine (SAM-e) for the treatment of major depressive disorder. J Clin Psychiatry. 2009;70 Suppl 5:18–22.
243. Papakostas GI, Mischoulon D, Shyu I, Alpert JE, Fava M. S-adenosyl methionine (SAMe) augmentation of serotonin reuptake inhibitors for antidepressant nonresponders with major depressive disorder: a double-blind, randomized clinical trial. Am J Psychiatry. 2010;167:942–8.
244. Alpert JE, Papakostas G, Mischoulon D, Worthington 3rd JJ, Petersen T, Mahal Y, et al. S-adenosyl-L-methionine (SAMe) as an adjunct for resistant major depressive disorder: an open trial following partial or nonresponse to selective serotonin reuptake inhibitors or venlafaxine. J Clin Psychopharmacol. 2004; 24:661–4.
245. Levkovitz Y, Alpert JE, Brintz CE, Mischoulon D, Papakostas GI. Effects of S-adenosylmethionine augmentation of serotonin-reuptake inhibitor antidepressants on cognitive symptoms of major depressive disorder. Eur Psychiatry. 2012;27:518–21.
246. Shippy RA, Mendez D, Jones K, Cergnul I, Karpiak SE. S-adenosylmethionine (SAM-e) for the treatment of depression in people living with HIV/AIDS. BMC Psychiatry. 2004;4:38.
247. Dording CM, Mischoulon D, Shyu I, Alpert JE, Papakostas GI. SAMe and sexual functioning. Eur Psychiatry. 2011;27:451–4.
248. Kennedy SH, Rizvi S. Sexual dysfunction, depression, and the impact of antidepressants. J Clin Psychopharmacol. 2009;29:157–64.
249. Ringdahl E, Pandit S. Treatment of knee osteoarthritis. Am Fam Physician. 2011;83:1287–92.
250. Soeken KL, Lee WL, Bausell RB, Agelli M, Berman BM. Safety and efficacy of S-adenosylmethionine (SAM-e) for osteoarthritis. J Fam Pract. 2002;51:425–30.
251. Harel Z, Harel S, Wald R, Mamdani M, Bell CM. The frequency and characteristics of dietary supplement recalls in the United States. JAMA Intern Med. 2013;15:1–3.
252. Price A, Gazewood J. Korean red ginseng effective for treatment of erectile dysfunction. J Fam Pract. 2003;52:20–1.

7 Complementary and Alternative Medicine and Lifestyle Changes and Prostate Cancer

Introduction

Prostate cancer cases in the USA will exceed 238,000 currently and will be the most diagnosed male cancer. It will be the second leading cause of cancer mortality, with approximately 30,000 deaths [1]. Despite all of the outstanding advances in the area of castrate-resistant prostate cancer (CRPC), there is always a need for ancillary treatment assistance, be it from lifestyle changes or complementary and alternative medicine (CAM). Currently, there is shift in the thinking I have tried to espouse over my career [2], which is the idea that concentrated antioxidants or supplements can increase cancer cell initiation and progression. Unless a dietary supplement can mimic the effects of a known anticancer agent or improve heart health, it is difficult to endorse it as a cancer preventive or ancillary treatment agent. And it is difficult to otherwise believe it will provide some form of assistance. James Watson, PhD, who shared the Nobel Prize in Physiology or Medicine for the discovery of the double-helix structure of DNA, was vocal as of late on this point based on past and existing research [3]. His argument is that antioxidants can contribute to metastatic cancer or undermine treatment. Since antioxidants appear to neutralize DNA- and RNA-damaging reactive oxygen species (ROS) that would normally trigger programmed cell death, then they arguably need to be reduced or stopped. This does make sense, in that the first approach with antioxidant supplements would be to first do no harm. Again, I agree with this approach and have advocated for this approach in urology for long periods of time; yet there is a counter argument to the Watson theory. It is possible that giving large quantities of some supplements may cause instability and generate free radicals instead of absorb them. And, although this theory is being tested with IV vitamins and minerals, it needs more preliminary evidence to be proven or advocated, and I have difficulty believing it will be generally successful in a treatment setting, but it may have some application for the reduction of some conventional treatment side effects or the disease itself. It is also possible that expecting CAM or dietary supplements to enhance treatment, especially in the advanced stages of the disease, is asking to overcome a daunting task. At the same time, I am discouraged when clinicians are dealing with advanced cancer patients and discuss CAM as being adverse to effective treatment responses when, in reality, the patient is not clear what the general prognosis is in this situation. In other words, advanced cancer patients should be able to also make objective decisions with their clinician, especially when realizing that regardless of the drug or treatment utilized, the overall prognosis is not good. In the meantime, a less is more philosophy, and utilizing some supplements for side effects of cancer treatment (e.g., androgen-deprivation therapy [ADT]), but not at the expense of treatment efficacy, again appears to be the best approach ("first do no harm") for most individuals being treated for prostate cancer.

M.A. Moyad, *Complementary & Alternative Medicine for Prostate and Urologic Health*,
DOI 10.1007/978-1-4614-8492-9_7, © Springer Science+Business Media New York 2014

Heart Health Is Tantamount to the Ideal Prostate, Men's, and Overall Health: Lessons from Pharmaceutical Prostate Cancer Prevention Trials

The mantra of heart health being tantamount to urologic and prostate health was highlighted in the opening chapter of this book and most other past written sources from this author [4].

Men have a consistently lower life expectancy in the USA and in most countries around the world and have a higher morbidity and mortality from heart disease, hypertension, cancer, and diabetes [5]. Yet it must be reiterated that heart-healthy changes are tantamount to overall men's health improvements, regardless of the part of the human anatomy that is receiving attention, including the penis and the prostate [6, 7]. Heart-healthy changes need to be advocated to men concerned about prostate cancer because it places probability and the overall research into perspective. Triaging preventive medicine for men's health is providing probability-based advice via evidence-based medicine and can impact all-cause mortality as well as potentially prevent prostate cancer.

One of the more fascinating features of large randomized clinical trials, especially for primary prevention, is that they appear to reflect the current health status and risk issues of not only the subjects being tested, but also perhaps the general population. The largest, most recent, and arguably the best-designed US and worldwide pharmaceutical-based cancer primary prevention trials for the prevention of prostate cancer exemplify the urgency for a different or changing perspective. For example, results of the Prostate Cancer Prevention Trial (PCPT) seem to have garnered attention and controversy regarding the use of finasteride daily versus placebo to reduce the risk of prostate cancer [8–11]. The debate over finasteride abounds, but another observation from this trial has not received adequate exposure in the medical literature. Over 18,000 healthy men were included in this randomized trial, and five men died from prostate cancer in the finasteride arm and five men died of prostate cancer in the placebo arm. However, 1,123 men in total died during this primary prevention trial [8]. Thus, prostate cancer was responsible for approximately less than 1 % of the deaths, while the majority of the overall causes of mortality were from CVD and other causes [8, 12, 13]. Additionally, the mean BMI, systolic blood pressure, and total and HDL cholesterol were the following: 27–28 (50 % overweight and approximately 25 % obese), 138–140 mm Hg (pre-hypertensive), and 212 mg/dL and 42–43 mg/dL (dyslipidemia or at risk). Despite 85 % of men with no history of CVD, approximately 50 % of the men reported some level of erectile dysfunction (ED) [12].

The international dutasteride high-risk prostate cancer prevention trial known as REDUCE (Reduction by Dutasteride of Prostate Cancer Events) had somewhat similar issues to the North American PCPT in terms of overt controversies [14–16], but what was not questioned, discussed, or even debated was the BMI and several other abnormal CVD parameter issues mentioned earlier were similar in the two trials. For example, on average men in REDUCE were overweight (BMI of 27–28) [14]. There were 8,231 men randomized and after the 4-year trial in this group of men there were 147 total deaths, primarily from cardiovascular events and none from prostate cancer. Of further note, men in the placebo arm of PCPT with low cholesterol (<200 mg/dL) had a 59 % ($p=0.02$) apparent reduction in risk of being diagnosed with aggressive prostate cancer (Gleason 8–10) compared to men with high cholesterol (≥200 mg/dL) [17], and men with coronary artery disease (CHD) at baseline in REDUCE were found to have a significantly higher risk of a prostate cancer diagnosis, and this included low-grade (OR = 1.34, $p=0.02$) and high-grade cancer (OR = 1.34, $p=0.09$) [18]. These notable but less recognized observations do not intend to belittle prostate cancer or these trials utilizing a specific chemoprevention agent, but again it places the overall risk of morbidity and mortality in a more proper perspective. Men inquiring about the advantages and disadvantages of finasteride and dutasteride for prostate cancer prevention need to be reminded that the number 1 risk to them in general is CVD, and in both clinical trials the researchers found good indications that heart health was tantamount to prostate health.

Lifestyle Changes Continue to Make a Difference with Prostate Cancer and Improve Conventional Treatment Outcomes

Whatever appears to improve heart health also appears to simultaneously improve prostate health. Encouraging patients to do whatever is practical and plausible to reduce their risk of CVD to as close to zero should be the mantra. This should provide the greatest potential to not only reduce the risk of prostate cancer, but other disease morbidity and even impact all-cause mortality. It is interesting that most major behavioral risk factors for CVD morbidity and mortality today appear to be correlated with a higher risk of prostate cancer or aggressive prostate cancer and/or fatal prostate cancer. For example, smoking is the single largest preventable cause of death and disease in the USA with approximately 443,000 deaths still occurring per year from tobacco-related disease, and approximately 20 % of adults smoke, which is a number that has remained constant the past several years [19, 20]. Smoking has been associated with a higher risk of being diagnosed with prostate cancer in recent meta-analyses [21], a higher risk of aggressive prostate cancer, and dying from prostate cancer [22, 23]. Similarly, obesity is associated with a higher risk of aggressive and fatal prostate cancer [24], and this is why it is no longer surprising that a higher risk of recurrence occurs posttreatment for prostate cancer [25]. It is also plausible that obesity is associated with a lower risk of localized prostate cancer, and a higher risk of advanced disease due to the artificial lowering of PSA or hemodilution impact associated with this condition [26, 27].

Weight gain ancillary issues abound. For example, ongoing evidence suggests an increased risk of certain cancers with insulin resistance, and this may include aggressive prostate cancer [28–31]. Increased growth factors occur with increased insulin levels, but long-term diabetes may result in insulin, IGF, and androgen reduction, which may be correlated with a lower prostate cancer risk in the short term ("diabetes paradox") [31]. The dramatic increase in the diabetes epidemic [32], along with the known 2–4 times increased risk of CVD events in diabetics over nondiabetics [33], should make type 2 diabetes prevention strategies a priority for simultaneous prostate cancer prevention. Only 15 years ago, 3 states in the USA had a diabetes prevalence of 6 % or higher, but now all 50 states in the USA have a rate of at least 6 % or higher [32]. Six states have rates of 10 % or more, along with Puerto Rico, and currently 19 million people in the USA have diabetes and 7 million are undiagnosed. Perhaps prostate cancer prevention strategies can help to modestly curb this epidemic. Exercise (aerobic and resistance) and dietary (caloric reduction) and other lifestyle changes have been shown to significantly prevent diabetes and metabolic syndrome in normal and high-risk individuals better than pharmacologic therapy [34–38].

Hypertension is a primary risk factor for CVD and stroke and almost a third of the US adult population has this condition [39]. Hypertension increases with age to approximately 70 % of individuals 65 years and older. Hypertension is a contributing factor in one out of every seven deaths, and 70 % of individuals who have a first heart attack or stroke have hypertension [40]. Treating hypertension has been correlated with dramatic reductions in the incidence of stroke (40 %), heart attacks (25 %), and heart failure (>50 %) [41]. However, the correlation between prostate cancer risk and hypertension and/or antihypertensive medications is weak [42]. Yet high blood pressure as part of a continuum of unhealthy parameters, such as observed with metabolic syndrome (central obesity, dyslipidemia, and insulin resistance), is becoming a potential risk factor for prostate cancer and other prostate issues [43]. It is also well known that alpha-blockers, originally discovered for blood pressure control, are now one of those most effective treatments for men with prostate issues (BPH) and lower urinary tract symptoms (LUTS) despite not having consistent positive or negative impacts on prostate cancer risk [44, 45]. In order to maintain prostate health, it is critical to prevent or control hypertension.

Regular vigorous exercise (3 h or more per week) is a potential strategy to significantly reduce prostate cancer death after diagnosis and simultaneously reduce all-cause mortality to a similar degree (50–60 %) in these same patients compared to men that perform only 1 h or less exercise per week [46]. Thus, it should not be a surprise that exercise may also contribute to a slightly lower risk of prostate cancer, from a review of past studies including a recent summary of 22 studies published over the past 12 years [47–49]. Patients should be told that the profound reduction in blood pressure, diabetes, depression, dyslipidemia, cancer, CVD, fatigue, obesity, and multiple other conditions would arguably be enough to garner exercise a Nobel Prize if it were a drug [4].

Patients should also be informed of the potential for exercise to profoundly enhance the effects of conventional medication. This has been a constant source of difficulty in the past to explain intuitively that one needs to continue to exercise daily despite utilizing an effective prescription drug. A truly novel prospective 10-year study of over 10,000 adults (mean age of 58 years) from the Veterans Affairs (VA) Medical Center in Palo Alto, CA, and Washington, DC, should help in educating men with dyslipidemia on the ancillary effects of exercise [50]. Researchers found a lower risk of dying from any cause when on a statin (cholesterol-lowering drug), but this was not the noteworthy news. Participants in this study had received an exercise test between 1986 and 2011. Over 2,300 patients died during this time and the risk of dying was significantly greater in the group that did not take a statin drug compared to those that did, but again this is also the noteworthy news. Next, researchers looked at the fitness level of those based on exercise testing and the use of a statin drug. The risk of death further decreased with fitness or improved health from exercise far beyond what the statin drug alone could provide. Men that were most fit in this study were able to reach slightly more than nine MET (metabolic equivalent tasks, a measure of the intensity of your exercise; higher numbers are better) peaks on an exercise machine, and this group experienced a 70 % reduction in overall mortality compared to the least fit! However, men who could do just 7.1–9 MET did almost as well (59 % reduction); even those who were able to perform 5.1–7.0 MET experienced a 36 % reduction! This is the noteworthy news! Think about this the next time a discussion with a patient occurs on the benefits of exercise in addition to proven conventional treatments. Again, the clinician reading this chapter or patient needs to ponder and appreciate what a 70 % advantage in reducing the risk of dying from all causes beyond what is already being provided by a lifesaving drug really means (arguably an immediate Nobel Prize in medicine)! A person gets 1 MET for sitting on the couch and breathing, 3–5 MET for just moving or carrying golf clubs, and 5–7 MET for a light jog or hike or brisk walk, and 7–9 MET for more intense exercises. A 10-min mile is approximately equivalent to 10 MET. In fact, exercising 30–60 min/day basically allows many individuals to reach this exercise capacity. Researchers also looked at men not taking statins and their fitness levels compared to other men not taking statins and found that the most fit had a 47 % reduction in the risk of overall mortality compared to the less fit [50]! This study also shows that individuals who simply cannot tolerate these drugs when everything has been tried should at least be exercising regularly to get some notable benefits. It should also be kept in mind that this is now the second paradigm-type study of men in medicine or urology that demonstrates the impact of exercise on proven health-promoting medicines. In the erectile dysfunction (ED) chapter on lifestyle changes, the clinical trial of PDE-5 inhibitors in association with exercise over 3 months was discussed, and the profound improvements that occurred for most ED parameters, including libido (an indication never approved by the FDA for PDE-5 inhibitors), were reviewed [51]. The mean age and BMI of the participants were 50 years and 27 (overweight), respectively. A significant improvement was observed in all aspects of the IIEF-15 except the orgasm domain for men who exercised 3 or more hours a week compared with the non-exercise pill-only group. Erectile function, confidence, sexual desire, intercourse satisfaction, and total satisfaction were all significantly improved in the exercise group

Table 7.1 Heart healthy = prostate healthy. A partial listing of miscellaneous lifestyle changes, medical conditions, or health parameters and their impact on prostate cancer risk, progression, and overall health

Lifestyle change/ health condition or parameter	Commentary on prevention or treatment of prostate cancer and overall health
Belly fat/obesity	Increases the risk of artificially lowering of PSA (hemodilution, false negatives) and more advanced or aggressive disease and one of the biggest risk factors for testosterone suppression. Also, may increase the risk of adverse events from conventional treatment options
Cholesterol/dyslipidemia	Dyslipidemia is associated with a higher risk of aggressive prostate cancer
Diabetes/glucose intolerance	Associated with a higher risk of aggressive disease in the long term
Diet/caloric control or reduction/fad diets	Reducing caloric intake to assist in preventing weight gain may reduce prostate cancer risk and PSA velocity (from BPH), which could reduce unneeded biopsies. 3500 calories = 1 pound (about 0.5 kg) of fat as weight loss begins and becomes more difficult with time (higher caloric reduction needed for weight loss). Thus, any diet that can remove 100–200 calories a day and causes heart-healthy parameter changes is arguably prostate healthy. Vegan, primarily plant based, Mediterranean, low glycemic, and even ketogenic diet plans could be considered based on the personality of the patient
Exercise (aerobic and resistance activity)	May reduce the risk of aggressive prostate cancer diagnosis and may reduce the risk of prostate cancer and overall mortality after a prostate cancer diagnosis/treatment. Weight lifting or resistance exercise appears to reduce fatigue and improve energy levels and quality of life in men receiving prostate cancer treatment. Weight lifting also increases metabolism and reduces the risk of type 2 diabetes. Exercise is not needed to lose weight in many patients but provides metabolic assistance and of course other overall health benefits. New research suggests “core exercises” and better heart health after primary treatment for prostate cancer (surgery, radiation, etc.) could improve time to continence, incontinence rates, reduce a variety of treatment side effects and improve quality of life
Hypertension/blood pressure	Part of the spectrum of metabolic syndrome that could increase the risk of prostate cancer. One primary class of BPH drugs (alpha-blockers) was originally derived from antihypertensive agents; thus, normal blood pressure is important for prostate health
Inflammation/inflammatory markers (hs-CRP, IL-6, etc.)	Higher numbers appear to be an independent predictor of cardiovascular events, diabetes, prostate cancer, and death from prostate cancer. Multiple organ systems under chronic inflammation from infectious and noninfectious sources have already been shown to increase the risk of cancer (hepatitis, esophagitis/acid reflux, inflammatory bowel disease, etc.)
Metabolic syndrome (low HDL, high triglycerides, high BMI or waist circumference, glucose intolerance, and high blood pressure)	Collectively appear to increase the risk of prostate cancer and progressive disease. Also, increase the risk of cardiovascular events
Smoking/tobacco	Increases the risk of aggressive and fatal prostate cancer and reduces the blood level of numerous antioxidants

taking PDE-5 medication over the PDE-5 alone group. Thus, the clinician today has wonderful motivating resources or research to utilize in discussions with patients. Whatever the drug utilized, it could be argued that exercise improves the efficacy of these conventional agents.

Thus, virtually every heart-healthy parameter of lifestyle change has now become associated with prostate health or prostate cancer. Obesity, a lack of exercise, high cholesterol, hypertension, glucose intolerance, inadequate diet, excessive alcohol intake, tobacco, etc. have all been linked to abnormal prostate health [4]. For example, Table 7.1 is a quick overview of general lifestyle changes, situations, or parameters that have been associated with the risk of prostate cancer and abnormal prostate issues, and all of them also impact cardiovascular risk [4].

Surgery/Radiation and Other Conventional Treatments for Prostate Cancer and Dietary Supplements (A Bad Combination Unless Heart Healthy): Less = More

Firstly, I have always had a policy of reducing dietary supplement intake before conventional medical treatment, especially surgery and radiation [4]. There are quality-control and blood-thinning issues that are virtually impossible to anticipate or predict. For example, small amounts of some dietary supplements could impact or increase the risk of bleeding events in some rare situations, including fish oil, which could have a qualitative effect on platelets, and no test is currently available to predict coagulation issues. A dose of fish oil as low as 1,800 mg/day in combination with a statin (another partial blood-thinning agent) significantly increased the risk of minor and serious bleeding events (subcutaneous, epistaxis, fundal, and cerebral hemorrhage) in one of the only randomized long-term clinical trials to ever address this issue [52]. The number of overall events was small compared to the control group (105 vs. 60; $p=0.006$), but the results in some of these rare cases were and could be catastrophic. In addition, when allowing the intake of herbal products that could also contain natural blood thinners ("coumarins," similar to coumadin) without identification on the bottle, the risk clearly outweighs the benefit for most patients. Thus, after complete recovery, or 1–2 months, potentially restarting dietary supplementation is an option. Clinicians should explain this safety issue with compassion because in my experience when it is handled without this approach, it can generate a response that does not encourage compliance from the patient, but rather conspiracy due to the lack of perceived general knowledge of CAM for healthcare professionals.

I have always been opposed to men taking megadoses of supplements when getting radiation treatment for prostate cancer unless they potentially mimic what could have provided benefit in the area of conventional medicine (e.g., cholesterol- or glucose-lowering or control, potential radiosensitizers) [53–57]. Taking numerous dietary supplements with radiation treatment does not appear to improve results and may in rare cases reduce efficacy, but more research is needed. Again, it is my opinion that no dietary supplement will improve the results of radiation treatment in my lifetime unless researchers try to copy what already might be working in the prescription drug world to improve outcomes after localized treatment, for example, aspirin, metformin, or statins (cholesterol lowering) [4, 53–57].

A retrospective review in utilizing the following dietary supplements with prostate cancer radiation treatment was published [58]:

- Green tea extract at 1,000–1,500 mg
- Melatonin at 20 mg a day at bedtime
- Vitamin C at 1,500–3,000 mg
- Vitamin E at 400–800 IU

A total of 134 men were treated with radiation therapy for primarily localized prostate cancer, and 69 patients received these high doses of dietary supplements. A total of 77 received hormone therapy, and all of the men on dietary supplements continued to use them for at least 24 months after radiation was completed. The follow-up period postradiation was 71–79 months. No significant differences were found in the patients receiving radiation alone in terms of pretreatment PSA, PSA nadir, time to reach nadir, and follow-up. Similar findings occurred in the group of men receiving hormone therapy. There was also no difference in urinary or sexual function between the men treated with hormone therapy in the dietary supplements group compared to the no supplements group. This study reflects the current thinking and past human radiation studies in cancer in terms of a lack of minimal or profound ancillary impact.

Why have patients risk even a 1 % chance that the supplements or CAM they are utilizing could compromise their conventional treatment success or cure? If a patient accepts the potential for cure or control of his prostate cancer with a conventional option, then to compromise this option even remotely undermines the very reason the patient chose this option with the doctor and the team he trusts in the first place. This needs to be explained compassionately and carefully, and in my experience most patients will accept this philosophy. When looking at the past two decades of cancer and radiation treatment and rigorous randomized trials that have been done in certain cancers with supplements like vitamin E and head and neck cancer, there were negative effects on treatment outcomes, especially in those with other unhealthy behaviors such as tobacco use [59–62]. Even though side effects may have been reduced, it came at the expense of treatment efficacy. There is also a concern with hormonal tumors and the ability of dietary supplements to provide cancer protection and simply worsen survival [63].

One counter argument to this thought is that the patient only wants to further enhance treatment outcomes or reduce side effects since there are efficacy issues with any conventional treatment for prostate cancer. This is true, but this is the point where lifestyle changes can be emphasized. The average weight or body mass index of a man with prostate cancer patient receiving surgery or radiation in the USA today classifies him as overweight or obese, and other comorbidity issues abound [4]. In other words, I find it interesting that reducing weight or waist size, aerobic and resistance exercise, improvements in diet, eliminating tobacco use, normal to low cholesterol or cholesterol reduction (statins), perhaps aspirin (for aggressive tumors), and controlling blood sugar (glucose) look more promising today to improve conventional treatment for prostate cancer than at any time I can remember in urology. Thus, I explain to patients compassionately that if they are trying for a prostate cancer cure, the smartest thing they can give their treating doctor and team is the gift of trying to become as healthy as possible before, during, and after treatment to only further increase the chances of success. For example, meta-analysis of aerobic exercise along with prostate cancer treatment and after treatment has found a reduction in fatigue [64]. Resistance exercise (weight lifting) just 2–3 times a week during and after radiation treatment also appears to provide quality-of-life benefits and a reduction in fatigue [65, 66]. Additional reduction in body fat and triglycerides and improvements in strength may also occur [66], which could translate into added treatment efficacy benefits and a reduction in cardiovascular disease (CVD).

Another common question over CAM and radiation for prostate cancer is the type of diet needed to reduce toxicity or enhance treatment effects. Yet, this has not been adequately addressed in clinical studies and there is considerable controversy. The primary mode of thought for a long time has been the use of a low residual (soft diet, generally low in fiber)-based diet during the entire time of radiation treatment, which could theoretically reduce bowel toxicity. One older retrospective observational study found a lower rate of gastrointestinal issues in men being treated for prostate cancer with radiation therapy compared to men that were not placed on this diet. The problem with this study is that whole pelvic radiation techniques were used and radiation treatment and targeting has changed dramatically since this time period [4, 67]. A brief review and partial summary of this older diet is listed in Table 7.2.

However, a randomized prostate cancer trial that included the reduction in insoluble fiber (a bulking agent) and lactose worked no better compared to the control diet [68]. And another retrospective observational study of 739 patients with no change in diet compared to 105 patients placed on a fairly strict antiflatulent diet to reduce intrafraction prostate motion actually found a significant increase in clinically relevant intrafraction motion increase of 43 % of those on the dietary intervention compared to 19 % ($p<0.0001$) of the control group [69]. The authors theorized that the change in diet may have caused bowel patterns to adjust or be altered dramatically and perhaps no change in diet during radiation treatment may be a better option. This is a philosophy that appears to make sense and should be discussed with patients. This same research group conducted a double-blind, placebo-controlled randomized trial of 1,000 mg of magnesium oxide per day or placebo during the treatment duration of intensity-modulated radiotherapy (IMRT) with the goal to reduce bowel changes that could impact intrafraction prostate motion [70]. No difference compared to placebo was found (46 patients per arm), and the secondary endpoints suggested a trend toward

Table 7.2 A soft diet ("low residue") that was utilized to reduce side effects of external beam radiation treatment for prostate cancer in an older often cited study

Dietary intervention	Options encouraged to consume	Options discouraged to consume
Beverages	Milk/milk drinks, coffee	Any alcoholic beverages
Breads	Enriched white and light rye breads or rolls, crackers	Breads or crackers with whole wheat flours, bran, or seeds
Cereals	Cooked refined wheat, cooked fine-cut oatmeal	Whole-grain cereals
Desserts	Candies, cakes, gelatin, pie, ice cream, yogurt, pudding	Coconut, seeds, nuts, tough skins
Fats	Butter, margarine, cream, oil, and vinegar salad dressing	Mayonnaise, Italian or French salad dressing
Meat, fish, eggs	Tender meat, eggs, cottage cheese, mild American cheese	Highly seasoned meat, fish, or chicken
Potatoes	Skinless potatoes, macaroni, noodles	Skin of potato, sweet potato, spaghetti, white, brown, or wild rice
Soups	Cream or broth based	Others and spicy veggie
Sugar/sweets	Candy, honey, jelly, syrup	Candy with fruits/nuts, seeds, skins
Vegetables	Juices, canned/cooked tender veggies without seeds/skin	All others
Miscellaneous	Gravy, smooth peanut butter	Relish, pepper, nuts, olives, salt pickles, popcorn, mustard, chili sauce, horseradish

It should be kept in mind that minimal changes in diet during radiation treatment also have as much evidence currently

worse quality of life and more potential toxicity in the magnesium oxide group, but the differences were not statistically significant.

Another issue is that IMRT and other sophisticated and well-targeted techniques today may simply negate the effects of any dietary changes in prostate cancer patients undergoing radiation therapy. It is for this reason that I am ambivalent in recommending dietary changes for men undergoing radiation treatment for prostate cancer. Perhaps the older low-residue or soft diet is still an option, but this discussion must be balanced with the newer data, which suggests no difference in potential treatment outcomes. However, there is some suggestion that diarrhea can be reduced utilizing or continuing the use of a psyllium fiber agent, which should also be discussed as a possible option [71, 72]. In other words, if a patient is already utilizing 1–2 teaspoons, for example, of psyllium or another soluble (and perhaps insoluble) fiber source, then continuing it throughout the period of radiation could provide some preventive advantages. More research is needed on the impact of insoluble fiber, but many heart-healthy food sources of fiber contain both types. Again, the data are so weak in this area of prostate cancer research that the conversation and decision should be doctor and patient determined, keeping in mind that no approach has more data compared to another at the current time.

Less Is More Overall for Prevention and Treatment (Learning from Past Cancer Supplement Studies)

One of the most surprising findings from a large phase 3 dietary supplement study occurred in the 1990s when the Alpha-Tocopherol, Beta-Carotene Cancer Prevention (ATBC) trial, a randomized 2×2 factorial prevention study of 50 mg of alpha-tocopherol and/or 20 mg of beta-carotene on over 29,000 male chronic smokers, was stopped [73]. Subjects receiving beta-carotene had a significant increase in lung cancer incidence and overall mortality compared to placebo. This study was designed originally because a plethora of epidemiologic research suggested beta-carotene could reduce the risk of lung cancer [74]. Yet, soon after the ATBC stopped, the Carotene and Retinol Efficacy Trial (CARET), another phase 3 randomized study of 30 mg of beta-carotene and 25,000 IU retinol in individuals with a history of past or current smoking or asbestos exposure, was also stopped for precisely the same reasons as ATBC [75]! A significant increase in lung cancer diagnoses and overall mortality occurred in the supplement versus the placebo arm. The third large prevention trial of beta-carotene, the Physicians' Health Study (PHS), did not show anything positive or negative, but PHS was not just conducted in smokers [76]. A total of 11 % were current and 39 % were former smokers, and 50 mg of beta-carotene was utilized every other day and the median blood level was 1.2 μg/mL, which was far lower compared to the median blood level in ATBC (3.0 μg/mL), or CARET (2.1 μg/mL). In other words, researchers received a real indication that an excess of certain supplements or antioxidants in certain populations could potentially increase the risk of cancer and early death. This was again a substantial change in the paradigm of thinking that really impacted my thoughts and beliefs forever.

Current and former smokers should be reducing their supplemental intake of beta-carotene regardless of their prostate cancer status. In fact, the results of the Age-Related Eye Disease Study 2 (AREDS2) phase 3 randomized trial were released years later, and they only highlighted the problem of overexposure of certain nutrients in some populations [77]. This clinical trial found that fish oil does not reduce the progression of macular degeneration. However, in this same trial the group that was utilizing 15 mg of beta-carotene in their supplement had a significant increase in the risk of lung cancer (23 vs. 11 cases or 2.0 % vs. 0.9 %; $p=0.04$), and most of the lung cancer cases were in former smokers. This finding was from secondary randomization excluding individuals who were smokers. It is now highly plausible that higher doses of beta-carotene dietary supplements (15 mg or more) increase the risk of lung cancer in former and current smokers. Former smokers should check their supplements to make sure they contain little or no beta-carotene. Current smokers should stop smoking and not ingest beta-carotene as a dietary supplement. Eating healthy foods high in beta-carotene has not been a safety issue in former and current smokers—only the supplements. I believe this is what is known as level 1 evidence that a dietary supplement in the wrong population of men and women can cause harm. Thus, with this in mind, perhaps one of the greatest examples in medical history that more is not better in terms of supplementation can be derived from urology and prostate cancer prevention, and this is known as the Selenium and Vitamin E Cancer Prevention Trial (SELECT).

Lessons from the SELECT Trial (Selenium and Vitamin E): Over-Antioxidation of the Population, Heart Unhealthy = Prostate Unhealthy, and More Issues

The ATBC, CARET, and AREDS2 dietary supplement trials were a surprise, but what would come next was an even more definitive sign that less is more, even in healthy individuals, when dealing with certain supplements. This would be especially true in populations already replete with these nutrients. SELECT randomized over 35,000 men into four groups: high-dose vitamin E (400 IU/day), high-dose selenium [200 micrograms (μg)/day], combination of vitamin E and selenium, or placebo [78]. The rapid time period to reach full recruitment was unprecedented; thus, it seemed that participants and healthcare professionals were both enthusiastic to test the theory that high-dose antioxidant supplementation could prevent prostate cancer (the primary endpoint) and perhaps other conditions. Yet, the trial was terminated early, after a median of 5.5 years, due to a lack of efficacy, although at the time a nonsignificant ($p=0.06$) increased risk of prostate cancer in the vitamin E arm and type 2 diabetes in the selenium group ($p=0.16$) was observed. Therefore, indications of a lack of effectiveness and potential harm existed in this healthy group of men.

And, to the credit of the SELECT research group, participant follow-up continued (54,464 added person-years), which provided more clarity about any further health impact after dietary supplement cessation [79]. What was revealed in this follow-up period was a concern and perhaps changed the perception of a lack of potential harm with dietary supplements in healthy populations forever. A significant ($p=0.008$; HR = 1.17) increased risk of prostate cancer was found in the vitamin E group, but not in the selenium or combination intervention arm. More concerning is that the risk of Gleason 7 or higher disease was greater for the three intervention arms compared to placebo, but did not reach statistical significance in any group. The HR and *p*-value for Gleason 7 and higher disease compared to placebo was 1.16 ($p=0.20$), 1.21 ($p=0.11$), and 1.23 ($p=0.08$) for vitamin E, selenium, and the combination. The increased risk of prostate cancer with vitamin E began to emerge after only 3 years and was found to be consistent for low- and high-grade disease types. It could be argued that had the trial been allowed to continue for several more years, there would have been a statistically significant increased risk of Gleason 7–10 prostate cancer in all groups except the placebo arm. This is speculative, but a trending plausible scenario.

The negative results from SELECT cannot be explained by bias or increased biopsy rates, but suggest that the dietary supplements themselves are the issue, and the confidence intervals have only continued to narrow over time [79]. Secondary endpoints that included other cancers and cardiovascular events did not find statistical differences compared to placebo with this additional analysis. This is indeed good news in light of such negativity from ingesting what many pundits would have perceived as benign over-the-counter dietary supplements.

Yet, the SELECT should still address the following question: Are any of the SELECT results a surprise when reviewing the history of these and other nutritional interventions in large dosages? It could easily be argued that not only were the results somewhat expected, but again they could have been even more disconcerting over time if the trial continued. And, even if any of these interventions would have prevented prostate cancer, it is highly questionable whether they would have still provided a tangible clinical advance in clinical medicine. Why? The controversy that plagued high-dose vitamin E and selenium supplements from past clinical trials was the lack or even negative impact these interventions have on the number one cause of death in men and women, cardiovascular disease [80, 81]. Even a past potential increased risk of all-cause mortality had been a concern with high-dose vitamin E supplementation based on meta-analysis [82].

One could argue that the synthetic vitamin E supplements utilized in the SELECT were the reason for negative findings, or in other words the classic "natural versus non-natural" debate, and this is a debate that often arises in meetings I attend. Yet, this cannot be the case because several past trials of "natural" vitamin E-derived supplements in high dose showed no overall effects [81, 83], and even a significant increased risk of specific cardiovascular events such as heart failure or hospitalization for heart failure from one large randomized trial [83]. So, it is highly doubtful that the form or type of vitamin E would have provided alternative results.

One might also argue that the frequency or daily use of vitamin E led to the negative observation and less frequent or intermittent dosing would have provided a better benefit-to-risk ratio. This also appears to be a weak argument because another large randomized trial of vitamin E and prostate cancer risk in healthy men, the Physicians Health Study II (PHS2), found no impact of 400 IU of vitamin E every other day compared to placebo [84], but a significant increased risk of hemorrhagic stroke was observed [85]. Additionally, for such an adverse event to occur in a completely healthy population from a primary prevention trial is concerning enough. One also has to ponder why two independent large phase 3 clinical trials (SELECT and PHS2), primarily initiated in the USA, utilizing high-dose vitamin E supplements for testing prostate cancer prevention were allowed to be conducted simultaneously at such an enormous financial burden with similar clinical endpoints. Why not conduct just one randomized trial and save a plethora of resources, time, enthusiastic volunteers, and money for another future and perhaps more relevant chemoprevention trial?

Some could argue that the dosage of vitamin E might have been the real issue or even the lack of adhering to phase I, II, and III trial principles, and this has some potential merit that I have agreed with for some time, along with other controversial issues from the initiation and design of SELECT [86]. One primary justification for SELECT was the Alpha-Tocopherol, Beta Carotene (ATBC) trial, which demonstrated a 35 % risk reduction of prostate cancer risk with vitamin E from a secondary endpoint, but the dosage utilized in ATBC was only 50 IU (approximately eight times lower compared to SELECT) and a higher rate of hemorrhagic stroke was also found with this lower dosage [73]. Men in ATBC were also chronic, 36 years on average, smokers, and continuous tobacco users are well known for multiple nutrient deficiencies, not just vitamin E [87]. Less than 10 % of SELECT males were smokers [78, 79], which leaves one to ponder the outcome of this trial if a lower, scientifically more evidence-based defendable dose had been utilized, or if a phase 1- and 2-type study was completed first, similar to conventional medicine protocol, before moving right to a phase 3 trial [88]. For example, why even the belief that more is better—400 IU trumps 50 IU? Isn't this one stereotype or prejudice applied to some patients that utilize a multitude of non–evidence-based dietary supplements? Since there were data to suggest that 50 IU of vitamin E might prevent prostate cancer in what researchers considered tantamount data to a phase I or II clinical trial, then, again, what is the justification for utilizing 400 IU in the phase 3 trial? This would not have seemed permissible if this were a conventional drug clinical trial in terms of dosage alterations based on past potentially effective prostate cancer prevention data [86]. In other words, PCPT or REDUCE would never, in my opinion, alter the dosage used in those trials because the past phase 1 and 2 data suggested the appropriate dosage to use in the phase 3 trial. Why treat dietary supplements differently?

Healthy and primarily non- or former smoking men (85 % of the participants) from a unique randomized trial (Supplementation en Vitamines et Mineraux Antioxydants or SU.VI.MAX) utilizing substantially reduced doses of vitamin E (30 IU) and other dietary supplements, including selenium, in combination (100 mg of ascorbic acid, 6 mg of beta-carotene, 100 μg selenium as enriched yeast, and 20 μg zinc gluconate) demonstrated the potential for notable benefit for prostate cancer prevention but also harm for men with higher baseline PSA levels [89, 90]. This trial included 13,017 healthy French adults and found a difference or potential benefit for men ($n=5,141$, age 45–60 years, 35 % nonsmokers, BMI of 25) in terms of a significant reduced cancer incidence and overall mortality and nonsignificant 18 % reduction in cardiovascular disease, but these benefits were not found for women ($n=7,876$, aged 35–60 years, 55 % nonsmokers, BMI of 23) in this same trial. Perhaps this is due to the lower baseline blood levels of antioxidants (especially beta-carotene and vitamin C) found in men compared to sufficient concentrations and more healthy behaviors and parameters found in women participating in this trial. Testing individual, multiple, or combination lower or reduced dosage, or what the authors cited as "nutritional" dosages of nutrients, appeared to be safer and perhaps more effective compared to larger dosage in those that appeared to have a lower intake of these nutrients from their diet and/or lifestyle. Less is more.

Other cited controversies by advocates of vitamin E supplements will arguably continue through time. For example, the modicum of positive data for the primary form of vitamin E derived from food, gamma-tocopherol, could have been tested as a dietary supplement based on some preliminary past evidence [91, 92]. Not only is this preliminary and would need phase 1 and 2 data, which it does not enjoy, but there is also some preliminary evidence to suggest that it could also have negative effects in excess [93]. Again, smokers with nutritional deficiencies have the most to benefit in this situation. Smoking cessation should be a more prominent goal over arguing and researching specific dietary supplementation in the dwindling population of current smokers that could be effective for prostate cancer prevention. And using data from smokers to equate what would happen to nonsmoker and former smokers is, again, a difficult argument.

What about the past issues with selenium dietary supplements? The impact of high-dose selenium supplements on cardiovascular and overall health from past clinical trials was arguably as concerning as past vitamin E clinical research [94] and included a potential significant increased risk of type 2 diabetes and non-melanoma skin cancer recurrence [95, 96]. Interestingly, this increased risk of skin cancer recurrence was the final conclusion surrounding the primary endpoint analysis of the landmark randomized selenium supplement trial (Nutritional Prevention of Cancer), which was utilized to justify initiating SELECT [95, 97].

In other words, it appeared that some researchers were more fascinated by the secondary endpoint reduction in prostate cancer risk compared to the primary endpoint increase in skin cancer risk.

A question to ponder in the first chapter of this book and when dealing with patients is: Why attempt to prevent prostate cancer with high-dose interventions that may actually increase the risk of other primary causes or even the number one cause of morbidity and mortality in men or women, regardless of its potential for a favorable impact on prostate cancer or another chronic disease? Again, primary prevention trials are simple excellent reflections of the current health status of populations from where recruitment originated. For example, the Prostate Cancer Prevention Trial (PCPT) and SELECT morbidity and mortality rates from cardiovascular events (primary causes of death in these two trials), regardless of the group assignment, were notable [8, 78, 79] and continue to demonstrate the ideal prostate cancer chemoprevention agent needs to potentially and simultaneously reduce the risk of cancer and some aspect of cardiovascular disease. This would appear to at least represent an advance in medicine, and not a lateral shift.

One of the most important lessons to learn from SELECT, and somewhat in defense of the researchers and designers of SELECT itself, was the chance of launching an externally uncontaminated clinical trial by the time of randomization was impossible. This is due to a novel phenomenon that I have termed the "over-antioxidation of the population." Interestingly, baseline serum selenium status in SELECT was 22 points higher (135 ng/mL vs. 113 ng/mL) compared to comparative trials from the 1990s in the USA [78, 79], which essentially equates to a population of men that are no longer deficient in this antioxidant or nutrient before they even begin to ingest selenium as a supplement. How could this occur?

In the USA and in multiple countries around the world, I have observed countless multiple nutrients being added to a diversity of foods, beverages, and supplements such as multivitamins, foods, and beverages at an uncontrolled rate over the past decade as preliminary research highlights some potential preliminary benefits in various laboratory and/or observational studies. This appears to be helpful in marketing and profit, but not for science, research, and safety. When any nutritional deficiency trial is designed and initiated over several years, the depleted participants being tested will now arguably be replete with the nutrients being tested even before the trial commences. This was one of the most important lessons of the SELECT that should be constantly taught and discussed among future healthcare professionals, researchers, and clinical trial designers. This should pose a serious challenge for any further nutrient prevention or treatment trial in the Western world. It is also my belief that multiple future supplement or nutritional interventional trials, including vitamin D, will also suffer from the same SELECT over-antioxidation or overexposure controversy, dilemma, or fate. Currently, it will be difficult to ever recommend any individual supplement of vitamin E or selenium to men trying to prevent prostate cancer, men with prostate cancer, men being treated for prostate cancer, or men that were treated for prostate cancer. If a supplement can increase the risk of prostate cancer in very little time, it can be argued that it can encourage the growth of existing prostate cancer in an even shorter time period, which is simply what occurred in the SELECT.

It could be argued that the lessons of the selenium and vitamin E trials are as lucid now as ever before in medicine, and these individual supplements should be abandoned in prostate cancer at these dosages. There is no further need to spend more time and resources on these compounds in prostate cancer or perhaps most of urology. However, this should not be construed that they have no place in rare situations in medicine where the benefit may outweigh the risk (similar to a prescription medicine). For example, 800 IU of d-alpha-tocopherol or vitamin E has been uniquely found to potentially benefit some nondiabetic non-cirrhotic NASH (nonalcoholic steatohepatitis) patients with aggressive histology from a major 96-week-duration phase 3–like clinical trial known as "PIVENS" (Pioglitazone versus Vitamin E versus placebo for the treatment of nondiabetic patients with Nonalcoholic Steatohepatitis) [98, 99]. Since there are few treatment options for this subset of patients, many expert reviews suggest the benefit outweighs risk [99]. Additionally, there are major phase 3 clinical trials with selenium ongoing, for example, to prevent bladder cancer recurrence (SELEBLAT; Selenium and Bladder Cancer Trial) [100], which may or may not change clinical practice based on the eventual outcomes.

SAM (Statins, Aspirin, and Metformin): An Acronym That Brings the SELECT and Other CAM Prostate Cancer Lessons to a Final Perspective

Based on the lesson learned from the SELECT, my full-time career in CAM and urology, and beyond, it has now become difficult to ignore three heart-healthy interventions that arguably appear to be more promising than any costly interventions that might selectively and precisely prevent prostate cancer, or any CAM option used for ancillary treatment. Cholesterol-lowering (statins) medications, aspirin, and metformin all continue to garner attention for being cost-effective, generic, generally safe, and heart healthy in the appropriate risk-stratified population (middle-aged and older men) [53–57, 101–107]. These heart-healthy agents have unique mechanisms of action that potentially reduce the number one cause of morbidity and mortality in men and women and may provide ancillary benefits in those being treated for prostate cancer, including reducing side effects of some standard treatments [107].

Statins or cholesterol-lowering medications may be associated with a lower risk of aggressive prostate cancer [108, 109] and could also be a partial explanation for noteworthy mortality rate reductions from prostate cancer in some countries such as the USA [110, 111]. Since most statins are now generic, the lost cost of these products is another attractive feature. It is disappointing that no prostate cancer prevention trial or ancillary treatment trial has been completed with cholesterol-lowering medications, but several studies are being proposed and initiated based on latest US government data [112]. It is also appealing that statins have side effect prognostic markers, for example, liver and muscle enzyme tests that can predict toxicity.

Aspirin may also reduce the risk of prostate cancer mortality, but these data are preliminary [55, 56, 101]. However, aspirin toxicity is more difficult to predict in clinical practice because hemorrhagic strokes, ulcers, or gastrointestinal bleeding events do not have laboratory tests to precisely predict outcomes. Still, based on cost and history of reducing the potential risk of colorectal cancer in high-risk patients [113] or hear disease, it should be of interest to potentially recommend in some prostate cancer patients that already are candidates for aspirin use based on their medical history.

Metformin is beginning to receive adequate attention in multiple cancers, and this generic low-cost drug, actually derived from the French Lilac, has over 100 clinical trials being designed and initiated in cancer [114]. In fact, the following cancers are currently testing metformin with and without conventional treatment:

- Brain tumors
- Breast cancer
- Colon cancer
- Endometrial
- Esophageal
- Head and neck cancer
- Leukemia (ALL, CLL)
- Liver injury prevention from chemo-induced injury
- Lung cancer (non-small cell)
- Lymphoma
- Melanoma
- Pancreatic cancer
- Prostate cancer

Preliminary observational research is impressive and requires further investigation with this gluconeogenesis and growth factor inhibitory and heart-healthy agent. For example, researchers at Sloan-Kettering in New York conducted a retrospective analysis of 2,901 consecutively treated patients for prostate cancer and radiation therapy, and 157 were using metformin, 162 were diabetic and not using metformin, and 2,582 were nondiabetic [57]. Mean age was approximately

70 years, and they were utilizing metformin for about 5 years at an average dosage of 500 μg twice a day (1,000 μg total). Prostate cancer–specific mortality (PCSM) rates were significantly reduced for those on metformin (2.7 %) compared to diabetic non-metformin (21.9 %) and nondiabetic patients (8.2 %). A total of 16 % compared to 33 and 25 % developed a PSA recurrence. Metformin use was associated with a reduction in the development of CRPC compared with diabetic non-metformin patients. Further analyses revealed that the largest benefit to metformin use appears to be in the high-risk recurrence group or those with more aggressive disease likely to return after regular treatment, and also a significant benefit in overall survival occurred with metformin use compared to the other groups. Metformin with conventional radiation treatment could reduce recurrence, distant metastasis, the risk of death from prostate cancer and all causes, and reduce the risk of developing CRPC. Only 157 individuals used metformin in this study but it was interesting enough to garner ongoing interest. The other potential health benefits of metformin are also interesting, such as the ability to promote neuronal growth in the brain and improve memory in laboratory studies, and this drug activates atypical protein kinase C-CBP pathway that directs neural stem cells to differentiate into mature neurons [115].

Statins, aspirin, and metformin (SAM) are not CAM, so why discuss these three interventions in this book? It is because they share many features that serve as teachable lessons including generic, low cost, originally derived from natural sources (fungus for statins, willow bark for aspirin, and French Lilac for metformin), good overall safety profile, and heart healthy. These three interventions provide a paradigm for what to achieve or potentially investigate in the area of CAM and prostate cancer, urology, and medicine. In fact, CAM options that tend to mimic the effects of one or more of these three interventions have the most potential to be utilized for prostate cancer prevention and ancillary treatment in my experience [116]. For example, statins were originally derived and extracted from red yeast rice (see section on "Red Yeast Rice" in this chapter), which is also a dietary supplement with an adequate history of cholesterol reduction. These are the types of CAM options that would be my primary choice to test in a clinical trial and that I believe have the most to offer along with conventional treatment for prostate cancer.

BPH Dietary Supplements/CAM (Beta-Sitosterol, Pumpkin Seed Oil, Pygeum, Saw Palmetto, Stinging Nettle) Versus Flaxseed

Since 5-alpha-reductase (5-AR) inhibitors have some adequate clinical research that they prevent nonaggressive prostate but may increase the risk of a rare aggressive prostate [8–10], it is not unusual for some advertisers of BPH supplements to suggest a preventive favorable effect with BPH supplements. Yet, despite some suggestion that the mechanisms of action of many of these herbal BPH supplements are somewhat similar to 5-AR inhibitors, this has not been proven. And, PSA reduction or prostate cancer prevention has not been consistently demonstrated with these agents [117–124]. It is my opinion that BPH CAM options do not prevent or treat prostate cancer and may have some weak 5-AR effects in large dosages in some cases. Regardless, despite men taking these supplements for "prostate health," and in the hope of prostate cancer prevention, it should be reiterated that this is not accurate.

However, flaxseed has some preliminary evidence that it could be used as an ancillary option for the treatment of BPH and cancer [125], but these trials utilized dietary flaxseed powder (30 g/day, or 3 rounded tablespoons) for prostate cancer and dietary and supplemental flaxseed for BPH [126, 127]. Flaxseed is one of the largest sources of plant omega-3 fatty acids (alpha-linolenic acid or ALA) and it is high in fiber. Some of the plant omega-3 (ALA) from flaxseed can be converted into marine longer chain forms of omega-3s (ALA into EPA, eicosapentaenoic acid) by the human body. The conversion rate is not predictable and is low in some cases, but there are exceptions. For example, flaxseed oil has been shown in some studies to increase blood levels of marine EPA by as much as 60 % [128].

The Lyon Diet Heart Study (one of the first published Mediterranean diet studies) is the one of the only randomized clinical trials completed with ALA supplementation that was actually designed not just observe laboratory changes, but actual clinical solid cardiovascular endpoints [129]. However, the actual source of ALA in this famous study was a canola-enriched margarine, which was given to recent heart attack patients along with a variety of other dietary changes. The group of patients getting the ALA margarine had a significant ($p=0.001$) 65 % reduced risk of cardiac death and nonfatal heart attacks. Also of interest was the 35 % increase in blood levels of EPA in the margarine group. It appears that canola or flaxseed or other sources of the plant omega-3 fatty acids have a good history of being heart healthy, but most of the positive studies have utilized dietary sources of plant omega and not supplemental sources. Again, this should be reiterated to patients excited about any of these plant omega-3 products (further information on omega-3 is found under the "Fish Oil" section of this chapter).

Fish Oil Supplements (Marine Sources of Omega-3)

Three omega-3 fatty acids have been shown to improve heart health and overall health [130, 131]. The primary omega-3 from plants again is known as ALA. The other two usually are derived from marine or fish and fish oil supplements and are known as EPA and DHA (docosahexaenoic acid). ALA can be converted into the body into EPA and some EPA and be converted to DHA. Again, as mentioned earlier, these three omega-3 fatty acids are not mutually exclusive. For example, in one of the most notable prostate cancer neoadjuvant or presurgical randomized clinical trials, men that consumed foods high in ALA (flaxseed powder) had significant increases in their blood EPA levels [125]. Yet, the data or research with fish oil to reduce the risk of prostate cancer or aid in treatment is inconsistent and should not be recommended for this purpose. There is a plethora of preliminary past data to suggest that fish oil may be beneficial for a variety of health conditions including:

- Heart health [132]
- Vision [133]
- Dry eye syndrome [134]
- Hearing [135]
- Skin tone [136]
- Muscle mass [137]
- Kidney stone risk [138]
- Improve results when combined with a cholesterol-lowering drug [52]
- Pregnancy outcomes for mom and baby [139]
- Hot flashes [140]
- Mental health [141]
- Alzheimer's disease [142]
- Diabetes [143]
- Erectile function [144]
- Fertility [145]

The problem with all of this positive preliminary data is that when it has been subject to some phase 3-like clinical trials, the effect of fish oil has been similar to placebo. For example, no impact of fish oil was found in a large trial on macular degeneration progression (AREDS2) [77], as well as a more definitive primary prevention heart health clinical trial in high-risk patients [146], or for prevention of postoperative atrial fibrillation [147], and from a comprehensive meta-analysis [148]. The positive data on fish oil for reducing the risk of prostate cancer mortality is derived primarily from dietary (not pills) observational studies [149]. In other words, perhaps the American Heart Association (AHA) recommendations are the most accurate for prostate cancer prevention and after diagnosis in terms of potential benefits and how to approach the issue of fish oil. Fish is an outstanding lean source of protein, one of the highest natural sources of vitamin D, and one of the highest natural sources of omega-3 fatty acids (EPA and DHA), which is why the AHA recommends two servings of oily and fatty EPA and DHA rich fish (salmon, anchovies, mackerel, sardines, trout, herring, etc.) and plant sources of omega-3 (this fact often gets missed) [150]. AHA also recommends 1,000 μg of fish oil for those with heart disease or those trying to reduce high triglycerides (the one FDA-approved indication). Thus, there is some indirect indication that select patients on androgen-deprivation therapy (ADT) could benefit from fish oil supplements in terms of muscle maintenance and triglyceride reduction [137, 140], which is discussed later in the chapter. Otherwise, most patients trying to prevent or treat prostate cancer with conventional therapy do not need fish oil supplements but should be encouraged to eat fatty and oily fish for heart health. Some patients claim that fish oil provides ancillary benefits, for example, a reduction in muscular or arthritic pain (anti-inflammatory), which helps them reduce their intake of pain medications, which is an area where the benefit may of course outweigh the risk.

Folic Acid History, Other B Vitamins, and Multivitamins

A fairly extensive overview of the history of folic acid is provided in this section in order to construe specifically who or who does not qualify for these supplements. The reader will notice that folic acid provides a powerful preventive role in certain areas of medicine, especially obstetrics and gynecology, but in other areas such as prostate cancer, the results are controversial and concerning based on its mechanism of action and clinical results. This is also true for other B vitamins in high dosages and multivitamins that harbor higher dosages of B vitamins including folic acid.

Folate or folic acid is a B vitamin, and some B vitamins can be recognized by their assigned numbers such as B_{12} (cobalamin), B_6 (pyridoxine), B_2 (riboflavin), and B_1 (thiamine) [151]. Other B vitamins are also known for their alternative nonnumerical names such as niacin (vitamin B_3), pantothenic acid (vitamin B5), biotin (vitamin B_7), and even folate (vitamin B_9). Folate is found in numerous diverse healthy nutritious food and beverage products [152]. Folic acid is actually the synthetic form of folate that is found in dietary supplements and added to some grain products, which are also known as "fortified foods." Folate is water soluble, hence the requirement for essentially daily or regular ingestion to maintain optimal serum (range: 5.4–40.0 ng/mL) and/or red blood cell (range: 280–903 ng/mL) concentrations [153, 154]. The primary benefit of folate is for the primary and secondary prevention of neural tube defects (NTDs), such as spina bifida [155–159], whose name was derived from the Latin words that translate to mean "split spine" [160]. The neural tube forms, shapes itself, and closes within the first month of conception, which highlights the need for folic acid consumption by the mother before and immediately after conception [161]. Research also preliminarily suggests that other medical conditions in the newborn, such as preterm birth, congenital heart defects, and other organ abnormalities such as orofacial cleft malformations, could be at least reduced to some significant degree by folic acid [162].

Experts recommend 400 micrograms (μg) of folic acid daily, which is a small amount in general (approximately 400 millionths of a gram), and it is 600 μg/day in pregnancy and 500 μg/day during lactation [163]. There are also a variety of other situations, conditions, and medications that may increase the demand for folate or the strict adherence to daily consumption of this compound. For example, a short partial list includes the following:

- Alcohol abuse [164]
- Antiepileptic drugs (AEDs)/anticonvulsants [165–167]
- Type 2 diabetes mellitus [168]
- Hispanic and African-American population [169]
- Kidney diseases and dialysis [170]
- Liver disease [171]
- Malabsorption syndromes (such as celiac disease, gastric bypass surgery) [171]
- Medications (other) [172]
- Obesity (body mass index [BMI] $\geq$ 30) [173, 174]
- Tobacco products [175]

For example, women taking AEDs are generally recommended to take 4,000 (or 4 μg) of folic acid daily because these medications are folic acid antagonists and have been shown to significantly reduce the absorption and efficacy of folic acid and increase the risk of NTDs [168]. Some experts also recommend that obese women take 800 μg/day of folic acid because research also suggests that lower amounts, such as 400 μg/day, may be clinically insufficient to maintain normal serum or RBC levels of folate [174].

Since folic acid requires regular ingestion for efficacy, it would be optimal to consume the recommended amount from a combination of diverse healthy food sources and from supplementation from an over-the-counter or prescription pill. Folic acid has no known side effects from food or pill sources when taken at the recommended dosages for women and should be taken with a meal to improve absorption and tolerability [162]. It is also of importance to mention that taking B vitamins in supplemental form, especially B_2, can cause the urine to turn a harmless fluorescent yellow color that could be concerning to an individual who had not been informed about this potential side effect.

Approximately half of all pregnancies in the USA are unplanned; thus, many women of childbearing age can potentially benefit from folic acid [176]. Folic acid is also beneficial for all individuals when consumed on a daily basis because it reduces the risk of macrocytic anemia [161, 177, 178]. Historically, there has also been a concern that folic acid supplementation can "mask" a vitamin B_{12} blood deficiency (approximately less than 300 pg/mL) [163], which also potentially can be further identified utilizing additional costly serum tests known as "methylmalonic acid" and "homocysteine."

However, there is minimal evidence to suggest that these tests are necessary, consistently supportive, or that the B_{12} potential "masking" concern is valid or an evidence-based issue [163]. Part of the reason may be due to the fact that only 6 μg (compared to 400 μg for folate) is needed to satisfy the RDA for B_{12}, which is easily obtained today in many foods, beverages, and multivitamins.

Focusing on healthy foods that contain a high amount of folate and taking a multivitamin or another pill daily with folic acid is one of best immediate methods to improve deficient or insufficient folic acid levels. For this reason, a list of healthy diverse food sources that contain an unusually large amount of folate (approximately 50–100 μg or more per serving) and other healthy compounds for the body are listed below [163, 179]:

- Beans (variety and contain healthy types of fiber)
- Black-eyed peas (good source of calcium—over 200 μg per 1 cup serving)
- Breakfast cereals (especially the healthier bran or high-fiber varieties)
- Granola/fiber/protein bars (a surprising source—watch the calorie content)
- Nutritional liquid beverages (a variety of vitamins and minerals and generally low in calories per 8 ounces)
- Spinach, collard greens, broccoli, kale, brussel sprouts (also one of the highest sources of eye-healthy compounds lutein and zeaxanthin), and other green and leafy vegetables
- Sunflower seeds (source of diverse beneficial minerals—B_1, B_3, B_5, B_6, vitamin E, iron, magnesium, and zinc and low in sodium)

Folic acid plays such a strong role in maternal and child health that it is perhaps one of the greatest preventive success stories in public health and preventive medicine, and it is utilized primarily as a dietary supplement. In fact, the potential novel benefits with folic acid appear to continue with more research. For example, there is now some observational data that suggest it has potential in contributing to a lower risk of autism or severe language delay at older ages [180, 181].

The Case Against Folic Acid, Excessive Dosages of B Vitamins and Multivitamins, and Prostate Cancer

Folic acid is involved in cell division or DNA and RNA synthesis, and several effective anticancer and other drugs from methotrexate, 5-FU, and trimethoprim-sulfamethoxazole arguably work by reducing the efficacy and utilization of folate [178]. These drugs can block dihydrofolate reductase, which is needed by folic acid to become active. Thus, it has been concerning in the past that excessive amounts of folic acid could theoretically increase the risk of some cancers, especially prostate cancer.

A large-scale meta-analysis has reviewed all of the randomized trial data on folic acid and other B-vitamin supplementation to reduce the risk of cardiovascular disease, cancer, or impact all-cause mortality [182]. It concluded that there was minimal to no impact of these supplements in reducing the risk of these conditions. In other words, currently it does not seem to impact the risk of most chronic diseases, despite the fact that it can reduce blood homocysteine levels by at least 25 %. Still, folic acid supplements may increase or encourage the growth of a variety of common tumors and precancerous lesions or polyps in high-risk individuals [183]. The cancer that receives the most attention in terms of a potential increased risk from folic acid is prostate cancer [184, 185]. Serum levels of folic acid also appear to be increasing in the elderly such that unmetabolized folic acid (UMFA) has become a concern in men and women [186]. UMFA may have the ability to cause immune suppression and is a reflection that aging along with fortification of foods does not require large intakes of folic acid from other sources.

Still, the controversy over the clinical significance of a potential increased risk of prostate cancer will and should continue without any resolution in the near future. A meta-analysis of randomized trials found a significant increased risk of prostate cancer [187]. Arguably, another larger meta-analysis of randomized trials in cancer suggested that there was no risk and that past meta-analysis were influenced by a higher rate of cancer from one clinical trial [188], where prostate cancer incidence in the folic acid arm was probably increased due to chance [184]. Although these researchers make a compelling argument for this case, the problem with this theory is that most of the major trials looking at prostate cancer incidence still found at least nonsignificant increases in risk that cannot be disregarded due to chance, and this is confirmed by another recent meta-analysis [189], including some recent population studies [190]. Still, there are also some data that will challenge this notion [191], which further enhance the nebulousness and controversy on this subject.

Yet, the sum of the data on folic acid is simply not demonstrating primarily a neutral or reduced effect, only an increase risk overall and the argument is whether or not it is statistically or clinically significant. This argument tends to miss the forest over the tree in men's health and especially prostate cancer, and until the risk is justified there has been no sound benefit for most men in taking higher doses of supplemental folic acid on overall health and wellness.

Thus, clinicians should not encourage supplemental folic acid use, especially in the elderly and in other cases such as men with a history of cancer concerned about fertility, despite some minimal positive or just non-impressive data in the area of fertility itself [192, 193], because other supplements are safer, just as effective, and do not appear to require megadosage (like folic acid) for a clinical impact. Some of the early and only clinical trials that involved folic acid were using dosages such as 5 μg/day (along with zinc), which is 12.5 times the recommended daily intake [192]. Again, food sources of folate can be recommended, because these have not been concerning overall, but the concentrated nutraceuticals do not follow the mantra right now of benefit exceeding risk. It appears that folic acid may even find some place in medicine in men's health in some future trial, perhaps eye health, but again will the benefit outweigh the risk?

Multivitamins are arguably the most concentrated and readily available form of B vitamins such as folic acid for men. Despite minimal scientific evidence, multivitamins are the largest selling and utilized supplements in the USA [194]. They are also the primary supplement utilized by men in notable prostate cancer screening studies [195], male health prevention trials or observational studies [13, 196], and by male physicians [197]. Why, because it is not a plethora of clinical research that could be propelling these sales? Perhaps it is the perception compared to the reality, but until some higher-quality evidence finds some realistic benefit with these supplements in megadoses, the potential for harm when taking them in excess (two or more pills daily) seems concerning [198]. For example, an increased risk of advanced and fatal prostate was found in one of the largest prospective epidemiologic studies of multivitamins (NIH-AARP study), and the greater use of other supplements was also associated with an even greater risk [199]. Men that were free of cancer were evaluated in this prospective cohort study selected from the 3.5 million AARP, 50–71 years old, who lived in one of the following six states or two of the following metropolitan areas, including:

- Atlanta, Georgia
- California
- Detroit, Michigan
- Florida
- Louisiana
- New Jersey
- North Carolina
- Pennsylvania

Individuals were sent a baseline questionnaire and asked how often they used three types of multivitamins in the past year leading up to filling out the questionnaire. Men were placed in the category of either never use, casual use (0–6 times a week), consistent use (7 times a week), or heavy use (more than 7 times per week). Men were also asked about the dose and frequency of individual vitamin and mineral supplements. The mean age of the men and BMI was 62 years and 27 (overweight), about 50 % of the men were physically active three or more times a week, 60 % were former smokers, and the average vitamin D intake was approximately 200 IU a day. About 5 % of the men in this study were heavy users of multivitamins (total of 13,854 men), and overall multivitamins were the most commonly ingested supplements (51 %), followed by vitamin C (40 %), vitamin E (37 %), and calcium (22 %). During 5 years of following the men in the NIH-AARP Diet and Health Study that included 295,344 men, a total of 10,241 were diagnosed with prostate cancer. This included a total of 8,765 localized and 1,476 advanced cancers, and 179 cases of fatal cancer (after 6 years of follow-up).

Overall no association was found between the use of multivitamins and the overall risk for localized prostate cancer [199]. However, an increased risk of advanced and fatal prostate cancer was found for the men reporting an intake of more than seven times a week for multivitamins. This concerning information was found to be even stronger for men that were heavy users of multivitamins and those who also had a family history of prostate cancer and/or who took additional individual supplements including beta-carotene, selenium, and zinc. For example, men that took multivitamins more than seven times a week had a nonsignificant increased risk of advanced and fatal cancer 1.3 and 2 times higher than the men never taking these pills, while men getting one multivitamin a day had a nonsignificant similar risk for advanced prostate cancer (to nonusers) and a 10 % lower risk of fatal prostate cancer compared to the nonusers of multivitamins. Men ingesting individual selenium supplements and more than seven multivitamin pills a week had an almost ($p=0.054$) significant 5.8 times higher risk of fatal prostate cancer. Men with a heavy use of multivitamins and also taking individual vitamin E or folic acid or other supplements (beta-carotene and zinc) had 1.6 to as much as 4.4 times the risk of fatal prostate cancer. The highest risk of fatal prostate cancer was found for the high-dose supplement takers and men with a family history of prostate cancer (16.4 times the risk of fatal prostate cancer). Let's review the findings in a simplistic table that shows the increased risk of advanced and fatal prostate cancer for men that were "heavy" users (more than seven times per week) of multivitamins from Table 7.3.

Lower doses of vitamin E were associated with less risk of getting prostate cancer overall including (none showed statistical significance) [199]:

- 400–799 IU/day = 1.1 times higher risk
- 200–399 IU/day = 1.2 times higher risk
- 100–199 IU/day = 1.3 times higher risk
- Less than or equal to 99 IU/day = normal risk

Another concern found in the study but apparently not statistically significant was that men in the high-use multivitamin group consumed almost 100 calories more per day than the other men in the lower supplement intake groups. A piece of positive news was for the men that never took multivitamins or those that took 1–6 multivitamins a week because they experienced no increased or decreased risk. Perhaps the best news from this study that did not receive much attention was for men taking one multivitamin a

Table 7.3 Heavy use (more than seven times a week) of multivitamins and other supplement use in the NIH-AARP study that caused some concern over megadoses of these same dietary supplements, especially in those with a family history of prostate cancer

Category of dietary supplement use[a]	Risk of advanced prostate cancer	Risk of fatal prostate cancer
Heavy users of multivitamins only	1.3 times higher ($p=0.21$)	2 times higher ($p=0.65$)
Heavy users of multivitamins and taking an individual selenium supplement	1.5 times higher ($p=0.36$)	5.8 times higher ($p=0.054$)
Heavy users of multivitamins and taking a vitamin E supplement	1.3 times higher ($p=0.55$)	1.9 times higher ($p=0.62$)
Heavy users of multivitamins and taking a folic acid supplement	1.2 times higher ($p=0.63$)	2.9 times higher ($p=0.14$)
Heavy users of multivitamins and taking a beta-carotene supplement	1.7 times higher (significant, $p=0.036$)	Unknown
Heavy users of multivitamins and taking a zinc supplement	Unknown	4.4 times higher (significant, $p=0.042$)
Heavy users of multivitamins and having a family history of prostate cancer	2.5 times higher (significant, $p=0.02$)	16.5 times higher (significant, $p=0.043$)

[a]Heavy user of a multivitamin again is tantamount to more than seven multivitamin pills a week. Also of concern was the finding that men that were heavy users of multivitamins who also took individual 800 IU of vitamin E or more per day had a significant ($p=0.019$) 1.4 times higher risk of being diagnosed with prostate cancer

day, which represented the largest numbers of men followed for fatal prostate cancer in the study. Men had a 10–20 % reduced risk of fatal prostate cancer in this group—the only group to demonstrate a lower nonsignificant risk of dying from prostate cancer in this study.

Several other large male observational studies have found somewhat similar results [200, 201]. It is interesting that some studies in breast cancer has somewhat mirrored these negative findings [202, 203]. Multivitamins are also replete with higher doses of B vitamins, which have also recently been found to potentially have no impact on health or increase the risk of prostate cancer from the largest and most recent meta-analysis of clinical trials [182, 185]. Some might argue that this is all due to reverse causation, and patients with more advanced and aggressive disease are perhaps more likely to take more vitamins and minerals as witnessed with some other cancers [204]. Regardless of the side of the argument that one supports, there is no consistent suggestion of benefit with a greater intake of multivitamins, and since there is a suggestion of either no impact or serious harm, it would have been prudent to wait for more clarity from more clinical studies [205].

Perhaps some level of greater insight was provided again in the SUVIMAX randomized, placebo-controlled trial that included several vitamins and minerals at very moderate or low dosages not usually utilized in clinical trials [89] and commonly found in children's formulations from my experience (mentioned earlier in the chapter). It appeared that taking a low-dose multivitamin minimally based formula could provide a potential benefit for some men. The researchers from this study suggested that men benefited because they had lower levels of these vitamins and minerals in their blood from less than optimal dietary patterns at the beginning of the study compared to the women that consumed a more healthy diet on average. A follow-up secondary observation to this study (8.8–9 years) found that this multivitamin reduced the risk of prostate cancer by 48 % in men with a low PSA (less than 3), but in men with a higher PSA, a multivitamin may have been associated with a higher risk of being diagnosed with prostate cancer [90]. In other words, if a man has an elevated PSA he should be careful about taking dietary supplements to reduce risk. This multivitamin did not impact PSA or IGF levels, suggesting that risk was impacted by other methods. It was also interesting in this study that older age (mean age of men, 51 years), higher body mass index (BMI), and men with higher PSA levels had significantly increased risks for prostate cancer. Side effects from the low-dose multivitamin were similar to placebo. Limitations in this study were prostate cancer as a secondary endpoint and no information was collected on family history of prostate cancer. It was this trial that suggested it would be wise not to still consume anything larger than a children's multivitamin or one adult multivitamin per day until some clinical trial can demonstrate that greater intakes are beneficial.

The most definitive trial to determine the impact of multivitamins on overall male health and prostate cancer would be the result of the first ever randomized primary prevention US trial of adult men known as the "Physicians Health Study II" (PHS2) [206]. This trial would arguably provide level 1 evidence to determine whether utilizing a multivitamin has merit in men's health with regard to total cancer and cardiovascular risk. PHS2 was a randomized, double-blind, placebo-controlled trial known, which included 14,641 healthy male physicians at least 50 years or older (average age of 64.3 years) [207]. A total of 1,312 of these men had a history of cancer at baseline. The study began in 1997 and continued to June 1, 2011. Men consumed one daily multivitamin (Centrum Silver) or placebo, and the primary endpoints were the total number of cancer cases and cardiovascular events diagnosed between the multivitamin and the placebo group. Men were followed for a median of 11.2 years, and there were 2,669 men diagnosed with cancer during this study, and over half the cases (1,373) were men diagnosed with prostate cancer, and there were 210 cases of colon cancer. Men taking a multivitamin daily compared to a placebo had an 8 % reduction in being diagnosed with cancer that was statistically significant ($p=0.04$). The daily multivitamin had no positive or negative statistical impact on prostate cancer, colorectal cancer, or other major cancers. There was no significant reduction in the risk of dying from any cause including cancer when the multivitamin was compared to the placebo. However, the daily multivitamin was associated with a significant 27 % ($p=0.02$) reduction in the risk of being diagnosed with cancer in the 1,312 men with a history of cancer. The researchers of this paper concluded their article by saying "In this large prevention trial of male physicians, daily multivitamin supplementation modestly but significantly reduced the risk of total cancer." Researchers also commented profoundly in the discussion section an important clinical take-home point, which was "The reduction in total cancer risk in PHS II argues that the broader combination of low-dose vitamins and minerals contained in the PHS II multivitamin, rather than an emphasis on previously tested high-dose vitamins and mineral trials, may be paramount for cancer prevention."

There were other fascinating findings from this study. For example, the physicians utilized in this study were for the most part one of the healthiest participants of a primary prevention trial I have reviewed [207]. Only 3–4 % were current smokers, and most were near a healthy weight or BMI, 60 % exercised regularly, 80 % drank alcohol in moderation, red meat intake was low, and fruit and vegetable intake was generally 4–5 servings per day. Why didn't this multivitamin significantly lower the risk of one major type of cancer like prostate or colon cancer? The answer is that multiple cancers were nonsignificantly reduced compared to placebo, and when they were all added together the results became significant or robust enough with all the cases, but one specific cancer did not necessarily provide a large significant risk reduction. For example, although the following specific cancers never reached statistical significance, there was a reduction in risk with the multivitamin compared to placebo in cancers such as:

- Colorectal cancer = 11 % reduction
- Lung cancer = 16 % reduction
- Bladder cancer = 28 % reduction
- Leukemia = 17 % reduction
- Leukemia death = 40 % reduction (almost reached significance or $p=0.053$)

In fact, there was almost a statistically significant reduction in cancer deaths, which were reduced 12 % ($p=0.07$), but one has to ponder what would have occurred if the study were permitted to continue for several more years.

The side effect rate with the multivitamin in PHS2 was similar to placebo overall, and in terms of gastrointestinal symptoms and most other adverse events [207]. Men were more likely to report getting rashes on the multivitamin (7 % increased risk that was significant, $p=0.03$), and a 10 % significantly ($p=0.01$) higher risk of reporting epistaxis, but there was a 9 % significant ($p=0.02$) lower risk of hematuria with the multivitamin compared to the placebo. Otherwise and overall there were no side effect concerns including bleeding issues.

It was interesting that men with a personal history ("baseline history") of cancer when they began the study had a 27 % reduction in the risk of being diagnosed with another cancer ($p=0.02$), and when eliminating the men that were diagnosed with leukemia or lymphoma the risk reduction was 34 %, but the reduction in risk of prostate cancer was 44 % in these men and this almost reached significance ($p=0.07$) [207]. So, in reality it is potentially possible that some men (those with a history of being diagnosed with another cancer) may reduce their risk of being diagnosed with prostate cancer if they take a multivitamin. Men that had no history of cancer at the start of the study experienced no significant reduction (adjusted HR=1.00) in the risk of prostate cancer.

Subgroup evaluation, albeit primarily nonsignificant, also provided some interesting findings or trends; for example, men with a parental history of cancer appeared to receive no benefit ($p=0.02$ for the interaction—the only significant subgroup finding), but again those with a baseline/personal history of cancer may have received a benefit [207]. Men 70 years or older at baseline experienced an 18 % reduction in risk of cancer in the multivitamin group compared to placebo, and men that were in their 50s or 60s only received a 0–4 % reduction ($p=0.06$ for interaction). Men that were of normal BMI had a slightly better risk reduction in the multivitamin group compared to men that were overweight or obese. It is also interesting that in the small group of current smokers, there was a 28 % nonsignificant reduction in cancer risk in the multivitamin group compared to the men that smoked but received the placebo. Men consuming seven or more fruits and vegetables daily appeared to benefit slightly more compared to those that consumed less. This finding, if accurate, may address the constant question I receive in lectures, which is the need for a multivitamin (or not) based on a strong history of already consuming a healthy diet with many nutrients. Perhaps, if the multivitamin does not contain megadoses of different items there appears to be no harm. Again, this is difficult to discern and, of course, during any subgroup analysis, the possibility for chance findings increases, but still this was interesting.

The most disconcerting result of the PHS2 appeared to be the criticism in the media from some medical experts. Some conventional doctors suggested that these findings, an 8 % significant reduction in total cancer, were not adequate enough to consume a multivitamin, or alternative statistics showed no difference. Some alternative medicine experts appeared to take the position that had another more appropriate megadose multivitamin supplement been used, there would have been a more profound risk reduction. It felt as if there were a polarizing game of politics being played out with conventional and alternative medical experts. Personally, there are three critical observations that were not objectively debated, and the first was that any pill with a similar side effect of a placebo that can reduce the risk of cancer over a little more than a decade and costs the consumer minimal money, arguably pennies a day, is worth a discussion and a consideration for use. Second, as is the mantra of this book, what was the impact of this multivitamin on the number one cause of death in men and women (cardiovascular disease)? There was no impact on cardiovascular events, except there was a significant reduction in the risk of fatal myocardial infarctions with the multivitamin over the placebo [$p=0.04$], which may or may not have been due to chance because of the small number of total events of this secondary endpoint [208]. Regardless, this multivitamin passed one of my primary requirements of any CAM (heart healthy

Table 7.4 Ingredients and dosages from the multivitamin used in the PHS clinical trial (compare this to your multivitamin or the multivitamin you recommend)

Vitamin A = 5,000 IU (50 % as beta-carotene)	Vitamin B_{12} = 25 mg	Copper = 2 mg
Vitamin C = 60 mg	Biotin = 30 mg	Manganese = 3.5 mg
Vitamin D = 400 IU	Pantothenic acid = 10 mg	Chromium = 130 mg
Vitamin E = 45 IU	Calcium = 200 mg	Molybdenum = 160 mg
Vitamin K = 10 mg	Iron = 4 mg	Chloride = 72.6 mg
Vitamin B_1 = 1.5 mg	Phosphorus = 48 mg	Potassium = 80 mg
Vitamin B_2 = 1.7 mg	Iodine = 150 mg	Boron = 150 mg
Niacin = 20 mg	Magnesium = 100 mg	Nickel = 5 mg
Vitamin B_6 = 3 mg	Zinc = 15 mg	Vanadium = 10 mg
Folic acid = 400 mg	Selenium = 20 mg	Silicon = 2 mg

Note: These dosages are similar to what might appear in a children's multivitamin today or at least a very low dose adult one pill a day multivitamin

or no impact on heart health and cannot be heart unhealthy). This should give the clinician another reason to feel comfortable discussing and potential recommending this low-cost, single-pill multivitamin. Third and final is the forgotten fact that the Centrum multivitamin used in this clinical trial might surprise clinicians and patients because it was the one commercially available in the 1990s when the study started. The diverse ingredients and dosages of the multivitamin used in PHS2 can be found in Table 7.4 [207].

There appear to be few adult male or female multivitamins available in the USA today that have such low levels of the vitamins and minerals used in the PHS2. It is for this reason I believe that taking a children's multivitamin for an adult man is the only recommendation I am comfortable with currently if a man wants to utilize a multivitamin. In Table 7.4, the dosages of most ingredients are generally low that they exemplify what is found in most children's multivitamins today from my experience. Another option would be to take Centrum Silver and accept the fact that some small changes have occurred in the number of nutrients offered and the dosages. The average adult multivitamin currently in the USA could reach as many as 4–5 pills, while the children's multivitamin also increases in size. The adult multivitamin utilized in the USA when I was a teenager (Unicap from Upjohn) was the size of the children's multivitamin today and had approximately eight ingredients. Again, sizes and dosages in the USA have appeared to increase so dramatically that the PHS2 study, in my opinion, actually suggested that a children's or low-dose multivitamin is safe for men and may reduce the risk of cancer, especially in older men. Thus, currently this is how I answer or discuss the question with individuals that seek my advice on what to take if they have or have not been diagnosed with prostate cancer.

Red Yeast Rice Extract (A Statin Drug Mimic)

Personal efforts to initiate a large-scale randomized trial of cholesterol-lowering agents have been unsuccessful to date. Many designs, including the evaluation of lipid reduction for the prevention of prostate cancer in average and high-risk patients, for men with prostate cancer on active surveillance, or as a neoadjuvant or adjuvant treatment, have been proposed over the past 20 years. Minimal interest in such a trial has been due to multiple obstacles, including perceived lack of a compelling scientific rationale, concerns over unpredictable toxicity, lack of funding, corporate instability, competition from generics, and a perception that other micronutrients (vitamin E, selenium, etc.) may be of more interest [209–211].

The field of dietary supplements has evolved and offers new opportunities for clinical trials to replace some pharmacologic agents that are not readily donated or funded for clinical trials.

Red yeast rice extract (RYR) is a dietary supplement that competes with low-dose lovastatin, pravastatin, and simvastatin in terms of potency, and is a realistic alternative for statin-intolerant patients [212–216].

RYR is a traditional Chinese herbal medicine first mentioned in 800 AD in the Tang Dynasty for blood circulation [217, 218]. It is produced by the fermentation of the fungal strain Monascus purpureus Went (red yeast) over moist and sterile rice. RYR is a common dietary compound and food colorant utilized in multiple Asian countries. In China, Japan, and several other countries, it is utilized as an additive and preservative for fish and meat. It has a strong red color, flavor, and aroma; thus, it is also utilized as a flavoring product in a number of recipes and dishes, and it is also used for brewing red rice wine. RYR is also known by multiple synonyms as a food product, including Hong Qu, Hung-Chu, Ang-kak, Ankak rice, Red Mold Rice, and Beni-Koji. It is also known as "xuezhikang" as a dietary supplement intervention in the medical literature.

Dr. Akira Endo found in the late 1970s that a Monascus yeast strain naturally produced a substance that inhibits cholesterol synthesis to block cell wall synthesis of bacterial intruders and named it "monacolin K" [219]. This compound was later isolated and is now known to be of the same molecular structure as lovastatin, the first marketed statin drug. Thus, theoretically RYR is the first known statin used in medical history. Like RYR, a fungus, three of the first prescribed statins utilized in the USA were derived from fungi (lovastatin, pravastatin, and simvastatin) [212, 220]. The amount of monacolin K in any capsule should equate to the amount of lovastatin it contains. For example, if a patient utilizes three capsules from a commercial product that contains 2.5 μg of monacolin K per capsule, then 7.5 μg lovastatin equivalent could be expected in terms of LDL reductions. There are at least 10 identified monacolins in RYR (K, J, JA, K, KA, L, LA, M, X, and XA).

Unlike numerous dietary supplements or CAM products, RYR has a vast amount of clinical data that would arguably give it FDA approval if it were treated as a drug. A meta-analysis of over 9,600 patients in 93 randomized trials involving three different commercial variants of RYR was published [221]. The mean reduction in total cholesterol, LDL, triglyceride, and increase in HDL was, respectively, the following: −35 μg/dL (−0.91 mmol/L), −28 μg/dL (−0.73 mmol/L), −36 μg/dL (−0.41 mmol/L), and +6 μg/dL (+0.15 mmol/L).

Xuezhikang was the commercial RYR product evaluated in a large, randomized, placebo-controlled clinical trial with robust endpoints [222, 223]. The China Coronary Secondary Prevention Study (CCSPS) enrolled 4,870 participants (3,986 men, 884 women) with a previous myocardial infarction (MI) and a baseline mean total cholesterol, LDL, triglyceride, and HDL of approximately 208 μg/dL (5.38 mmol/L), 129 μg/dL (3.34 mmol/L), 165 μg/dL (1.85 mmol/L), and 46 μg/dL (1.19 mmol/L). Subjects received RYR 600 μg twice daily (1,200 μg total, monacolin K 2.5–3.2 μg/capsule) or matching placebo and followed for 4.5 years. The trial was conducted from May 1996 to December 2003 in 65 hospitals in China. The primary endpoint was nonfatal MI or death from coronary or cardiac causes. Secondary endpoints included total mortality from CV disease, total all-cause mortality, need for coronary revascularization procedure, and alterations in lipid levels. Fasting blood samples were drawn at baseline, 6–8 weeks after randomization, and at 6-month intervals. The mean LDL reduction compared to placebo was 18 % ($p<0.001$).

Two interim analyses occurred, and the second one demonstrated a significant difference for the primary endpoint [222, 223]. A total of 98 % of the participants completed the study. Multiple clinical endpoints were significantly reduced with the exception of a nonsignificant reduction in fatal MI. Lipids were significantly reduced as well as a 56 and 33 % reduced cancer mortality ($p=0.01$) and all-cause mortality ($p=0.0003$). Potential anticancer benefits found in the overall trial with RYR were also found among the elderly (significant reduction in cancer deaths) [26, 36] and included a 51 % reduction in cancer incidence [224]. No serious adverse events were observed during this trial. Total adverse events and treatment cessation numbers were similar for RYR and placebo. The number needed to treat

(NNT) to prevent a primary endpoint over the 4.5 year duration of the trial is 21, which compares with any prevention trial (primary or secondary).

Laboratory studies suggest that RYR has direct effects on androgen-dependent LNCaP cells and androgen-independent cells over expressing androgen receptors [225]. RYR inhibited prostate cancer growth compared to a prescription lovastatin. And whole RYR inhibited proliferation to a greater extent than monacolin K and pigment-enriched fractions isolated from RYR ($p<0.001$). This suggests that other monacolins or ingredients apart from monacolin K in RYR may also have activity against prostate cancer. RYR also significantly reduced androgen-dependent and androgen-independent xenograft tumors in SCID mice ($p<0.05$) [226]. Intact whole RYR again provided more inhibition than monacolin K alone. RYR also significantly ($p<0.05$) reduced gene expression of several androgen-synthesizing enzymes (AKR1C3, HSD3B2, and SRD5A1) in both androgen-dependent and androgen-independent tumors. A significant ($p<0.001$) correlation was observed between tumor volume and serum cholesterol. Identical findings have been demonstrated in colon cancer cell lines [227]. RYR has pleiotropic actions on a variety of pathways and markers beyond LDL cholesterol [228–231], which is similar to statin drugs and could have an impact on prostate cancer proliferation and progression [232, 233].

The active surveillance (formerly known as "watchful waiting") population is ideal for an initial prostate cancer clinical trial of RYR [108, 234, 235]. Repeat biopsy, PSA kinetic data, and even imaging can be achieved without the interference of other treatments. Such a trial has been initiated in Toronto, Canada, by this author and Dr. Laurence H. Klotz, MD, and is known as "REALITY" (Reduction in Active Surveillance Lipid Indices Through Yeast of red rice). Men will receive 3,600 μg daily of RYR with a potency of monacolin K that is approximately 2.5 μg per capsule (600 μg of RYR per capsule) based on previous clinical trials. It is expected that compliant participants will experience a 20–35 % LDL reduction [236, 237]. Active surveillance patients will be followed for at least 1 year and have at least two biopsies in this 12-month period. Level of LDL is not predictive for response, and therefore will not be an eligibility or inclusion criterion.

Quality control (QC) with RYR is an issue that needs to be considered [238, 239]. Different commercial products of RYR have different concentrations of monacolins. Some contain a potentially harmful by-product of yeast fermentation known as "citrinin" [239]. Obviously, citrinin needs to be eliminated and monacolin K specifically reported for any clinician to feel comfortable utilizing this product for clinical trials or just patient care. The irony in the U SA currently is that manufacturers of RYR are not allowed to standardize monacolin K levels because it suggests a drug mimic, which the FDA could enforce. This ruling makes little sense because it only confuses the clinician and patient when trying to find a suitable alternative to statin drugs.

Contraindications for RYR should be at least identical to lovastatin, including hepatic or renal abnormalities, and allergies to yeast or fungus. RYR should be taken with or especially after meals, since lovastatin absorption is significantly improved under these circumstances [240–242]. Higher concentrated fiber sources such as pectin or oat bran should not be consumed with RYR because of the potential for the reduced absorption of monacolin K.

Overall, RYR has been a safe product in clinical trials and could be a good proxy for statins in a prostate prevention or ancillary treatment trial. Hopefully, more agents that mimic potentially effective prescription drugs will be available in the near future. The need is great because safe chemoprevention of prostate cancer, for example, appears to have hit stasis. And other agents for neoadjuvant or adjuvant use are costly and have their own set of toxicity issues.

Vitamin C (Ascorbic Acid)

Vitamin C supplements at a dosage of 500 μg compared to placebo were found to be safe in a large randomized US trial primarily addressing this issue, but it did not have any impact on prostate cancer risk [84]. This clinical trial ended any excitement for vitamin C as a stand-alone prostate cancer preventive agent. On the other hand, there has always been interest in vitamin C given in IV form in megadoses to cancer patients because in the alternative medicine arena this is not uncommon. One of the first ever phase 1 dose-escalating trial of IV vitamin C to determine if it is safe and if it could inhibit the growth of cancer cells in 24 patients with advanced forms of certain cancers was already published [243]. This was a safety and tolerability study using cohorts that were sequentially infused with 0.4, 0.6, 0.9, and 1.5 g vitamin C/kg body weight three times a week over a 90- to 120-min period. Patients had normal renal function. The average duration of treatment was 10 weeks with a maximum of 30 weeks. Median age was 61 and 24 patients with advanced tumors that had originated from various localized sites (breast, head and neck, liver, lung, lymphoma, ovarian, pancreatic prostate, renal, sarcoma, etc.) were included. No patients had an objective treatment response and all patients eventually progressed. There was a suggestion of physical quality-of-life maintenance for patients that completed this study. The recommended phase II dose will be 1.5 g/kg along with first-line chemotherapy for advanced stage non–small cell lung cancer based on safety and practicality. Intravenous vitamin C given in large doses appeared to be safe and free of toxic effects, including kidney stones, but provided no treatment impact by itself. Perhaps in combination with conventional therapies, and used earlier in the course of the disease, there may be a better chance of a treatment response or simply a quality-of-life response. The impact of these IV vitamin C treatments on increasing oxalate levels and kidney stone risk is controversial [244], and with the dietary supplements in large doses there is a realistic concern in the healthy patients at doses of 1,000 μg or more [245].

One option is to switch to a calcium ascorbate oral form of vitamin C (ascorbic acid) for patients that want to take oral vitamin C [4]. Our past research suggested a minimal or reduced oxalate change in the pill form (it was not tested in an IV form). Yet in individuals with advanced cancer, the argument over oxalate should not be as paramount as whether or not there is a quality or quantity of life benefit. This question needs to be further answered because these infusions are usually not of a low cost to the patient from my observational experience. Case studies abound in terms of potential benefits in select cancer patients [246], but strong clinical research has not yet supported the routine use of this method in most cancer patients. More answers in this area are really needed now, but currently the decision should be between the patient and the clinician he or she trusts until more research is conducted.

Vitamin D and/or Calcium

Vitamin D appears to have as many issues as multivitamins or any other dietary supplement for prostate cancer when some clinicians and patients want to believe that more is better. The tendency for patients to ingest higher amounts of this supplement is enticing, but in the area of prostate cancer vitamin D has not been consistently impressive, and several studies of no impact or potential harm have been demonstrated at higher blood levels [247]. Vitamin D is important for bone health, but the amount needed has been embellished and exaggerated. Vitamin D tends to mimic the function of a hormone, which is why caution should be followed because the potential for a U-shaped risk curve does exist (similar to alcohol and other hormones) for male health [248]. Perhaps indirect evidence is providing some clues because one of the largest and longest randomized trials in women found that excessively high blood levels of vitamin D from supplementation compared to placebo were actually associated with an increased risk of falls and fractures [249]. The normal level of vitamin D should arguably be from 30 to 40 ng/mL (75–100 nmol/L) based on expert opinion from a review of past clinical trials accessing multiple outcomes [250]. A total of 1,000 IU (25 μg) of vitamin D is adequate to increase blood levels of vitamin D over time (5–10 ng/mL or more over 6–12 months), and a suggestion of outright deficiency (less than 10 ng/mL or 25 nmol/L) from consistent reliable blood testing may lead to slightly greater intakes. However, even vitamin D blood tests have a history of uncertainty based on the assay utilized (RIA, ELISA, HPLC, etc.) [251, 252]. Monitoring vitamin D in men, especially higher-risk bone loss patients—for example, men on ADT for prostate cancer—may be appropriate, but in general for men's health the vitamin D test may provide more harm than good until more tangible clinical endpoints are followed in healthy individuals [252, 253]. Even a large-scale high-dose trial (100,000 IU in general over 18 months) to prevent upper respiratory tract infections in otherwise healthy adults showed no benefit over placebo [254]. Perhaps it was the lack of patients with deficient levels that caused these findings, or it could be that vitamin D blood levels are simply a marker of healthy behavior rather than this vitamin's impact itself [4]. A young, lean individual, with no prediabetes or diabetes, a low cholesterol, and who consumes fish and exercises outside regularly is more likely to have a higher blood level of vitamin D compared to an older, physically inactive obese or prediabetic or diabetic man with a high cholesterol level [4, 255–259]. One of the best indicators of a lower vitamin D level is weight gain because vitamin D remains in adipose tissue instead of blood circulation. So, is it really the vitamin D supplement providing the majority of the benefit for men's health or the finding that higher vitamin D levels could be found on average in more healthy men? I believe it is more of the latter observation, but this does not imply that individuals with overt deficiency would not benefit from supplementation.

Again, the highest concentration of vitamin D is found in some of the heart-healthiest fish, so patients receive a dual benefit by consuming fish high in omega-3 compounds and vitamin D such as salmon. Wild salmon contains as much as three times the amount of vitamin D compared to farmed salmon [260]. Patients inquiring about the differences and similarities between farmed and wild fish should be given an objective review. Both types of fish are high in omega-3 fatty acids, which are heart healthy, and both tend to have a low level of mercury and other environmental contaminants in some studies [261], but contamination standards for farmed salmon need to be more stringent and transparent. Both types of fish are generally healthy to consume, and the demand and cost for fish globally cannot be sustained without farmed fish becoming another viable option.

Patients and clinicians often suggest that individuals residing in areas with more sun exposure experience higher blood levels of vitamin D. Theoretically, this makes sense, of course, but has not been substantiated through past research that has demonstrated low or insufficient blood levels of vitamin D in people residing in Florida and southern Arizona [262, 263]. Yet, these mean blood levels of between 20 and 30 ng/mL are encouraging. Perhaps regular sun avoidance via clothing, wide brimmed hats, aging, and obesity are both independently or synergistically involved in lowering vitamin D levels in some of these geographic areas.

Fortification of some foods and beverages have not yet been an immediate solution to the vitamin D deficiency rates, and recent studies suggest that the regular daily intake of vitamin D in older individuals may increase blood levels greater than weekly or monthly oral intakes of equivalent doses [264]. Keep in mind that the ongoing excitement and enthusiasm for vitamin D, in my opinion, will translate into an overcompensation of vitamin D added to food and beverage products in the next few years. Again, another reason to encourage following moderate and evidence-based intakes of this vitamin or the less is more philosophy as the hype exceeds the expectations.

There are two forms (vitamin D_2 or ergocalciferol and vitamin D_3 or cholecalciferol) of vitamin D that the clinician should be familiar with, and both are generally low cost and are adequate, but vitamin D_3 is the one humans synthesize when exposed to UVB light [4]. Vitamin D_2 is a plant or a fungus/yeast-derived product, and it is synthetically produced from radiating a compound (ergosterol) from the mold ergot [256, 265]. Vitamin D_3 is produced commercially and synthetically in a similar method that it utilized to synthesize intrinsically in human and animal skin when exposed to UVB light. Wool sources of 7-dehydrocholesterol are used (from cholesterol) and irradiated to produce active vitamin D_3. Vegetarians and vegans may choose not to utilize vitamin D_3 supplements because it is derived from an animal source and understandably should then be directed toward vitamin D_2. Some companies are currently trying to produce a plant-derived vitamin D_3. Multivitamins have either vitamin D_2 or D_3, but many companies are now utilizing primarily vitamin D_3. Cod liver oil supplements contain vitamin D_3.

A historical note and other commentary should place vitamin D megadosing in perspective. Rickets, a defect in bone growth in infancy and childhood, was first identified in 1650 [266]. It was not until 1922 that medical research demonstrated that a compound in cod liver oil prevented and cured this condition. Vitamin D_2 was also created and added to milk in the USA and Europe in the 1930s that essentially eliminated rickets or osteomalacia. Currently, fortification with vitamin D_2 or D_3 has continued to keep rickets an anomaly in North America. The minimum amount of vitamin D needed to prevent rickets is 100 IU (2.5 μg) per day in infants with minimal to no sun exposure.

Historically, 400 IU (10 µg) of vitamin D was recommended for better health because it closely approximated the amount of vitamin D in a teaspoonful of cod liver oil [267].

The latest Institute of Medicine (IOM) guidelines on vitamin D only increased suggested intakes from 400 to 600 to 800 IU (800 IU in ages 70+) for adults because of the concern for toxicity (e.g., hypercalcemia, hypercalciuria, nephrolithiasis) and the lack of profound data to advocate for higher amounts [268, 269]. It is also for this reason I generally do not recommend more than 1,000 IU/day, and this is the dosage that more commonly achieves a blood level of 30–40 ng/mL over a long period of time (6–12 months) [270, 271]. Perhaps the IOM report will be completely correct in the near future because again with the excess of vitamin D being added to foods, multivitamins, and calcium supplements, I will have to adopt the 600–800 IU IOM standard in the near future. Healthcare professionals need to keep in mind that in general, 100 IU (2.5 μg) of vitamin D_3 per day can raise the vitamin D blood test 1 ng/mL or just 2.5 nmol/L after 2–3 months, regardless of age [272, 273]. Vitamin D_2 is less predictable and produces approximately half or more of the response rate compared to vitamin D_3 in the elderly [272], which again is another reason to encourage vitamin D_3 intake if there are no issues with animal-derived products.

Over the past few decades, the "normal" blood level of vitamin D or 25-OH vitamin D was based on the amount required to keep parathyroid hormone (PTH) from becoming abnormally elevated [256]. However, PTH can vary based on renal function, exercise level, time of day, and even diet. There has been no consensus on the optimal level of vitamin D intake to reduce PTH, and this is why laboratories report a wide normal range of vitamin D such as 20–40 ng/mL or 50–100 nmol. This is a large variation. Again, a consistent clinical numerical answer of a blood level of vitamin D in the range of 30–40 ng/mL was found (ideally they reported 36–40 ng/mL, but this is too narrow for clinical purposes) [250].

Why not extend the ideal laboratory values of normalcy well beyond 30–40 ng/mL? If no acute toxicity (hypercalcemia/hypercalciuria) is associated with blood levels of 70 or 80 ng/mL and higher, or only 500 nmol/L or more than 20,000 IU of vitamin D per day causes adverse events [274], then why not recommend higher blood levels? Higher must be better? More must be better? This simply cannot be the case, and no history lesson is needed here if the reader has already covered this book or chapter replete with the plethora of examples in and out of urology that more is not better. In fact, there is even a suggestion from several epidemiological studies and reviews that long-term significant increases in vitamin D could be detrimental and increase the risk of prostate cancer and more aggressive disease, perhaps by downregulating vitamin D receptors needed for cellular differentiation (megadoses of calcium may have the same impact) [275–280].

Thus, most patients do not need vitamin D testing, with the potential exception of ADT patients in some cases where profound deficiency is suspected. A total of 1,000 IU per day for 6–12 months is needed in most cases and is safe. There is no strong suggestion that vitamin D prevents prostate cancer or the progression of this disease and in fact may encourage tumor growth at high doses. In the meantime, it should be clearly explained to patients that vitamin D is necessary for bone health and is important for muscle coordination, balance, strength, and reducing body sway, and it is for these reasons it may also prevent falls and fractures [281–284]. Yet, it is just as important to know that resistance exercise may work as well or even better to increase bone mineral density and reduce fractures [285]. In fact, novel randomized studies are preliminarily suggesting that many men and perhaps women may not need calcium and vitamin D supplementation if they regularly perform aerobic and resistance exercise [286, 287]. It is, of course, my hope that this finding can be definitely proven one day soon.

What About Calcium?

First I agree with the latest IOM report that men and women really do not require more than roughly 1,000–1,200 μg of calcium per day total (from food and supplements) [268, 269]. It is for this reason men need to calculate their average daily intake of calcium from food with the help of a reputable Internet site, or more ideally a nutritionist. If 1,000 μg/day is already being achieved with food, then higher intakes can be associated with toxicity from hypercalcemia, hypercalciuria, calcification of blood vessels, kidney stones, and other concerns. Men need calcium, but higher amounts from supplements have raised serious issues of an increased risk of cardiovascular events [288], which is preliminarily suggestive but not proven. Yet, does it matter that clinicians wait for more evidence? Not really, because more has not been proven to be better, but normalization of intake is best. Every man concerned about bone health should be told to print out the top food sources of calcium from an Internet site and place it on the refrigerator door (yogurt, milk, fortified soy, almond milk, kale, cheese, etc.) [4].

There is a concern with a higher risk or progression of prostate cancer with higher calcium intakes. This has not only been preliminarily found for calcium from dietary sources, but calcium supplements [289, 290]. These concerning past studies have found a concern primarily for individuals with higher than recommended intakes (for example >2,000 μg/day). And, excessive calcium intakes tend to be a marker for unhealthy behaviors and greater caloric intakes. Are there any data from randomized trials that suggests a concern for prostate cancer patients? Researchers directing one of the largest calcium supplement trials to reduce colon polyps published their findings on prostate cancer risk [291]. The original clinical trial began in 1988 and randomly assigned 930 (total of 672 men) individuals to receive 1,200 μg a day of calcium carbonate or placebo for 4 years. No patients had a history of prostate cancer in the study. The male participants in this study had the following features: mean age, PSA, and time of calcium supplementation were 62 years, 1.8 ng/mL, and 44 months (3.5–4 years), and there was 10 years of follow-up. A total of 24 prostate cancers were diagnosed during the 4-year treatment phase, and 46 cases of prostate cancer were diagnosed during the 6-year follow-up after the trial. Average Gleason score was 6, and 11 tumors were diagnosed as non-localized. The risk of prostate cancer was reduced approximately 2 years after the calcium supplement study commenced and also significantly persisted approximately 2 years after the treatment ended. The conclusion of the authors was the following: "In this randomized controlled clinical trial, there was no increase in prostate cancer risk associated with calcium supplementation and some suggestion of a protective effect." Interestingly, one of the only other randomized trials to access calcium supplementation was the Prostate Cancer Prevention Trial (PCPT) that found a significant reduction in PSA velocity in men taking calcium supplements, and no other dietary supplement was found to possess this potential activity [292]. Obviously, more research is needed, but some men need to take calcium supplements for bone health because they are receiving inadequate amounts from dietary sources, and this could provide an ancillary benefit. One needs to be careful of the continuous addition of calcium in dietary sources, so supplementation should be reserved for those that simply cannot achieve normalized intakes from diet.

Men on ADT for prostate cancer treatment need more attention than most urologic patients because of the increased risk of accelerated bone loss. Whether or not men are also consuming adequate levels of calcium regardless of prostate cancer status has not been adequately researched. A cross-sectional study of 372 men with prostate cancer and without bone metastases was conducted [293]. Approximately 72 % were receiving ADT and 28 % had a radical prostatectomy with no ADT. Daily calcium intake was assessed with a questionnaire and bone mineral density (BMD) was also assessed through dual-energy X-ray absorptiometry (DEXA) at the lumbar spine and hip. An abnormal daily calcium intake was defined as less than 1,000 μg a day and was found in 93 % of the men regardless of treatment status. Osteoporosis was identified in approximately 50 % of the men (55 % receiving ADT and 35 % after surgery). The average daily calcium intake was significantly ($p < 0.001$) lower and approximately 610 μg in those men with osteoporosis compared to 683 μg in those without this condition. In a multivariate analysis, daily calcium intake was an independent risk factor for osteoporosis along with patient age and ADT and length of time on this treatment. This would suggest that a lack of adequate calcium intake is an issue in many prostate cancer patients. This is concerning because the risk of bone mineral density (BMD) reductions increase with the duration of the treatment [294]. One study from North America found that only 18 % of patients on ADT actually received calcium and vitamin D recommendations when initiating ADT [295].

Men need to be told to approximate their dietary daily intake of calcium, also keeping in mind that calcium is found in many multivitamins. If they are receiving close to 1,000–1,200 μg/day from diet there is no need for supplementation. Otherwise if their dietary intake falls short, they can try and increase it and/or add a calcium supplement. It should also be of interest to men and women that there is some randomized trial research to suggest that normalizing calcium intakes can reduce the risk of colon polyps and colon cancer [296, 297], and in urology normalizing calcium intake, especially from food sources, has strong data from a large randomized trial for the reduction of recurrent nephrolithiasis [298].

Zinc

Overall, past studies have demonstrated the potential for high doses of zinc to increase prostate carcinoma risk and potential raise the risk of a variety of adverse events (see BPH CAM Chapter 3) [2, 299], but perhaps one of the most detailed epidemiologic investigations to implicate large intakes of zinc supplements as one apparent etiology of prostate cancer was published [300]. This research was taken from the Health Professionals Follow-Up Study. A total of approximately 47,000 US men participated in this prospective investigation. During 14 years of follow-up, a total of 2,901 new cases of prostate cancer were recorded and 434 of these cases were diagnosed as advanced prostate cancer. Researchers found zinc supplement doses equal to or less than 100 μg/day were not related to a risk of prostate cancer. However, compared to nonusers of these supplements, men that ingested greater than 100 μg/day of zinc supplements per day had a significantly increased risk of being diagnosed with advanced prostate cancer (RR = 2.29). Additionally, men that consumed zinc supplements for 10 or more years also had a significantly higher risk of being diagnosed with advanced prostate cancer (RR = 2.37). In this cohort, approximately 32 % of the total zinc intake was from dietary supplements, which represented the largest source of zinc. Other sources, which were much lower, were from beef (11 %) and breakfast cereals (5 %). However, zinc from food sources was not related to prostate cancer risk. Men consuming zinc supplements also consumed more supplemental calcium, multivitamins, vitamin E supplements, lycopene, iron, copper, folate, and fish, but consumed less red meat and were less likely to have had a history of prostate-specific antigen (PSA) screening compared to nonusers of zinc supplements. Researchers also attempted to identify any other confounding factors in this study. One analysis restricted the study population to men reporting lower levels of calcium supplement intake and adjusting for intakes of iron, copper, folate, BPH, and other factors, but this had no impact on the final observations. Therefore, zinc supplements themselves were still the most likely etiology from this study.

Other epidemiologic work has been mixed on the subject, but the concern for toxicity has been fairly persistent [2, 299]. An older phase 3 randomized trial for macular degeneration found an increased risk of genitourinary hospitalizations for men taking 80 μg or more of zinc [301, 302], but a follow-up to this study did not [77]. Regardless, it takes minimal zinc to normalize blood levels (10–15 μg) and persistent higher or megadosages (40 μg and higher) could create a copper deficiency-generated anemia unless copper is of course supplemented [4]. The future of high-dose zinc supplementation for prostate cancer prevention in nonsmokers or former smokers in my opinion appears nonexistent. Additionally, it is important to appreciate that low zinc levels could be a marker for less optimum health, which is why it is fairly common in obesity or tobacco use, and perhaps other comorbidities [303]. Low-dose zinc may have a future in medicine, for example, for eye health [77] or for common cold treatment [304], but again the concern will always revolve around detrimental health changes with high doses of zinc.

Miscellaneous: PSA Doubling Times and Dietary/Supplement Interventions, Pomegranate Juice, and ADT and Other Options

Covering all nutrients and supplements that have received some laboratory or clinical research would require more than one text. However, there are a few interesting nutrients or supplements that deserve some brief review in prostate cancer. For example, pomegranate juice and/or dietary supplement extract. One older human study that received a tremendous amount of attention is a two-stage clinical study of men with rising PSA following surgery or radiation therapy [305]. Patients had a PSA of greater than 0.2 or less than 5 ng/mL and a Gleason score of 7 or less. Each patient had at least three PSA values over at least 6 months before the study began, so that PSA doubling time could be assessed. Patients were instructed to drink 8 ounces of pomegranate juice daily. The pomegranates in this study were hand-picked, washed, chilled (to 4 °C) and stored. The fruit was crushed, squeezed, and treated with the enzyme pectinase to liberate the juice and other products, which utilized the inner and outer peels and the actual seeds of the fruit.

Pomegranate juice is known for its compounds known as "polyphenols," and a subclass of these compounds is known as the flavonoids such as anthocyanins, catechins, and phenols, which make up 40 % of the total polyphenols in the juice [4, 305, 306]. For example, another popular flavonoid known as "quercetin" is also found in this fruit. The polyphenols found in the highest concentration and potency is "punicalagin," which is an ellagitannin (similar to ellagic acid) that is apparently also responsible for the majority of the antioxidant capacity of the juice.

Finally, the juice in this study was filtered, pasteurized, concentrated, and stored (at −20 °C) until it was needed in the study [305]. The authors of this study also reported that each 8-ounce drink of pomegranate juice contained "570 μg total polyphenol gallic acid equivalents." This study recruited 48 patients over a 13-month period in two stages, but 2 patients left the study before the first evaluation, so 46 patients were evaluated for the treatment response, and out of these patients:

- 68 % were originally treated with radical prostatectomy
- 10 % treated with external beam radiation
- 10 % with seed implants
- 7 % with surgery and radiation
- 5 % with cryotherapy

At the beginning of the study, the average PSA was 2.23 ng/mL (±2.58 ng/mL), and the median PSA was 1.05 ng/mL. A total of 94 % of these patients had a Gleason score of 5–7, and 6 % had a Gleason score of 4. An "objective response" in this study was considered a PSA reduction of 50 % or more from the highest PSA value. A "progressive disease" was considered a 100 %

increase in PSA (from a minimum potential value of 1.0 ng/mL) compared to the best observed PSA, or it is also defined as anyone having recurrence or advanced prostate cancer during the study. If a patient had a "stable disease" then they could not qualify for having an objective or progressive disease.

Why was this study considered a two-stage study by the authors [305]? Here is the reason:

- Stage 1—A total of 24 patients are treated with the 8 ounces of pomegranate juice per day, and if more than 1 patient had an objective response or stable disease, then another 22 patients would be treated for a total of 46 patients.
- Stage 2—This stage would end after all the 46 patients were treated, and after this stage if less than 4 patients had an objective response, the pomegranate juice treatment would be considered "ineffective." However, if four or more patients had an objective response, then the response rate of 20 % considered by the authors to be the effective rate would be enough to encourage further testing of pomegranate juice in a phase 3 randomized trial.

It is also interesting how the researchers decided on 8 ounces of pomegranate juice a day compared to any other amount. The authors mention in the paper that the dose was based on the antioxidant effect in studying human males at the following daily doses: 0 ounces (0 mL), 3 ounces (90 mL), 6 ounces (180 mL), 8 ounces (240 mL), 12 ounces (360 mL), and 15 ounces (450 mL). The authors state that the results of these studies that are "not published" demonstrated that the intake of pomegranate juice by healthy males shows a slow but increasing antioxidant capacity with an increasing dose from 0 to 15 ounces for 1 week. The researchers then mention that based on these findings of a significant "clinical antioxidant effect and with no significant effect on serum triglycerides and glucose," they chose the dosage of 6–8 ounces (180–240 mL) as the "optimal dosage." This is interesting because I believe the high caloric and sugar content of this juice is enough to raise triglycerides and blood sugar if one ingests too much. In other words, the one potential drawback with some of these high-antioxidant juices like pomegranate is the approximately 140–160 calories a day for some products with just 8 ounces of the juice. This is a large amount of calories compared to other juices, and, for example, compared to a cola drink, which is about 100 calories per 8 ounces. In fact, I decided to purchase a number of juices at the local grocery and health food stores in my neighborhood, and a comparison of calories reveals that very few juices have as many calories or even alcoholic drinks have as many calories.

The results were quite interesting and should be discussed with patients [305]. In stage 1 of the study, a total of 24 patients received 8 ounces of pomegranate juice per day, and 2 patients ended up having an objective response, with a PSA reduction of 85 and 50 %. The first responder took 6 months to respond and then had the large reduction, which did not return to "peak" value until 21 months. The second responder continues to have a 57 % reduction in "peak" PSA at almost 3 years after the study (33 months). So, this fits the criteria just barely to go on to stage 2, because remember the researchers wanted more than one objective responder in stage 1 and since a total of two responses occurred they moved on to stage 2.

The manuscript also mentioned "…6 of the first 24 patients progressed by PSA criteria" [305]. This is concerning because this means 25 % of the patients experienced progression. So there were more PSA failures than responders in the first stage of the study. When combining the entire group of 46 patients, the following results were published:

- 35 % (16 patients) of the patients had a reduction in PSA, and the average reduction was 27 % with a range of 5–85 % (median reduction of 18 %).
- Four patients had objective responses (PSA reduction of more than 50 %), which met the authors' criteria of having pomegranate juice tested in a phase 3 study. Remember, if less than four patients had a response the juice would be declared "ineffective" for patients in this specific situation, so it barely met these criteria by having just four responders.
- The authors discussed PSA doubling time and the impact of the juice on this situation. A total

of 28 patients had enough data for analysis at this point. Also, the authors discuss other time points and improvements in PSA doubling times. However, the most impressive finding is the 33-month time point of the study, which showed an average PSA doubling time of 54.7 ± 102 months (median 28.7 months) with the juice compared to the doubling time of the 42 patients before the juice which was 15.6 ± 10.8 months (median 11.5 months). A difference that was statistically very significant ($p<0.001$). A total of 83 % of the patients had an improvement in PSA doubling time during the study ($p<0.0001$), but the baseline stage of the patient's prostate cancer demonstrated "some correlation" with the altered PSA doubling time, but this finding did not reach statistical significance. The authors of the study also reported that there were no side effects with pomegranate juice, and no patient developed metastatic disease, which would have been unusual in most of these patients after only a few years after recurrence with such a low PSA.

The juice was also tested in the lab against a human prostate cell line (LnCaP) and significantly reduced cell growth and increased cell death and significantly increased levels of a potentially healthy compound (nitric oxide) and functioned as an antioxidant [305]. Yet, it must be kept in mind that this study used no placebo group or control group. In other words, these men were only compared to themselves which is a concern, because recent placebo studies of men with rising PSA after treatment have found an improvement in doubling times in as many as 70 % of the men taking a sugar pill. Additionally, I have always been concerned about a treatment that is believed to be effective with no side effects. Regardless, these researchers provided a lot of information in this one study to ponder, and along with other studies on pomegranate juice, it is time to summarize some overall thoughts on pomegranate juice for the readers in terms of a potential good and bad news scenario.

If a PSA doubling time changes after surgery or radiation failure, for example, does this really have any meaning? One strong area of research to highlight the benefits and detriments of PSA doubling time probably is derived from the University of Pittsburgh School of Medicine along with Johns Hopkins researchers and others [307]. This research group utilized 209 patients (started with 222) that had a rising PSA after surgery was completed for localized prostate cancer. Men had to have a PSA between 0.4 and 5 ng/mL with a PSA doubling time of equal to or less than 12 months based on two PSA values at least 2 weeks apart. There were 107 patients given a placebo and 102 patients given a 10 μg once a day oral experimental drug known as "atrasentan" (failed to achieve FDA approval for castrate-resistant prostate cancer). The baseline PSA value or the PSA number right before this study began was lower in the placebo group (average of 1.4 ng/mL) compared to the drug group (average of 1.8 ng/mL), and this difference was statistically significant ($p=0.012$). When the patients were compared during treatment they had at least three PSA values to compare, and the researchers collected blood and acquired a PSA every 12 weeks for 1 year. During the clinical trial, there was no difference in PSA doubling time (PSADT) between the placebo and drug group ($p=0.363$). The percentage of patients with a PSADT of greater than 1 year was 55 % with the placebo and 51 % with the drug! However, what was really interesting was the finding that PSADT increased for most patients on either side of the study (drug or placebo). Here is a summary of these findings:

- A total of 76 out of 107 patients taking placebo or 71 % of placebo patients had an improved PSADT.
- A total of 68 out of 102 patients or 64 % of the treated patients had an improved PSADT.
- PSA velocity also increased or improved significantly in both the placebo ($p<0.001$) and drug-treated ($p=0.017$) groups. The authors of this study concluded their presentation by stating, "The fact that over 70 % of patients receiving placebo experienced lengthened PSADT suggests that, in the absence of a control arm, changes in PSADT from baseline are not a reliable measure of treatment effect in trials in early prostate cancer. PSADT data from trials in this population should be interpreted with caution."

In other words, unless there is a comparison group of individuals in a study of PSADT to determine the effect of a treatment, it is really difficult to determine how effective this treatment really is in any situation [307]. Another issue concerning PSADT is that perhaps it is a great predictor of prognosis if one has the luxury of follow-up time and PSA values [308]. It is difficult to determine the impact of PSADT unless adequate time has elapsed to give a clinician some idea as to what the average PSADT really is in the patient's specific situation. Another study from Johns Hopkins and others highlights this issue. Researchers completed a retrospective study of 379 patients treated with a radical prostatectomy between 1982 and the year 2000 that experienced a PSA recurrence or a rising PSA sometime after surgery. The median follow-up after PSA recurrence was 11 years. Interestingly, men with a PSADT of greater than 15 months were more likely to die of non-prostate cancer causes compared to men with worse PSADT (less than 15 months) where the primary cause of death (90 % of patients) was prostate cancer. Thus, PSADT is one of many measurements that allow clinicians and patients to learn more about prognosis, especially if the patient has been followed for long periods of time and has had numerous PSA levels.

Pomegranate juice and dietary supplement extract appear preliminarily promising, but until it is actually compared to something such as a placebo, tomato juice, or a drug in a clinical trial, it is difficult to determine efficacy. This is also true of a recent two-dose pomegranate dietary supplement that exhibited similar effects on PSA doubling time that were significant [309], but since there was no placebo group and since high and low doses exhibited similar impacts, it could be argued that it would work no better than placebo. However, the other side of the argument is the improvement in doubling time demonstrates these supplements have efficacy. These are the issues when no control or placebo group exists. Still, the researchers and manufacturers of pomegranate should be given credit for funding these studies and utilizing some research to support some of their claims, but this has also come with controversy. My concern with most studies of concentrated high caloric juices is that it adds too many calories to an already worsening obesity epidemic, so patients should be instructed to either wait for the results of a long-term placebo trial or utilize the capsules at 1,000 μg a day [309], because of the smaller or really minimal caloric contribution. In my opinion, anytime a vegetable and especially a fruit is processed, the consumer has a higher probability of spending more money, getting more calories and not necessarily the same nutrition or fiber that could promote weight loss, but in fact weight or waist gain. Thus, if one believes in the pomegranate or any juice data, examine the possibility of dilution or a low caloric option and many of these manufacturers offer these options.

Does sexual activity have an impact on the risk of prostate cancer? This is a question often asked but rarely studied. Researchers wanted to answer this question from one of the largest prospective epidemiologic studies in the USA [310]. This study comes from information taken during the ongoing Health Professionals Follow-up Study (HPFS) of 29,342 US men aged 46–81 years (average age 55–62 years old), who provided information on the history of the frequency of ejaculation (from sexual intercourse, nocturnal emission, and masturbation) on a self-administered questionnaire in 1992 and responded to questionnaires every 2 years to the year 2000. Participants were asked to report the average number of ejaculations they experienced per month during the ages of 20–29 years, 40–49 years, and during the past year. A total of 222,426 person-years of follow-up documented a total of 1,449 new cases of prostate cancer (953 localized and 147 advanced cases). Ejaculation frequency was generally not related to cancer risk except for higher numbers of reported ejaculations. Men reporting 21 or more ejaculations per month versus men reporting 4–7 ejaculations per month had the following reduced risk of prostate cancer:

- 11 % reduction at ages 20–29 years
- 32 % reduction at ages 40–49 years
- 51 % reduction for previous year
- 33 % reduction averaged across a lifetime

Ejaculation frequency was not significantly associated with the risk of advanced prostate cancer. The researchers in this study commented that in the past there have been numerous theories on the risk of prostate cancer as it relates to sexual activity. For example, some theories suggest that increased sexual activity could be related to higher testosterone levels and this could cause an increase in prostate cancer. Also, increased sexual activity may increase the risk of sexually transmitted diseases (STD), which may increase the risk of prostate cancer, but currently no STD has been clearly related to the risk of prostate cancer. Other opposite theories are that infrequent ejaculations increase the risk of prostate cancer because carcinogens are not eliminated frequently from the prostate (so-called not use it and you may lose it theory). In addition, there is the "use it or lose it theory" or those that have more ejaculations can reduce their risk of prostate cancer because of the regular elimination of carcinogens or cancer causing compounds in the prostate. This is similar to the higher fluid intake and reduced risk of bladder cancer theory because more frequent urination reduces the exposure time of a carcinogen on the bladder tissue, but this has mixed data and also needs more evaluation [311]. At least it is healthy to maintain hydration. One problem with the large ejaculation study was that the participants from the HPFS are mostly Caucasians; therefore, it is difficult to comment on the impact of ejaculations in minority groups.

A comprehensive review of the dietary and supplement and other CAM options for prostate cancer prevention and for ancillary treatment effects (or not) from this chapter and other author sources [4] are listed in Table 7.5.

Table 7.5 Diet, dietary supplements, other CAM, and the respective impact on prostate cancer and general health

CVD parameter/ interventions	Correlation with prostate cancer risk
Alcohol	In excess may reduce the efficacy of prostate medications (finasteride) and may increase the risk of prostate cancer and all-cause mortality. In moderation (1–2 drinks a day in men or an amount that will not cause weight gain and 1 drink in women) appears to be heart healthy and may reduce the risk of BPH/LUTS
Aspirin (low dose or 81 mg, generic) (originally derived from willow bark)	Determine if a man concerned about prostate cancer qualifies for aspirin based on CVD risk working with his physicians and utilizing risk scores such as Framingham or Reynolds Risk Score. Low-dose aspirin may reduce the risk of prostate cancer mortality in men with aggressive prostate cancer. Aspirin has been shown to lower the risk of colorectal cancer in those at high risk, but the data in prostate cancer is preliminary in terms of benefit
Beta-carotene dietary supplements (15 mg or higher)	Appears to increase the risk of lung cancer in smokers and former smokers from three large randomized trials (ATBC, CARET, AREDS2). May also increase the risk of all-cause mortality in smokers. Former and current smokers should eliminate beta-carotene from supplements (including multivitamins) and receive beta-carotene from food and beverage sources only
BPH/LUTS dietary supplements (saw palmetto, beta-sitosterol, Pygeum africanum, pumpkin seed oil, stinging nettle, etc.)	No impact on prostate cancer thus far. STEP and CAMUS trial showed no impact of 320–960 mg of saw palmetto on BPH and no hint of this herbal from this and other studies to impact prostate cancer. PSA changes have not been consistently been reduced on any of these agents. Most contain a plant sterol, beta-sitosterol, that may slightly lower cholesterol levels
Calcium	1,000–1,200 mg a diet from dietary sources is the best option and may provide some cancer (colon, etc.) and bone preventive effects. Higher doses have been linked to an increase risk of prostate cancer and aggressive disease and may increase the risk of kidney stones and calcification of the arteries (controversial). If a calcium supplement is needed, calcium carbonate, citrate, and phosphate are all effective in potentially slowing loss. Calcium carbonate has been the most clinically tested in prostate cancer, but calcium citrate is arguably the safest in urology because it does not appear to increase the risk of kidney stones in previous calcium oxalate stone formers. Yet, constipation is an issue with calcium supplements in some individuals. Calcium carbonate and phosphate should be taken with food for better absorption, but calcium citrate can be utilized with or without food but may require more pills because it is a less concentrated form of calcium

(continued)

Table 7.5 (continued)

CVD parameter/ interventions	Correlation with prostate cancer risk
Coenzyme Q10 (ubiquinone)	May provide a slight benefit in reducing the side effects of cholesterol-lowering drugs (statins) at 100–300 mg per day, but there is no other role for this supplement in prostate cancer prevention treatment and could impact blood-thinning medications
Curcumin (derived from turmeric)	Preliminary clinical results suggest it has an anti-inflammatory effect (some efficacy in arthritis) and its impact in cancer prevention is controversial. Higher doses could deter compliance but awaiting the results of several clinical trials with conventional treatment
Fish oil/omega-3 fatty acids from marine (EPA and DHA) and plant sources (ALA)	Marine (oil and fatty fish) and plant dietary sources high in omega-3 compounds may reduce the risk of prostate cancer or aggressive disease. For example, flaxseed has some preliminary positive research at 30 g (3 rounded tablespoons) per day. Fish oil or omega-3 dietary supplements do not have adequate data to recommend for prevention or treatment of prostate cancer. They may provide some benefit in patients to reduce side effects of androgen-deprivation therapy (ADT)
Flaxseed or soy	Most of the positive research is from food sources and not dietary supplements. Soy protein powder isolate is an outstanding source of protein at just 10–25 g/day. And, flaxseed is not only high in plant omega-3 but also in fiber and actually has clinical research to espouse its potential use in prostate cancer
Folic acid supplements/ high-dose B-vitamin supplements	Folic acid in excessive dosages has been preliminarily associated with a higher risk of prostate cancer and/or an increased risk of progressive disease (this is controversial). Prostate cancer has the most evidence compared to any other cancer that individual folic acid supplements could increase risk and interfere with treatment. A maximum of 400 μg should be found in your multivitamin. There are no issues with dietary sources of folate, but only large intakes from dietary supplements
Ginger	Has been used at 500–1,000 mg a day to reduce nausea with conventional antiemetics from chemotherapy (utilized 3 days before and after chemotherapy). Could be an option in this situation
Lycopene	No current defined role in prostate cancer prevention and treatment. Lycopene from food sources (fruits and veggies) is heart healthy. Lycopene from dietary supplements has mixed data and is not generally recommended
Metformin (generic prescription drug originally derived from the French Lilac)	Reduces IGF-1, type 2 diabetes risk in high-risk patients, weight gain, and gluconeogenesis, which all may increase the risk of prostate cancer. Dosage of 850 mg BID and a low glycemic index diet (low carbohydrates) utilized in androgen-deprivation therapy (ADT) patients demonstrated preliminary reductions in weight, waist, and blood pressure and controlled glucose levels along with a low glycemic index diet in a 6-month trial. Preliminary observational evidence suggests it may reduce the risk of being diagnosed with prostate cancer and reducing the risk of prostate cancer progression
Multivitamin	One pill of day of a low-dose multivitamin or children's multivitamin in adults is safe and may lower overall cancer risk, but more than one multivitamin a day may increase risk of aggressive prostate cancer. Centrum Silver was tested against placebo in a randomized trial (Physician's Health Study II), and after a median of 11.2 years there was no increase or decrease risk of prostate cancer found, but a significant reduced risk (8 %) in total cancer was observed in men and it had no positive or negative effect on total cardiovascular events. Thus, it was as safe as a placebo overall
Pomegranate capsules and/or juice (also any other caloric drinks)	Low- and high-dosage (1 or 3 g) capsules appear to have similar effects on PSA doubling times in men failing primary treatment for prostate cancer. This still raises the question of how much better these capsules or juice work than placebo. The juice or capsules need a long-term placebo-controlled study. Be careful of the caloric content of these and other juices that could be as high as 140–160 calories per 8 ounces. Look for no-calorie or low-calorie options if an advocate of this approach
Probiotics	Have no current role in prostate cancer, but perhaps in bladder cancer. Fiber is a prebiotic that is adequate for establishing healthy gut flora
Protein powders (whey, casein, egg white, soy, brown rice, pea, etc.)	Works with most dietary programs to provide adequate daily protein (0.8 g minimum per kilogram), appetite suppression, stimulates muscle protein synthesis, and may improve cardiovascular health. Concentrated protein isolates can provide up to 25 g of protein per 100–125 calories (perfect for most diets and better than most protein bars on the market)

(continued)

Table 7.5 (continued)

CVD parameter/ interventions	Correlation with prostate cancer risk
Radiation and diet and supplements and other conventional localized or locally advanced treatment options	No current dietary regimen is standard to reduce side effects from radiation treatment. In fact, dramatically changing diet during the time of radiation should be questioned. Statins, aspirin, and metformin are being studied with radiation to potentially enhance success (e.g., radiosensitizers), and CAM options should mimic some of these agents with their own products
Red yeast rice extract (RYR)	This "natural" statin (cholesterol-lowering supplements) similar to the pharmacologic drug "lovastatin" is being tested in men on active surveillance for prostate cancer in one clinical trial (REALITY). It already has been demonstrated to be an option for statin-intolerant patients at 1,200–3,600 mg/day based on the monacolin K content (effective lovastatin natural agent)
Resveratrol	Compound found the skin of grapes that is being touted as an antiaging supplement. It needs more clinical trials and needs to demonstrate some improvement in heart health markers to be advocated. In the meantime, a glass of red wine makes more sense compared to supplementation
Selenium dietary supplements	High-dose selenium supplements may increase the risk of type 2 diabetes and non-melanoma skin cancer recurrence. Dosages from 200 to 800 mg have not shown any efficacy in men for prevention, high-risk prevention (HGPIN), or men diagnosed with prostate cancer. There is some suggestion that it may reduce the risk of prostate cancer in men with overt selenium deficiency, but it may increase PSA velocity in men with already adequate intake of selenium. A total of 20–70 mg/day is more than adequate and can be derived from food and/or a low-dose multivitamin
Shark cartilage	No efficacy currently in cancer treatment
Statins (primarily generic prescription drug originally derived from a fungus/yeast)	Associated with a lower risk of aggressive and advanced prostate cancer
Tea (black, green, oolong, etc.)	Low calorie and can be utilized with most health diets. Whether or not they reduce the risk of prostate cancer is controversial and there is not role for tea dietary supplements in prostate cancer. However, the beverage may be part of a lower caloric dietary regimen that could aid in prostate cancer prevention and treatment
Vitamin C (oral or intravenous)	Could increase the risk of kidney stones in higher dosages (1,000 mg or more) and has no impact on prostate cancer as a dietary supplement. IV forms are being studied for quality-of-life improvement, but whether or not it can be used to extend life in prostate cancer patients is controversial
Vitamin D supplements	Potentially a U- or J-shaped curve with higher blood levels showing an increased risk and normalization of deficient or insufficient levels showing a reduction in risk. Functions more like a hormone and may have a role in reducing bone loss from androgen-deprivation therapy (ADT), but whether or not it has any other role in prostate cancer remains to be determined. The RDA is only 600–800 IU/day and overt deficiency or insufficiency of a man on ADT should prompt further vitamin D treatment (1,000 IU/day for example) to normalize blood levels. Vitamin D_3 is mostly derived from animal sources and vitamin D_2 is derived from plant sources. Both are effective, but vitamin D_3 is produced by the human body when exposed to UVB light
Vitamin E supplements	High-dose vitamin E supplements (400 IU) significantly increase the risk of prostate cancer and may increase the risk of aggressive disease. Only small amounts are needed to normalize the blood test (10–20 IU), which can be derived from a multivitamin
Zinc supplements	High-dose (80 mg or more) individual zinc supplements have not been shown to reduce risk and may actually increase risk and may increase risk of other urologic conditions

Note: Always inquire if the CAM or dietary intervention is at least heart healthy or heart neutral, but it should never be adverse to heart health

Androgen-Deprivation Therapy Side Effects and Solutions

The controversy over androgen-deprivation therapy (ADT) for prostate cancer has shifted over time. Side effects appear to have become the more tangible issue compared to clinical efficacy in numerous scenarios [312–314]. A variety of side effects have been attributed either indirectly or directly to ADT in an acute or chronic situation [315–319].

A partial list of the potential common and uncommon side effects experienced by men on ADT therapy for prostate cancer is briefly listed in Table 7.6.

Mild anemia associated with ADT (continuous or intermittent) is usually normochromic normocytic type (not microcytic or macrocytic) [320, 321], which is somewhat similar to what is experienced in the aging male [322, 323], except it occurs in the first months with ADT compared to decades with normal aging. An acute reduction in hemoglobin occurs in most patients on ADT with a mean of 10 % or greater decrease in hemoglobin and RBC counts, but with minimal changes in MCV (mean corpuscular volume) and no changes in MCH (mean cell hemoglobin), MCHC (mean cell hemoglobin concentration), or iron levels and other nutrient levels [324]. Thus, most patients with localized or locally advanced or nonmetastatic prostate cancer do not require treatment with diet, dietary supplements (not iron, B12, or folate), or prescription medications for this side effect. If ADT is discontinued, then the anemia should resolve with testosterone normalization.

Table 7.6 A partial list of the potential common and uncommon side effects experienced by men on ADT therapy for prostate cancer

Anemia
Cholesterol/lipid changes
Cognitive changes/depression
Erectile dysfunction/decreased libido
Fatigue
Hot flashes
Osteoporosis
Weight gain and glucose/insulin changes
Other changes, such as muscle/joint discomfort, loss of body hair, increased density of scalp hair, dry skin

Preliminary evidence suggests that the hemoglobin changes on average are not as dramatic in men if they perform regular resistance exercises [285]. The only concern is men with bone metastasis need to be evaluated for the possibility or not of initiating a strength training or resistance exercise regimen due to the potential for increase bone fragility or fracture.

Accelerated bone loss is an issue with ADT, but it was arguably exaggerated in the past based on little to no suggested CAM intervention or preventive therapy. Older investigations utilized patients with more advanced disease generally not on minimal forms of preventive therapy for bone loss, and rates per year of spinal bone loss were reported to be as high as 5–8.5 % and in the hip as high as 2–6.5 % [325]. This would greatly exceed what occurs in female menopause. However, research on Japanese patients with prostate cancer has found a low rate of osteoporosis (approximately 10–12 %) [326, 327], which could be attributed to healthy lifestyle change(s). ADT-treated patients have significantly reduced bone mineral density (BMD) numbers, T- and Z-scores compared to hormone-naïve Japanese patients, but research continues to demonstrate no significant increase of osteoporosis prevalence in these men on ADT for a mean of approximately 31 months. Again, it is plausible that heart-healthy lifestyle changes common among the older Japanese population are responsible for this benefit [328]. Additionally, deficiencies of calcium and vitamin D and a lack of resistance activity are just some of the many factors that could equate to a misrepresentation of the true rate of bone loss on ADT. More recent US and international research has suggested a reduced risk of bone loss in men receiving calcium and vitamin D supplementation while on ADT [329, 330]; unfortunately, only a minority (10–20 %) of patients are following these recommendations, primarily due to a lack of education on this issue from their providers [295, 331, 332].

One large randomized trial can highlight the change in philosophy that should occur with CAM and ADT bone loss. A large 3-year trial of denosumab given every 6 months ($n=734$)

compared to placebo ($n=734$) in men receiving ADT for nonmetastatic prostate cancer was published [333]. Participants were instructed to utilize 1,000 μg or more of calcium and 400 IU of vitamin D. This represents one of the first long-term randomized studies to provide the placebo arm with realistic and relevant dietary supplementation or CAM options. Median serum vitamin D levels at baseline were approximately 24–25 ng/mL and increased to 31 ng/mL (normal range) after 36 months. Only 14–15 % of participants began the trial with osteoporosis (T-score below −2.5) at any site and the median time on ADT at baseline of 20–21 months. The primary endpoint was the percent change in BMD at the lumbar spine at 24 months, and secondary endpoints included percent change in BMD at the femoral neck and total hip at 24 months and at all three anatomic locations at 36 months, along with incidence of new fractures. After 24 months, there was a significant loss in lumbar spine BMD at 24 months in the placebo group, but this loss was just 1 % and minimally changed at 36 months. There were also significant reductions in femoral neck and total hip, but this loss was only 2–3 % at 36 months. The largest percentage of bone loss occurred in the distal radius. Fracture at any anatomic location was lower with denosumab compared to placebo, but the difference was not found to be statistically significant at 36 months. No significant differences were found in the time period to first fracture (non-vertebral or vertebral) between the groups. The authors reported that more than one fracture at any location occurred in significantly more patients on placebo compared to denosumab and a significantly higher rate of vertebral fractures. Yet these were secondary endpoints, and more participants in the placebo group had a history of vertebral fracture (+2.6 %) and a history of osteoporotic fracture (+4.5 %) at baseline. The 36-month clinical difference of 2.4 % more new vertebral fractures (3.9 % vs. 1.5 %) in the placebo group cannot be due to the intervention alone, but may also have been due to the slight inequality between groups as it related to vertebral and overall fractures at baseline in favor of denosumab. The difference between most clinical endpoints for the calcium and vitamin D group compared to pharmacologic treatment was minimal at 36 months. Furthermore, a less than 4 % total fracture percentage in the placebo arm (vs. 1.9 %) over 3 years is low considering that no aggressive lifestyle and supplemental preventive therapy before ADT was initiated. How much difference would have existed if the placebo group were also assigned to regular resistance and aerobic exercises during this study period or before initiating ADT? Preliminary studies suggest some patients have been able to maintain bone mineral density without supplementation [285]. Denosumab appears to be an option for accelerated spinal and hip bone loss despite aggressive CAM intervention and perhaps for those men that cannot adequately maintain distal radius density with aggressive lifestyle changes. Regardless, a clinical trial of nonmetastatic patients on ADT with adequate calcium and vitamin D status with aerobic and resistance exercise may compare favorably to pharmacologic intervention over 1 year or more.

Sarcopenia could improve significantly if men on ADT perform upper and lower body resistance exercises at least twice a week, regardless of the time period on ADT [334]. Diverse amino acid or protein supplementation via low-calorie powders or liquids also has the potential to provide ancillary benefits to resistance exercise for those trying to prevent sarcopenia. Clinical studies in the elderly have already documented increased lean body mass (LBM), reduction in fat mass, increased handgrip strength, leg strength, and muscle protein synthesis with essential amino acid supplementation for several months [335–338]. Minor IGF-I increases can also occur with protein supplementation (similar to resistance exercise), but the overall health benefit appears to trump any specific physiologic concern. This is tantamount to the original concern and subsequent debunking of the myth that resistance exercise can exacerbate lymphedema in breast cancer [339]. Protein powders from animal sources (whey, casein, egg white) or plant sources (soy, brown rice, pea, hemp) allow for up to 25 g of protein on 100–125 calories [4]. This form of concentrated protein works for most diet plans and allows other benefits such as the suppression of appetite along with the stimulation of muscle protein synthesis.

More concerning options in prostate cancer patients such as DHEA dietary supplementation and growth hormone replacement have failed to provide tangible consistent qualitative benefits in elderly patients [340, 341]. One of the most interesting older studies of GH supplementation found no added benefit, especially if elderly patients engaged in strength training via resistance exercise initially for 14 weeks before supplementing with this hormone [342]. Clinicians could advocate more heart-healthy and cost-effective interventions that are more promising. For example, fish oil is another supplement that has recently garnered new data in the area of sarcopenia prevention by potentially reducing some inflammatory markers [137].

The potential for increased cardiovascular events and overall deaths on ADT is controversial [343]. A meta-analysis of randomized trials suggests no increase in cardiovascular mortality and a potential for a lower risk of all-cause mortality [344]. Cardiovascular disease (CVD) is either the number one or number two potential cause of death in men and those with prostate cancer or on ADT [319]. Thus, this debate may be moot because all men on ADT still should attempt to reduce their CVD risk as much as possible. A combination of lifestyle changes and a low-dose statin, if needed, could arguably provide this type of needed protection during ADT. Men on ADT utilizing statins compared to non-statins while on ADT found significant increases in HDL, the prevention of a significant increase in LDL, but still a significant increase in triglycerides [345]. Perhaps the concern of weight gain and triglyceride increases should also be addressed, beyond lifestyle changes and statins in men on ADT. Fish oil is FDA approved to lower triglycerides, and there is some consistent data to suggest that it may lower the risk of insulin resistance [346–351], but this has not been researched in ADT patients. Weight and especially waist loss and a low glycemic index diet may be the best method to combat increasing triglycerides and insulin resistance [4]. There are some clinical data to suggest a reduction in diabetes in ADT patients on vitamin D or the normalization of vitamin D intake [352]. Yet, prediabetes and diabetes and weight gain could increase the chance of vitamin D deficiency (reverse causation). The American Heart Association (AHA) recommendations are 1,000 μg of the main components of fish oil (EPA and DHA) daily in individuals with heart disease and the inclusion of plant sources of omega-3s [353], but again fish oil needs efficacy studies in the ADT population.

Resistance exercise or weight lifting controls or reduces glucose and insulin in ADT and others [334, 354], and it significantly improved triglycerides from another clinical trial of ADT patients also receiving radiation therapy [66]. Triglycerides, glucose, and insulin sensitivity could improve in ADT patients with an increase in muscle mass or reduction in body fat, because triglycerides are stored in adipose tissue and metabolism is further reduced with declining muscle mass [319, 354].

Fatigue was significantly reduced in a 12-week randomized trial of aerobic and resistance exercise of ADT patients [334]. Increases in muscle mass and increases in metabolism and energy levels were also noted [354]. Interestingly, the reduction in fatigue in cancer patients is a consistent finding in clinical trials [4]. Part of the benefit could also be derived from the socialization or attention received in a social training program because this could also improve mental health. Another large randomized trial of American ginseng (Panax quinquefolius) compared to placebo found a potential reduction in reported fatigue from cancer patients assigned to 1,000 or 2,000 μg a day of this herbal compound after 4–8 weeks [355]. Side effects were similar to placebo.

It is also of interest that a combined resistance and aerobic exercise in men on ADT ($n=29$) compared to a non-exercise group ($n=28$) reported a significant maintenance of sexual activity over 12 weeks [356]. This also included a major interest in sex (17 % vs. 0 %; $p=0.02$). This is a highly remarkable potential finding since ADT is known to cause general suppression in libido and sexual activity. It is plausible that resistance and aerobic exercise could provide a novel method whereby some ADT patients have a chance of maintaining or improving sexual health despite a lack of testosterone.

Treatment of hot flashes is arguably more extensively studied in breast cancer compared to any other cancer [357, 358]. The lessons learned should be applied to the prostate carcinoma research, including the use of a hot flash diary for patients in clinical studies and in clinical practice [4]. One major trial involving prostate cancer patients addressed pharmacologic interventions compared to nonintervention in men on ADT with hot flashes [359]. A total of 311 men that had already received 6 months of ADT were randomly assigned to one of three regimens daily for 12 weeks: 75 μg of venlafaxine, 100 μg cyproterone acetate, or 20 μg of medroxyprogesterone acetate. Patients also completed a 1-week hot flash diary before each clinical visit. Participants included in the analysis reported that 80 % of their hot flashes on average were moderate to severe before the randomization period (using a hot flash diary at home to assess vasomotor symptoms). The change in median hot flash score was −47 % for venlafaxine, −94 % for cyproterone, and −84 % for medroxyprogesterone, and the reduction was significant ($p<0.0001$) for each medication from baseline, but there was a significant improvement for the other two medications over venlafaxine. Approximately a quarter to a third of hot flashes in these two groups were eliminated. The authors concluded that medroxyprogesterone should be considered the standard treatment for hot flashes in men on ADT that need treatment because cyproterone is a treatment for prostate cancer that could interfere with ADT. The benefits of different progesterone delivery methods on ADT hot flashes are impressive and consistent [359, 360].

However, a total of only 22 % of men that had received ADT for 6 months actually spontaneously requested hot flash treatment, which provided difficulty in recruitment for this study [359]. Approximately one out every five men either felt they needed hot flash pharmacologic treatment or requested it. The authors commented, "In our view, this justifies the recommendation not to systematically prevent hot flashes in all patients on initiation of an androgen-suppressing treatment." Men should utilize a diary for only 1–2 weeks, and based on the results the clinician should discuss the need for lifestyle and/or pharmacologic intervention in case the patient does not have knowledge about treatment or is not comfortable discussing the subject. Multiple lifestyle changes from exercise, weight loss, and paced respiration could be beneficial for some men along with some dietary supplements, but for those with moderate to severe or very severe hot flashes expecting a CAM to provide resolution alone for this common condition in ADT is not realistic, but could be synergistic (as is true for most ADT issues).

A final interesting observation from this clinical trial was the significant benefit on the emotional functional scale with patients that only occurred in the venlafaxine group and appeared within the first 4 weeks [359]. This is another reason to individualize treatment for ADT side effects and consider men with a need for mental and emotional improvement on ADT with moderate to severe hot flashes to be treated with venlafaxine or another similar class medication compared to progesterone or perhaps a dietary supplement that could improve mental health (SAM-e, fish oil, etc.). Following the research on menopausal symptom relief in women should again be a guide for men on ADT. For example, omega-3 intake and supplementation suggests a potential to reduce hot flash frequency (not intensity) and the potential to improve mental health [140, 361–363], but again this is preliminary, but for many patients the benefit will outweigh the risk.

Another emerging area of interest is combining effective dietary changes with a generic heart-healthy prescription for weight loss from ADT. A 6-month trial of 850 μg BID of metformin with a low glycemic index diet caused significant reduction in waist size ($p=0.05$), weight ($p<0.001$), BMI ($p<0.001$), and systolic blood pressure ($p=0.01$) compared to the control arm [107]. In the metformin group, there was also significant reduction in hemoglobin A1c ($p<0.01$). The excitement for the use of metformin in prostate cancer ancillary treatment was mentioned earlier in the chapter, but if it is indeed effective in reducing weight in those on ADT (apart from standard dietary change and exercise), then this would represent a novel dual approach of side effect reduction and potential treatment effect. How well the patients would have performed on the low glycemic diet alone is not known.

Table 7.7 is a summary of some potential solutions to almost every side effect of ADT utilizing CAM mentioned in this chapter and other author

Table 7.7 Summary of lifestyle changes and other minimal or CAM interventions to prevent and treat some of the side effects of ADT

Lifestyle changes and/or CAM options	Potential benefit while on ADT
Acupuncture	May reduce moderate to severe hot flashes in some patients when other options are not working (traditional needle or electrostimulated forms appear to both have some efficacy)
Aerobic exercise every other day and weight lifting/resistance exercise just 2–3 times a week (note: metastatic disease patients may not qualify for weight lifting due to a potential increased risk of fracture)	– Improves heart and mental health – Reduces bone loss – Reduces weight gain – May improve anemia – Reduces bone loss – Reduces sarcopenia – Reduces fatigue – Improves cardiovascular health – Maintains sexual health and interest in sex
Aspirin (low dose, 81 mg)	– May improve heart health in those at high risk – May reduce inflammatory markers
Body moisturizer (with UVA and UVB blocker)	– Use after bathing/showering and drying off if there are dry skin problems from low testosterone. Additionally, it can protect the skin from ultraviolet light. These body moisturizers are now widely available
Heart-healthy diet (Mediterranean diet, etc.)	– Improves heart and mental health
Calcium and vitamin D supplementation	– Reduces bone loss – May reduce risk of insulin insensitivity – May reduce the risk of falls (provides muscular balance and vitamin D receptors in muscle tissue) – If dietary intake of calcium is already 1,000–1,200 mg, there is no current need to take calcium supplementation
Cholesterol lowering (statin over the counter statin equivalent such as red yeast rice extract)	– Reduces risk of elevated LDL and triglycerides – Reduces inflammatory markers – May promote bone health (controversial)
Diary	– Records number and intensity of hot flashes – Records any other issues with ADT and provides this record to his physician
Fish oil and plant sources of omega-3 fatty acids	– Reduce triglycerides – May reduce insulin resistance – May reduce sarcopenia – May reduce hot flash frequency (1,000–2,000 mg/day) – May improve mental health
Flaxseed	– 2 to 3 rounded tablespoons per day can maintain digestive regularity and could provide some hot flash reduction (controversial but at least very heart healthy)
Ginseng (Panax quinquefolius or Panax ginseng based on new clinical research)	– May reduce fatigue at doses of 1,000–2,000 mg/day over 4–8 weeks
Korean red ginseng (Panax ginseng) or L-arginine aspartate + pycnogenol or L-citrulline	– Could be used to promote sexual health but may cause a slight reduction in blood pressure. See the erectile dysfunction chapter for information and dosages – Panax ginseng may also reduce fatigue
Metformin (generic prescription drug derived originally from the French Lilac)	– 850 mg BID with a low glycemic diet could reduce weight and waist size and lower blood pressure and hemoglobin A1c – Also being studied for a treatment benefit for prostate cancer patients
Protein or amino acid powder supplementation (whey, casein, and egg white are animal-derived and soy, brown rice, and pea are plant-derived. Animal-derived tend to have a better taste profile and flexibility to be added to beverages, but plant protein development may also compete soon in these areas)	– May reduce sarcopenia with resistance activity – May improve calcium absorption – May reduce weight gain – May reduce fatigue by maintaining muscle mass – Works with most weight-loss programs and provides appetite suppression

Note: Any women's menopausal agents that provide a benefit could be beneficial for men on ADT ("male menopause")

sources [4]. It is interesting that research now suggests that CAM could mitigate many of these issues without and with conventional side effect therapies.

The Future of Side Effect Reduction and CAM

The potential for CAM options to reduce side effects of conventional therapy for prostate cancer is promising and needs more attention [4]. Most of the research exists for other forms of cancer or noncancerous conditions, but still would apply to prostate cancer patients (similar to the hot flash data). For example, 500–1,000 μg of ginger in dietary supplement form may be an effective nausea-reducing agent along with conventional medicine from the results of a large randomized trial [364]. Alpha-lipoic acid has impressive data for reducing peripheral neuropathy in diabetics at 600 μg/day [365] and could have potential for this same condition as a result of chemotherapy. Weight loss is a potential option with this same CAM intervention at higher dosages [366]. It is of interest that one mechanism of action for weight loss could be activation of AMPK (adenosine monophosphate-activated protein kinase) [366], which is similar to what is described for metformin [103, 104, 107]. The potential for CAM and dietary or supplemental options to provide some ancillary benefit for almost any side effect from prostate cancer treatment is a testament to the future of these interventions when used appropriately [4].

Conclusion

Heart healthy = prostate healthy! Less is more! It is of interest that the themes of this chapter continue to echo through urology. For example, three major clinical trials of selenium supplements for prostate cancer prevention or treatment have now been completed (apart from the SELECT of vitamin E and/or selenium). And, dosages of 200–800 μg of selenium were utilized in these studies [367–370], and researchers found no impact except a hint of potential prevention in a deficient subset of participants [366] and a potential increase in PSA kinetics and growth or prostate cancer in men with higher blood levels of selenium that were given high doses (800 μg) of selenium supplements [370]. These findings are symbolic of the message in this chapter, which is chasing high doses of antioxidants to solve prostate cancer may be simply providing impetus for more disease.

The irony of past observations in prostate cancer and this chapter is that it appears men with higher risk of prostate cancer because of family history appear to be utilizing several dietary supplements that actually place them at a potentially even higher risk of prostate cancer [371]. In other words, many "prostate health" supplements are in fact prostate unhealthy in large dosages. Thus, the need for objective education is critical especially at a time where there is more data on CAM than ever before.

If researchers are going to spend a decade or more of their life pursuing a preventive or treatment breakthrough while utilizing large sums of taxpayer money for this cause, and patients are going to give up enormous time for the sake of science, then it appears to be time to "first do no harm" and think of heart-healthy regimens or CAM products that could simultaneously prevent or reduce the progression of cardiovascular disease and prostate cancer simultaneously. This method allows researchers, healthcare professionals, and patients to focus on the forest and the tree(s) and appears to allow the highest probability of overall and specific success stories [372–374].

References

1. Siegel R, Naishadham D, Jemal A. Cancer statistics 2013. CA Cancer J Clin. 2013;63:11–30.
2. Moyad MA. Zinc for prostate disease and other conditions: a little evidence, a lot of hype, and a significant potential problem. Urol Nurs. 2004;24:49–52.
3. Watson J. Oxidants, antioxidants and the current incurability of metastatic cancers. Open Biol. 2013;3:120144.
4. Moyad MA. Promoting wellness for prostate cancer patients. 4th ed. Ann Arbor, MI: Spry; 2013.

5. Pinkhasov RM, Shteynshlyuger A, Hakimian P, Lindsay GK, Samadi DB, Shabsigh R. Are men shortchanged on health? Perspective on life expectancy, morbidity, and mortality in men and women in the United States. Int J Clin Pract. 2010;64:465–74.
6. Moyad MA. Lifestyle changes to prevent BPH: heart healthy=prostate healthy. Urol Nurs. 2003;23: 439–41.
7. Moyad MA. The optimal male health diet and dietary supplement program. Urol Clin North Am. 2012;39:89–107.
8. Thompson IM, Goodman PJ, Tangen CM, Lucia MS, Miller GJ, Ford LG, et al. The influence of finasteride on the development of prostate cancer. N Engl J Med. 2003;349:215–24.
9. Scardino PT. The prevention of prostate cancer–the dilemma continues. N Engl J Med. 2003;349:297–9.
10. Lebdai S, Bigot P, Azzouzi AR. High-grade prostate cancer and finasteride. BJU Int. 2010;105:456–9.
11. Svatek RS, Lee JJ, Roehrborn CG, Lippman SM, Lotan Y. Cost-effectiveness of prostate cancer chemoprevention: a quality of life–years analysis. Cancer. 2008;112:1058–65.
12. Thompson IM, Tangen CM, Goodman PJ, Probstfield JL, Moinpour CM, Coltman CA. Erectile dysfunction and subsequent cardiovascular disease. JAMA. 2005;294:2996–3002.
13. Kristal AR, Arnold KB, Schenk JM, Neuhouser ML, Goodman P, Penson DF, et al. Dietary patterns, supplement use, and the risk of symptomatic benign prostatic hyperplasia: results from the prostate cancer prevention trial. Am J Epidemiol. 2008;167:925–34.
14. Andriole GL, Bostwick DG, Brawley OW, Gomella LG, Marberger M, Montorsi F, et al. Effect of dutasteride on the risk of prostate cancer. N Engl J Med. 2010;362:1192–202.
15. Azzouni F, Mohler J. Role of 5-alpha-reductase inhibitors in prostate cancer prevention and treatment. Urology. 2012;79:1197–205.
16. Walsh PC. Chemoprevention of prostate cancer. N Engl J Med. 2010;362:1237–8.
17. Platz EA, Till C, Goodman PJ, Parnes HL, Figg WD, Albanes D, et al. Men with low serum cholesterol have a lower risk of high-grade prostate cancer in the placebo arm of the prostate cancer prevention trial. Cancer Epidemiol Biomarkers Prev. 2009;18: 2807–13.
18. Thomas II JA, Gerber L, Banez LL, Moreira DM, Rittmaster RS, Andriole GL, et al. Prostate cancer risk in men with baseline history of coronary artery disease: results from the REDUCE Study. Cancer Epidemiol Biomarkers Prev. 2012;21:576–81.
19. US Department of Health and Human Services. How tobacco smoke causes disease: the biology and behavioral basis for smoking-attributable disease: a report of the Surgeon General, GA: US Department of Health and Human Services, CDC. 2010. http://www.cdc.gov/tobacoo/data_statistics/sgr/2010/index.htm. Accessed 1 May 2013.
20. Centers for Disease Control and Prevention (CDC). Current cigarette smoking among adults-United States, 2011. Morb Mortal Wkly Rep. 2012;61:889–94.
21. Huncharek M, Haddock KS, Reid R, Kupelnick B. Smoking as a risk factor for prostate cancer: a meta-analysis of 24 prospective cohort studies. Am J Public Health. 2010;100:693–701.
22. Zu K, Giovannucci E. Smoking and aggressive prostate cancer: a review of the epidemiologic evidence. Cancer Causes Control. 2009;20:1799–810.
23. Kenfield SA, Stampfer MJ, Chan JM, Giovannucci E. Smoking and prostate cancer survival and recurrence. JAMA. 2011;305:2548–55.
24. Cao Y, Ma J. Body mass index, prostate cancer-specific mortality, and biochemical recurrence: a systematic review and meta-analysis. Cancer Prev Res. 2011;4:486–501.
25. Joshu CE, Mondul AM, Menke A, Meinhold C, Han M, Humphreys EP, et al. Weight gain is associated with an increased risk of prostate cancer recurrence after prostatectomy in the PSA era. Cancer Prev Res (Phila). 2011;4:544–51.
26. Discacciatl A, Orsini N, Wolk A. Body mass index and incidence of localized and advanced prostate cancer–a dose response meta-analysis of prospective studies. Ann Oncol. 2012;23:1665–71.
27. Woodard G, Ahmed S, Podelski V, Hernandez-Boussard T, Presti Jr J, Morton JM. Effect of Roux-en-Y gastric bypass on testosterone and prostate-specific antigen. Br J Surg. 2012;99:693–8.
28. Tsugane S, Inoue M. Insulin resistance and cancer: epidemiological evidence. Cancer Sci. 2010;101: 1073–9.
29. Albanes D, Weinstein SJ, Wright ME, Mannisto S, Limburg PJ, Snyder K, et al. Serum insulin, glucose, indices of insulin resistance, and risk of prostate cancer. J Natl Cancer Inst. 2009;101:1272–9.
30. Yun SJ, Min BD, Kang HW, Shin KS, Kim TH, Kim WT, et al. Elevated insulin and insulin resistance are associated with the advanced pathological stage of prostate cancer in Korean population. J Korean Med Sci. 2012;27:1079–84.
31. Grossmann M, Wittert G. Androgens, diabetes and prostate cancer. Endocr Relat Cancer. 2012;19:F47–62.
32. Centers for Disease Control and Prevention (CDC). Increasing prevalence of diagnosed diabetes-United States and Puerto Rico, 1995–2010. MMWR. 2012;61:918–21.
33. Snell-Bergeon JK, Wadwa RP. Hypoglycemia, diabetes, and cardiovascular disease. Diabetes Technol Ther. 2012;14 Suppl 1:S51–8.
34. Grontved A, Rimm EB, Willett WC, Andersen LB, Hu FB. A prospective study of weight training and risk of type 2 diabetes mellitus in men. Ann Intern Med. 2012;6:1–7.
35. Knowler WC, Barrett-Connor E, Fowler SE, Hamman RF, Lachin JM, Walker EA, et al. Reduction in the incidence of type 2 diabetes with lifestyle intervention or metformin. N Engl J Med. 2002;346:393–403.

36. Orchard TJ, Temprosa M, Goldberg R, Haffner S, Ratner R, Marcovina S, et al. The effect of metformin and intensive lifestyle intervention on the metabolic syndrome: the Diabetes Prevention Program randomized trial. Ann Intern Med. 2005; 142:611–9.
37. Diabetes Prevention Program Research Group. 10-year follow-up of diabetes incidence and weight loss in the Diabetes Prevention Program Outcomes Study. Lancet. 2009;374:1677–86.
38. Perreault L, Pan Q, Mather KJ, Watson KE, Hamman RF, Kahn SE, Diabetes Prevention Program Research Group. Effect of regression from prediabetes to normal glucose regulation on long-term reduction in diabetes risk: results from the Diabetes Prevention Program Outcomes Study. Lancet. 2012;379: 2243–51.
39. CDC. Vital signs: prevalence, treatment, and control of hypertension-United States, 1992–2002 and 2005–2008. MMWR. 2011;60:103–8.
40. Rogers VL, Go AS, Lloyd-Jones DM, Adams RJ, Berry JD, Brown TM, et al. Heart disease and stroke statistics-2011 update: a report from the American Heart Association. Circulation. 2011;123:e18–209.
41. Neal B, McMahon S, Chapman N. Effects of ACE inhibitors, calcium antagonists, and other blood pressure-lowering drugs. Lancet. 2000;356: 1955–64.
42. Bhaskaran K, Douglas I, Evans S, van Staa T, Smeeth L. Angiotensin receptor blockers and risk of cancer: cohort study among people receiving antihypertensive drugs in UK General Practice Research Database. BMJ. 2012;344:e2697.
43. De Nunzio C, Aronson W, Freedland SJ, Giovannucci E, Parsons JK. The correlation between metabolic syndrome and prostatic diseases. Eur Urol. 2012;61:560–70.
44. Loeb S, Gupta A, Losonczy L, Tosoian J, Walsh PC. Does benign prostatic hyperplasia treatment with alpha-blockers affect prostate cancer risk? Curr Opin Urol. 2013;23(1):2–4.
45. Roehrborn CG. BPH progression: concept and key learning from MTOPS, ALTESS, COMBAT, and ALF-ONE. BJU Int. 2008;101 Suppl 3:17–21.
46. Kenfield SA, Stampfer MJ, Giovannucci E, Chan JM. Physical activity and survival after prostate cancer diagnosis in the Health Professionals Follow-up Study. J Clin Oncol. 2011;29:726–32.
47. Oliveria SA, Lee IM. Is exercise beneficial in the prevention of prostate cancer? Sports Med. 1997;23:271–8.
48. Torti DC, Matheson GO. Exercise and prostate cancer. Sports Med. 2004;34:363–9.
49. Young-McCaughan S. Potential for prostate cancer prevention through physical activity. World J Urol. 2012;30:167–79.
50. Kokkinos PF, Faselis C, Myers J, Panagiotakos D, Doumas M. Interactive effects of fitness and statin treatment on mortality risk in veterans with dyslipidemia: a cohort study. Lancet. 2013;381:394–9.
51. Maio G, Saraeb S, Marchiori A. Physical function and PDE5 inhibitors in the treatment of erectile dysfunction: results of a randomized controlled study. J Sex Med. 2010;7:2201–8.
52. Yokoyama M, Origasa H, Matsuzaki M, Matsuzawa Y, Saito Y, Ishikawa Y, et al. Effects of eicosapentaenoic acid on major coronary events in hypercholesterolaemic patients (JELIS): a randomised open-label, blinded endpoint analysis. Lancet. 2007;369:1090–8.
53. Moyad MA, Merrick GS, Butler WM, Wallner KE, Galbreath RW, Butler EG, et al. Statins, especially atorvastatin, may improve survival following brachytherapy for clinically localized prostate cancer. Urol Nurs. 2006;26:298–303.
54. Gutt R, Tonlaar N, Kunnavakkam R, Karrison T, Welchselbaum RR, Liauw SL. Statin use and risk of prostate cancer recurrence in men treated with radiation therapy. J Clin Oncol. 2010;28:2653–9.
55. Zaorsky NG, Buyyounouski MK, Li T, Horwitz EM. Aspirin and statin nonuse associated with early biochemical failure after prostate radiation therapy. Int J Radiat Oncol Biol Phys. 2012;84:e13–7.
56. Choe KS, Correa D, Jani AB, Liauw SL. The use of anticoagulants improves biochemical control of localized prostate cancer treated with radiotherapy. Cancer. 2010;116:1820–6.
57. Spratt DE, Zhang C, Zumsteg ZS, Pei X, Zhang Z, Zelefsky MJ. Metformin and prostate cancer: reduced development of castration-resistant disease and prostate cancer mortality. Eur Urol. 2013;63:709–16.
58. Braun DP, Gupta D, Birdsall TC, Sumner M, Staren ED. Effect of naturopathic and nutritional supplement treatment on tumor response, control, and recurrence in patients with prostate cancer treated with radiation therapy. J Altern Complement Med. 2013;19:198–203.
59. Bairati I, Meyer F, Gelinas M, Fortin A, Nabid A, Brochet F, et al. A randomized trial of antioxidant vitamins to prevent second primary cancers in head and neck cancer patients. J Natl Cancer Inst. 2005;97:481–8.
60. Bairati I, Meyer F, Gelinas M, Fortin A, Nabid A, Brochet F, et al. Randomized trial of antioxidant vitamins to prevent acute adverse effects of radiation therapy in head and neck cancer patients. J Clin Oncol. 2005;23:5805–13.
61. Bairati I, Meyer F, Jobin E, Gelinas M, Fortin A, Nabid A, et al. Antioxidant vitamin supplementation and mortality: a randomized trial in head and neck cancer patients. Int J Cancer. 2006;119:2221–4.
62. Meyer F, Bairati I, Fortin A, Gelinas M, Nabid A, Brochet F, et al. Interaction between antioxidant vitamin supplementation and cigarette smoking during radiation therapy in relation to long-term effects on recurrence and mortality: a randomized trial among head and neck cancer. Int J Cancer. 2008;122:1679–83.
63. Lawenda BD, Kelly KM, Ladas EJ, Sagar SM, Vickers A, Blumberg JB. Should supplemental antioxidant administration be avoided during

chemotherapy and radiation therapy? J Natl Cancer Inst. 2008;100:773–83.
64. Cramp F, Byron-Daniel J. Exercise for the management of cancer-related fatigue in adults. Cochrane Database Syst Rev. 2012;11, CD006145.
65. Mustian KM, Peppone L, Darling TV, Palesh O, Heckler CE, Morrow GR. A 4-week home-based aerobic and resistance exercise program during radiation therapy: a pilot randomized clinical trial. J Support Oncol. 2009;7:158–67.
66. Segal RJ, Reid RD, Courneya KS, Sigal RJ, Kenny GP, Prud'Homme DG, et al. Randomized controlled trial of resistance or aerobic exercise in men receiving radiation therapy for prostate cancer. J Clin Oncol. 2009;27:344–51.
67. Liu L, Glicksman AS, Coachman N, Kuten A. Low acute gastrointestinal and genitourinary toxicities in whole pelvic irradiation of prostate cancer. Int J Radiat Oncol Biol Phys. 1997;38:65–71.
68. Pettersson A, Johansson B, Persson C, Berglund A, Turesson I. Effects of a dietary intervention on acute gastrointestinal side effects and other aspects of health-related quality of life: a randomized controlled trial in prostate cancer patients undergoing radiotherapy. Radiother Oncol. 2012;103:333–40.
69. Lips IM, Kotte AN, van Gils CH, van Leerdam ME, van der Heide UA, van Vulpen M. Influence of antiflatulent dietary advice on intrafraction motion for prostate cancer radiotherapy. Int J Radiat Oncol Biol Phys. 2011;81:e401–6.
70. Lips IM, van Gils CH, Kotte AN, van Leerdam ME, Franken SP, van der Heide UA, et al. A double-blind placebo-controlled randomized clinical trial with magnesium oxide to reduce intrafraction prostate motion for prostate cancer radiotherapy. Int J Radiat Oncol Biol Phys. 2012;83:653–60.
71. Murphy J, Stacey D, Crook J, Thompson B, Panetta D. Testing control of radiation-induced diarrhea with a psyllium bulking agent: a pilot study. Can Oncol Nurs J. 2000;10:96–100.
72. Muehlbauer PM, Thorpe D, Davis A, Drabot R, Rawlings BL, Kiker E. Putting evidence into practice: evidence-based interventions to prevent, manage, and treat chemotherapy- and radiotherapy-induced diarrhea. Clin J Oncol Nurs. 2009;13:336–41.
73. The ATBC Study Group. The effect of vitamin E and beta-carotene on the incidence of lung cancer and other cancers in male smokers. N Engl J Med. 1994;330:1029–35.
74. Peto R, Doll R, Buckley JD, Sporn MB. Can dietary beta-carotene materially reduce human cancer rates? Nature. 1981;290:201–8.
75. Omenn GS, Goodman GE, Thornquist MD, Balmes J, Cullen MR, Glass A, et al. Effects of a combination of beta-carotene and vitamin A on lung cancer and cardiovascular disease. N Engl J Med. 1996;334:1150–5.
76. Hennekens CH, Buring JE, Manson JE, Stampfer M, Rosner B, Cook NR, et al. Lack of effect of long-term supplementation with beta carotene on the incidence of malignant neoplasms and cardiovascular disease. N Engl J Med. 1996;334:1145–9.
77. The Age-Related Eye Disease Study 2 (AREDS2) Research Group. Lutein + zeaxanthin and omega-3 fatty acids for age-related macular degeneration: the age-related eye disease study 2 (AREDS2) randomized clinical trial. JAMA. 2013;309:2005–15.
78. Lippman SM, Klein EA, Goodman PJ, Lucia MS, Thompson IM, Ford LG, et al. Effect of selenium and vitamin E on risk of prostate cancer and other cancers: the Selenium and Vitamin E Cancer Prevention Trial (SELECT). JAMA. 2009;301:39–51.
79. Klein EA, Thompson Jr IM, Tangen CM, Crowley JJ, Lucia MS, Goodman PJ, et al. Vitamin E and the risk of prostate cancer: the Selenium and Vitamin E cancer prevention trial (SELECT). JAMA. 2011;306:1549–56.
80. Eidelman RS, Hollar D, Hebert PR, Lamas GA, Hennekens CH. Randomized trials of vitamin E in the treatment and prevention of cardiovascular disease. Arch Intern Med. 2004;164:1552–6.
81. Lee IM, Cook NR, Gaziano JM, Gordon D, Ridker PM, Manson JE, et al. Vitamin E in the primary prevention of cardiovascular disease and cancer: the Women's Health Study: a randomized controlled trial. JAMA. 2005;294:56–65.
82. Miller III ER, Pastor-Barriuso R, Dalal D, Riemersma RA, Appel LJ, Guallar E. Meta-analysis: high-dosage vitamin E supplementation may increase all-cause mortality. Ann Intern Med. 2005; 142:37–46.
83. Lonn E, Bosch J, Yusuf S, Sheridan P, Pogue J, Arnold JM, et al. Effects of long-term vitamin E supplementation on cardiovascular events and cancer: a randomized controlled trial. JAMA. 2005;293:1338–47.
84. Gaziano JM, Glynn RJ, Christen WG, Kurth T, Belanger C, MacFadyen J, et al. Vitamins E and C in the prevention of prostate and total cancer in men: the Physicians' Health Study II randomized controlled trial. JAMA. 2009;301:52–62.
85. Sesso HD, Buring JE, Christen WG, Kurth T, Belanger C, MacFadyen J, et al. Vitamins E and C in the prevention of cardiovascular disease in men: the Physicians' Health Study II randomized controlled trial. JAMA. 2008;300:2123–33.
86. Moyad MA. Selenium and vitamin E supplements for prostate cancer: evidence or embellishment? Urology. 2002;59(4 Suppl 1):9–19.
87. Lodge JK. Vitamin E, bioavailability in humans. J Plant Physiol. 2005;162:790–6.
88. Duffield-Lillico AJ, Begg CB. Reflections on the landmark studies of beta-carotene supplementation. J Natl Cancer Inst. 2004;96:1729–30.
89. Hercberg S, Galan P, Preziosi P, Bertrais S, Mennen L, Malvy D, et al. The SU.VI.MAX Study: a randomized, placebo-controlled trial of the health effects of antioxidant vitamins and minerals. Arch Intern Med. 2004;164:2335–42.
90. Meyer F, Galan P, Douville P, Bairati I, Kegle P, Bertrais S, et al. Antioxidant vitamin and mineral supplementation and prostate cancer prevention in the SU.VI.MAX trial. Int J Cancer. 2005;116:182–6.

91. Weinstein SJ, Wright ME, Pietinen P, King I, Tan C, Taylor PR, et al. Serum alpha-tocopherol and gamma-tocopherol in relation to prostate cancer risk in a prospective study. J Natl Cancer Inst. 2005;97:396–9.
92. Helzlsouer KJ, Huang HY, Alberg AJ, Hoffman S, Burke A, Norkus EP, et al. Association between alpha-tocopherol, gamma-tocopherol, selenium, and subsequent prostate cancer. J Natl Cancer Inst. 2000;92:2018–23.
93. Weinstein SJ, Peters U, Ahn J, Friesen MD, Riboli E, Hayes RB, et al. Serum alpha-tocopherol and gamma-tocopherol concentrations and prostate cancer risk in the PLCO Screening Trial: a nested case-control study. PLoS One. 2012;7:e40204.
94. Navas-Acien A, Bleys J, Guallar E. Selenium intake and cardiovascular risk: what is new? Curr Opin Lipidol. 2008;19:43–9.
95. Duffield-Lillico AJ, Slate EH, Reid ME, Turnbull BW, Wilkins PA, Combs Jr GF, et al. Selenium supplementation and secondary prevention of nonmelanoma skin cancer in a randomized trial. J Natl Cancer Inst. 2003;95:1477–81.
96. Stranges S, Marshall JR, Natarajan R, Donahue RP, Trevisan M, Combs GF, et al. Effects of long-term selenium supplementation on the incidence of type 2 diabetes: a randomized trial. Ann Intern Med. 2007;147:217–23.
97. Clark LC, Combs Jr GF, Turnbull BW, Slate EH, Chalker DK, Chow J, et al. Effects of selenium supplementation for cancer prevention in patients with carcinoma of the skin: a randomized controlled trial. JAMA. 1996;276:1957–63.
98. Sanyal AJ, Chalasani N, Kowdley KV, McCullough A, Diehl AM, Bass NM, et al. Pioglitazone, vitamin E, or placebo for nonalcoholic steatohepatitis. N Engl J Med. 2010;362:1675–85.
99. Pacana T, Sanyal AJ. Vitamin E and nonalcoholic fatty liver disease. Curr Opin Clin Nutr Metab Care. 2012;15:641–8.
100. Goossens ME, Buntinx F, Joniau S, Ackaert K, Ameye F, Billiet I, et al. Designing the selenium and bladder cancer trial (SELEBLAT), a phase III randomized chemoprevention study with selenium on recurrence of bladder cancer in Belgium. BMC Urol. 2012;12:8.
101. Rothwell PM, Fowkes FG, Belch JK, Ogawa H, Warlow CP, Meade TW. Effect of daily aspirin on long-term risk of death due to cancer: analysis of individual patient data from randomized trials. Lancet. 2011;377:31–41.
102. Solomon KR, Freeman MR. The complex interplay between cholesterol and prostate malignancy. Urol Clin N Am. 2011;38:243–59.
103. Jalving M, Gietema JA, Lefrandt JD, de Jong S, Reyners AK, Gans RO, et al. Metformin: taking away the candy for cancer? Eur J Cancer. 2010;46:2369–80.
104. Avci CB, Harman E, Dodurga Y, Susluer SY, Gunduz C. Therapeutic potential of an anti-diabetic drug, metformin: alteration of miRNA expression in prostate cancer cells. Asian Pac J Cancer Prev. 2013;14:765–8.
105. Colquhoun AJ, Venier NA, Vandersluis AD, Besla R, Sugar LM, Kiss A, et al. Metformin enhances the antiproliferative and apoptotic effect of bicalutamide in prostate cancer. Prostate Cancer Prostatic Dis. 2012;15:346–52.
106. Moyad MA. Re: a prospective, randomized pilot study evaluating the effects of metformin and lifestyle intervention on patients with prostate cancer receiving androgen deprivation therapy. Eur Urol. 2012;61:623–4.
107. Nobes JP, Langley SE, Klopper T, Russell-Jones D, Laing RW. A prospective, randomized pilot study evaluating the effects of metformin and lifestyle intervention on patients with prostate cancer receiving androgen deprivation therapy. BJU Int. 2012;109:1495–502.
108. Murtola TJ, Visakorpi T, Lahtela J, Syvala H, Tammela TLJ. Statins and prostate cancer prevention: where we are now, and future directions. Nat Clin Pract Urol. 2008;5:376–87.
109. Moyad MA. Heart health=urologic health and heart unhealthy=urologic unhealthy: rapid review of lifestyle changes and dietary supplements. Urol Clin N Am. 2011;38:359–67.
110. Colli JL, Amling CL. Exploring causes for declining prostate cancer mortality rates in the United States. Urol Oncol. 2008;26:627–33.
111. Colli JL, Amling CL. High cholesterol levels are associated with reduced prostate cancer mortality rates during periods of high but not low statin use in the United States. Urol Oncol. 2009;27:170–3.
112. Statins and prostate cancer. http://www.clinicaltrials.gov. Accessed 10 May 2013.
113. Burn J, Gerdes AM, Macrae F, Mecklin JP, Moeslein G, Olschwang S, et al. Long-term effect of aspirin on cancer risk in carriers of hereditary colorectal cancer: an analysis from the CAPP2 randomised controlled trial. Lancet. 2011;378:2081–8.
114. Metformin and cancer. http://www.clinicaltrials.gov. Accessed 10 May 2013.
115. Wang J, Gallagher D, DeVito LM, Cancino GI, Tsui D, He L, et al. Metformin activates an atypical PKC-CBP pathway to promote neurogenesis and enhance spatial memory formation. Cell Stem Cell. 2012;11:23–35.
116. Moyad MA, Klotz LH. Statin clinical trial (REALITY) for prostate cancer: an over 15-year wait is finally over thanks to a dietary supplement. Urol Clin North Am. 2011;38:325–31.
117. Wilt TJ, Macdonald R, Ishani A. B-sitosterol for the treatment of benign prostatic hyperplasia: a systematic review. BJU Int. 1999;83:976–83.
118. Wilt TJ, Ishani A, MacDonald R, Stark G, Mulrow CD, Lau J. Beta-sitosterols for benign prostatic hyperplasia. Cochrane Database Syst Rev. 2000;2, CD001043.
119. Wilt T, MacDonald R, Ishani A, Rutks I, Stark G. Cernilton for benign prostatic hyperplasia. Cochrane Database Syst Rev. 2000;2, CD001042.
120. Hong H, Kim CS, Maeng S. Effects of pumpkin seed oil and saw palmetto oil in Korean men with symptomatic benign prostatic hyperplasia. Nutr Res Pract. 2009;3:323–7.

121. Wilt T, Ishani A, MacDonald R, Rutks I, Stark G. Pygeum africanum for benign prostatic hyperplasia. Cochrane Database Syst Rev. 2002;1, CD001044.
122. Bent S, Kane C, Shinohara K, Neuhaus J, Hudes ES, Goldberg H, et al. Saw palmetto for benign prostatic hyperplasia (BPH). N Engl J Med. 2006;354: 557–66.
123. Barry MJ, Meleth S, Lee JY, Kreder KJ, Avins AL, Nickel JC, et al. Effect of increasing doses of saw palmetto extract on lower urinary tract symptoms: a randomized trial. JAMA. 2011;306:1344–51.
124. Safarinejad MR. Urtica dioica for treatment of benign prostatic hyperplasia: a prospective, randomized, double-blind, placebo-controlled, crossover study. J Herb Pharmacother. 2005;5:1–11.
125. Demark-Wahnefried W, Polascik TJ, George SL, Switzer BR, Madden JF, Ruffin 4th MT, et al. Flaxseed supplementation (not dietary fat restriction) reduces prostate cancer proliferation rates in men presurgery. Cancer Epidemiol Biomarkers Prev. 2008;17:3577–87.
126. Zhang W, Wang X, Liu Y, Tian H, Flickinger B, Empie MW, et al. Effects of dietary flaxseed lignan extract on symptoms of benign prostatic hyperplasia. J Med Food. 2008;11:207–14.
127. Denmark-Wahnefried W, Robertson CN, Walther PJ, Polascik TJ, Paulson DF, Vollmer RT. Pilot study to explore effects of low-fat, flaxseed-supplemented diet on proliferation on benign prostatic epithelium and prostate-specific antigen. Urology. 2004;63: 900–4.
128. Harper CR, Edwards MJ, DeFilipis AP, Jacobson TA. Flaxseed oil increases the plasma concentrations of cardioprotective (n-3) fatty acids in humans. J Nutr. 2006;136:83–7.
129. DeLorgeril M, Renaud S, Mamelle N, Salen P, Martin JL, Monjaud I, et al. Mediterranean alpha-linolenic acid-rich diet in the secondary prevention of coronary heart disease. Lancet. 1994;343: 1454–9.
130. Moyad MA. An introduction to dietary/supplemental omega-3 fatty acids for general health and prevention: Part I. Urol Oncol. 2005;23:28–35.
131. Moyad MA. An introduction to dietary/supplemental omega-3 fatty acids for general health and prevention: Part II. Urol Oncol. 2005;23:36–48.
132. Vrablik A, Prusikova M, Snejdrlova M, Zlatohlavek L. Omega-3 fatty acids and cardiovascular disease risk: do we understand the relationship. Physiol Res. 2009;58 Suppl 1:S19–26.
133. Olson JH, Erie JC, Bakri SJ. Nutritional supplementation and age-related macular degeneration. Semin Ophthalmol. 2011;26:131–6.
134. Rand AL, Asbell PA. Nutritional supplements for dry eye syndrome. Curr Opin Ophthalmol. 2011;22:279–82.
135. Gopinath B, Flood VM, Rochtchina E, McMahon CM, Mitchell P. Consumption of omega-3 fatty acids and fish and risk of age-related hearing loss. Am J Clin Nutr. 2010;92:416–21.
136. Neukam K, De Spirt S, Stahl W, Bejot M, Maurette JM, Tronnier H, et al. Supplementation of flaxseed oil diminishes skin sensitivity and improves skin barrier function and condition. Skin Pharmacol Physiol. 2011;24:67–74.
137. Smith GI, Atherton P, Reeds DN, Mohammed BS, Rankin D, Rennie MJ, et al. Dietary omega-3 fatty acid supplementation increases the rate of muscle protein synthesis in older adults: a randomized controlled trial. Am J Clin Nutr. 2011;93:402–12.
138. Siener R, Jansen B, Watzer B, Hesse A. Effect of n-3 fatty acid supplementation on urinary risk factors for calcium oxalate stone formation. J Urol. 2011;185: 719–24.
139. Klemens C, Berman D, Mozurkewich E. The effect of perinatal omega-3 fatty acid supplementation on inflammatory markers and allergic diseases: a systematic review. BJOG. 2011;118:916–25.
140. Freeman MP, Hibbein JR, Silver M, Hirschberg AM, Wang B, Yule AM, et al. Omega-3 fatty acids for major depressive disorder associated with the menopausal transition: a preliminary open trial. Menopause. 2011;18:279–84.
141. Tajalizadekhoob Y, Sharifi F, Fakhrzadeh H, Mirarefin M, Ghaderpanahi M, Badamchizade Z, et al. The effect of low-dose omega 3 fatty acids on the treatment of mild to moderate depression in the elderly: a double-blind, randomized, placebo-controlled study. Eur Arch Psychiatry Clin Neurosci. 2011;261:539–49.
142. Winslow BT, Onysko MK, Stob CM, Hazlewood KA. Treatment of Alzheimer disease. Am Fam Physician. 2011;83:1403–12.
143. Brostow DP, Odegaard AO, Koh WP, Duval S, Gross MD, Yuan JM, et al. Omega-3 fatty acids and incident type 2 diabetes: the Singapore Chinese Health Study. Am J Clin Nutr. 2011;94:520–6.
144. Meldrum DR, Gambone JC, Morris MA, Meldrum DA, Esposito K, Ignarro LJ. The link between erectile and cardiovascular health: the canary in the coal mine. Am J Cardiol. 2011;108:599–606.
145. Showell MG, Brown J, Yazdani A, Stankiewicz MT, Hart RJ. Antioxidants for male subfertility. Cochrane Database Syst Rev. 2011;1, CD007411.
146. Risk and Prevention Study Collaborative Group. N-3 fatty acids in patients with multiple cardiovascular risk factors. N Engl J Med. 2013;368:1800–8.
147. Mozaffarian D, Marchioli R, Macchia A, Silleta MG, Ferrazzi P, Gardner TJ, et al. Fish oil and postoperative atrial fibrillation: the Omega-3 fatty acids for prevention of post-operative atrial fibrillation (OPERA) randomized trial. JAMA. 2012;308: 2001–11.
148. Rizos EC, Ntzani EE, Bika E, Kostapanos MS, Elisaf MS. Association between omega-3 fatty acid supplementation and risk of major cardiovascular disease events: a systematic review and meta-analysis. JAMA. 2012;308:1024–33.
149. Szymanski KM, Wheeler DC, Mucci LA. Fish consumption and prostate cancer risk: a review and meta-analysis. Am J Clin Nutr. 2010;92:1223–33.

150. American Heart Association Web site. http://www.heart.org. Accessed 1 May 2013.
151. Konings EJ. Water-soluble vitamins. J AOAC Int. 2006;89:285–8.
152. Obican SG, Finnell RH, Mills JL, Shaw GM, Scialli AR. Folic acid in early pregnancy: a public health success story. FASEB J. 2010;24:4167–74.
153. ZemLin AE, Essack Y, Rensburg M, Keller T, Brinkmann T. Stability of red blood cell folate in whole blood and haemolysate. Clin Lab. 2010;56:391–6.
154. National Reference Laboratory. http://www.aruplab.com/guides/ug/tests/ugf.jsp. Accessed 5 Feb 2013.
155. MRC Vitamin Study Research Group. Prevention of neural tube defects: results of the Medical Research Council Vitamin Study. Lancet. 1991;338:131–7.
156. Czeizel AE, Dudas I. Prevention of the first occurrence of neural-tube defects by periconceptional vitamin supplementation. N Engl J Med. 1992;327:1832–5.
157. Recommendations for the use of folic acid to reduce the number of cases of spina bifida and other neural tube defects. MMWR Recomm Rep. 1992;41(RR-14):1–7.
158. Shaw GM, Schaffer D, Velie EM, Morland K, Harris JA. Periconceptional vitamin use, dietary folate, and the occurrence of neural tube defects. Epidemiology. 1995;6:219–26.
159. LumLey J, Watson L, Watson M, Bower C. Periconceptional supplementation with folate and/or multivitamins for preventing neural tube defects. Cochrane Database Syst Rev. 2001;3, CD001056.
160. http://www.babylon.com/define/112/Latin-Dictionary.html. Accessed 6 Feb 2012.
161. Zeisel SH. Importance of methyl donors during reproduction. Am J Clin Nutr. 2009;89:673S–7.
162. Botto LD, Olney RS, Erickson JD. Vitamin supplements and the risk for congenital anomalies other than neural tube defects. Am J Med Genet C Semin Med Genet. 2004;125C:12–21.
163. Institute of Medicine, Food and Nutrition Board. Folate. In: Dietary reference intakes for thiamin, riboflavin, niacin, vitamin B6, folate, vitamin B12, pantothenic acid, biotin, and choline. Washington, DC: National Academy Press; 2000. pp. 196–305.
164. Mason JB, Choi SW. Effects of alcohol on folate metabolism: implications for carcinogenesis. Alcohol. 2005;35:235–41.
165. Ornoy A. Valproic acid in pregnancy: how much are we endangering the embryo and fetus? Reprod Toxicol. 2009;28:1–10.
166. Yerby MS. Management issues for women with epilepsy. Neural tube defects and folic acid supplementation. Neurology. 2003;61:S23–6.
167. Pittschieler S, Brezinka C, Jahn B, Trinka E, Unterberger I, Dobesberger J, et al. Spontaneous abortions and the prophylactic effect of folic acid supplementation in epileptic women undergoing antiepileptic therapy. J Neurol. 2008;255(12):1926–31.
168. Wilson RD, Davies G, Desilets V, Rid GJ, Summers A, Wyatt P, et al. The use of folic acid for the prevention of neural tube defects and other congenital anomalies. J Obstet Gynaecol Can. 2003;25:959–73.
169. Tinker SC, Cogswell ME, Devine O, Berry RJ. Folic acid intake among U.S. women aged 15–44 years, National Health and Nutrition Examination Survey, 2003–2006. Am J Prev Med. 2010;38:534–42.
170. Ferechide D, Radulescu D. Hyperhomocysteinemia in renal diseases. J Med Life. 2009;2:53–9.
171. Gonzalez-Casas R, Jones EA, Moreno-Otero R. Spectrum of anemia associated with chronic liver disease. World J Gastroenterol. 2009;15:4653–8.
172. Prey S, Paul C. Effect of folic or folinic acid supplementation on methotrexate-associated safety and efficacy in inflammatory disease: a systematic review. Br J Dermatol. 2009;160:622–8.
173. Chen CP. Syndromes, disorders and maternal risk factors associated with neural tube defects (I). Taiwan J Obstet Gynecol. 2008;47:1–9.
174. Mojtabai R. Body mass index and serum folate in childbearing age women. Eur J Epidemiol. 2004;19:1029–36.
175. Kim DB, Oh YS, Yoo KD, Lee JM, Park CS, Ihm SH, et al. Passive smoking in never-smokers is associated with increased plasma homocysteine levels. Int Heart J. 2010;51:183–7.
176. Borrero S, Moore CG, Qin L, Schwarz EB, Akers A, Creinin MD, et al. Unintended pregnancy influences racial disparity in tubal sterilization rates. J Gen Intern Med. 2010;25:122–8.
177. Rosenberg IH. A history of the isolation and identification of folic acid (folate). Ann Nutr Metab. 2012;61:231–5.
178. Pietrzik K, Bailey L, Shane B. Folic acid and L-5-methyltetrahydrofolate: comparison of clinical pharmacokinetics and pharmacodynamics. Clin Pharmacokinet. 2010;49:535–48.
179. U.S. Department of Agriculture's Nutrient Database Web site. http://www.nal.usda.gov/fnic/cgi-bin/nut_search.pl. Accessed 17 May 2013.
180. Roth C, Magnus P, Schjolberg S, Stoltenberg C, Suren P, McKeague IW, et al. Folic acid supplements in pregnancy and severe language delay in children. JAMA. 2011;306:1566–73.
181. Suren P, Roth C, Bresnahan M, Haugen M, Horning M, Hirtz D, et al. Association between maternal use of folic acid supplements and risk of autism spectrum disorders in children. JAMA. 2013;309:570–7.
182. Clarke R, Halsey J, Lewington S, Lonn E, Armitage J, Manson JE, et al. Effects of lowering homocysteine levels with B vitamins on cardiovascular disease, cancer, and cause-specific mortality. Meta-analysis of 8 randomized trials involving 37,485 individuals. Arch Intern Med. 2010;170:1622–31.
183. Cole BF, Baron JA, Sandler RS, Halle RW, Ahnen DJ, Bresaller RS, et al. Folic acid for the prevention of colorectal adenomas: a randomized clinical trial. JAMA. 2007;297:2351–9.

184. Figueriredo JC, Grau MV, Haile RW, Sandler RS, Summers RW, Bresalier RS, et al. Folic acid and risk of prostate cancer: results from a randomized clinical trial. J Natl Cancer Inst. 2009;101:432–5.
185. Collin SM, Metcalfe C, Refsum H, Lewis SJ, Zuccolo L, Smith GD, et al. Circulating folate, vitamin B12, homocysteine, vitamin B12 transport proteins, and risk of prostate cancer: a case-control study, systematic review, and meta-analysis. Cancer Epidemiol Biomarkers Prev. 2010;19:1632–42.
186. Balley RL, Millis JL, Yetley EA, Gahche JJ, Pfeiffer CM, Dwyer JT, et al. Unmetabolized serum folic acid and its relation to folic acid intake from diet and supplements in a nationally representative sample of adults aged > or =60 y in the United States. Am J Clin Nutr. 2010;92:383–9.
187. Wien TN, Pike E, Wisloff T, Staff A, Smeland S, Klemp M. Cancer risk with folic acid supplements: a systematic review and meta-analysis. BMJ Open. 2012;2(1):e000653.
188. Vollset SE, Clarke R, Lewington S, Ebbing M, Halsey J, Lonn E, et al. Effects of folic acid supplementation on overall and site-specific cancer incidence during the randomized trials: meta-analyses of data on 50,000 individuals. Lancet. 2013;381(9871): 1029–36.
189. Qin X, Cui Y, Shen L, Sun N, Zhang Y, Li J, et al. Folic acid supplementation and cancer risk: a meta-analysis of randomized controlled trials. Int J Cancer. 2013. doi:10.1002/ijc.28038.
190. Bassett JK, Severi G, Hodge AM, Baglietto L, Hopper JL, English DR, et al. Dietary intake of B vitamins and methionine and prostate cancer incidence and mortality. Cancer Causes Control. 2012;23:855–63.
191. Roswall N, Larsen SB, Frilis S, Outzen M, Olsen A, Christensen J, et al. Cancer Causes Control. 2013;24:1129–35.
192. Wong WY, Merkus HM, Thomas CM, Menkveld R, Zielhuis GA, Steegers-Theunissen RP. Effects of folic acid and zinc sulfate on male factor subfertility: a double-blind, randomized, placebo-controlled trial. Fertil Steril. 2002;77:491–8.
193. Murphy LE, Mills JL, Molloy AM, Qian C, Carter TC, Strevens H, et al. Folate and vitamin B12 in idiopathic male infertility. Asian J Androl. 2011;13:856–61.
194. Rock CL. Multivitamin-multimineral supplements: who uses them? Am J Clin Nutr. 2007;85(Suppl):277S–9.
195. Barqawi A, Gamito E, O'Donnell C, Crawford ED. Herbal and vitamin supplement use in a prostate cancer screening population. Urology. 2004;63: 288–92.
196. Zheng Selin J, Rautiainen S, Lindblad BE, Morgenstern R, Wolk A. High-dose supplements of vitamins C and E, low-dose multivitamins, and the risk of age-related cataract: a population-based prospective cohort study of men. Am J Epidemiol. 2013;177:548–55.
197. Muntwyler J, Hennekens CH, Manson JE, Buring JE, Gaziano M. Vitamin supplement use in a low-risk population of US male physicians and subsequent cardiovascular mortality. Arch Intern Med. 2002;162:1472–6.
198. Giovannucci E, Chan AT. Role of vitamin and mineral supplementation and aspirin use in cancer survivors. J Clin Oncol. 2010;28:4081–5.
199. Lawson KA, Wright ME, Subar A, Mouw T, Hollenbeck A, Schatzkin A, et al. Multivitamin use and risk of prostate cancer in the National Institutes of Health-AARP Diet and Health Study. J Natl Cancer Inst. 2007;99:754–64.
200. Stevens VL, McCullough ML, Diver WR, Rodriguez C, Jacobs EJ, Thun MJ, et al. Use of multivitamins and prostate cancer mortality in a large cohort of US men. Cancer Causes Control. 2005;16:643–50.
201. Neuhouser ML, Barnett MJ, Kristal AR, Ambrosone CB, King IB, Thornquist M, et al. Dietary supplement use and prostate cancer risk in the Carotene and Retinol Efficacy Trial. Cancer Epidemiol Biomarkers Prev. 2009;18:2202–6.
202. Larsson SC, Akesson A, Bergkvist L, Wolk A. Multivitamin use and breast cancer incidence in a prospective cohort of Swedish women. Am J Clin Nutr. 2010;91:1268–72.
203. Berube S, Diorio C, Brisson J. Multivitamin-multimineral supplement use and mammographic breast density. Am J Clin Nutr. 2008;87:1400–4.
204. Rosen J, Gardiner P, Saper RB, Fillppelli A, White LF, Pearce EN, et al. Complementary and alternative medicine use among patients with thyroid cancer. Thyroid. 2013. Epub ahead of print.
205. Ng K, Meyerhardt JA, Chan JA, Niedzwiecki D, Hollis DR, Saltz LB, et al. Multivitamin use is not associated with cancer recurrence or survival in patients with stage III colon cancer: findings from CALGB 89803. J Clin Oncol. 2010;28:4354–63.
206. Christen WG, Gaziano JM, Hennekens CH. Design of Physicians' Health Study II-a randomized trial of beta-carotene, vitamins E and C, and multivitamins, in prevention of cancer, cardiovascular disease, and eye disease, and review of results of completed trials. Ann Epidemiol. 2000;10:125–34.
207. Gaziano JM, Sesso HD, Christen WG, Bubes V, Smith JP, MacFadyen J, et al. Multivitamins in the prevention of cancer in men: the Physicians' Health Study II randomized controlled trial. JAMA. 2012;308:1871–80.
208. Sesso HD, Christen WG, Bubes V, Smith JP, MacFadyen J, Schvartz M, et al. Multivitamins in the prevention of cardiovascular disease in men: the Physicians' Health Study II randomized controlled trial. JAMA. 2012;308:1751–60.
209. van Adelsberg J, Gann P, Ko AT, Damber JE, Logothetis C, Marberger M, et al. The VIOXX in Prostate Cancer Prevention study: cardiovascular events observed in the rofecoxib 25 mg and placebo treatment groups. Curr Med Res Opin. 2007;23: 2063–70.

210. Thompson IM, Tangen CM, Klein EA, Lippman SM. Phase III prostate cancer prevention trials: are the costs justified? J Clin Oncol. 2005;23:8161–4.
211. Klein EA, Thompson IM, Lippman SM, Goodman PJ, Albanes D, Taylor PR, et al. SELECT: the next prostate cancer prevention trial. Selenium and Vitamin E Cancer Prevention Trial. J Urol. 2001;166:1311–5.
212. Nijjar PS, Burke FM, Bloesch A, Rader DJ. Role of dietary supplements in lowering low-density lipoprotein cholesterol: a review. J Clin Lipidol. 2010;4:248–58.
213. Becker DJ, Gordon RY, Halbert SC, French B, Morris PB, Rader DJ. Red yeast rice for dyslipidemia in statin-intolerant patients: a randomized trial. Ann Intern Med. 2009;150:830–9.
214. Venero CV, Venero JV, Wortham DC, Thompson PD. Lipid-lowering efficacy of red yeast rice in a population intolerant to statins. Am J Cardiol. 2010;105:664–6.
215. Halbert SC, French B, Gordon RY, Farrar JT, Schmitz K, Morris PB, et al. Tolerability of red yeast rice (2400 mg twice daily) versus pravastatin (20 mg twice daily) in patients with previous statin intolerance. Am J Cardiol. 2010;105:198–204.
216. Sikka P, Kapoor S, Bindra VK, Sharma M, Vishwakarma P, Saxena KK. Statin intolerance: now a solved problem. J Postgrad Med. 2011;57:321–8.
217. Red yeast rice. Med Lett Drugs Ther. 2009;51:71–2.
218. Lin Y-L, Wang T-H, Lee M-H, Su N-W. Biologically active components and nutraceuticals in the Monascus-fermented rice: a review. Appl Microbiol Biotechnol. 2008;77:965–73.
219. Endo A. Monacolin K, a new hypocholesterolemic agent produced by a Monascus species. J Antibiot (Tokyo). 1979;32:852–4.
220. Landers P. Stalking cholesterol. How one scientist intrigued by molds found first statin. Feat of Japan's Dr. Endo led to heart-care revolution but brought him nothing. Nature as a drug laboratory. Wall Street Journal, January 9, 2006, pp. A1, A8.
221. Liu J, Zhang J, Shi Y, Grimsgaard S, Alraek T, Fonnebo V. Chinese red yeast rice (Monascus purpureus) for primary hyperlipidemia: a meta-analysis of randomized controlled trials. Chin Med. 2006;1:4.
222. Lu Z, Kou W, Du B, et al. Effects of Xuezhikang, an extract from red yeast Chinese rice, on coronary events in a Chinese population with previous myocardial infarction. Am J Cardiol. 2008;101:1689–93.
223. China Coronary Secondary Prevention Study Group. China coronary secondary prevention study (CCSPS)-Lipid regulating therapy with xuezhikang for secondary prevention of coronary heart disease. Chin J Cardiol (Chin). 2005;33:109–15.
224. Ye P, Lu ZL, Du BM, Chen Z, Wu YF, Yu XH, et al. Effects of xuezhikang on cardiovascular events and mortality in elderly patients with a history of myocardial infarction: a subgroup analysis of elderly subjects from China coronary secondary prevention study. J Am Geriatr Soc. 2007;55:1015–22.
225. Hong MY, Seeram NP, Zhang Y, Heber D. Chinese red yeast rice versus lovastatin effects on prostate cancer cells with and without androgen receptor overexpression. J Med Food. 2008;11:657–66.
226. Hong MY, Henning S, Moro A, Seeram NP, Zhang Y, Heber D. Chinese red yeast rice inhibition of prostate tumor growth in SCID mice. Cancer Prev Res (Phila). 2011;4:608–15.
227. Hong MY, Seeram NP, Zhang Y, Heber D. Anticancer effects of Chinese red yeast rice versus monacolin K alone on colon cancer cells. J Nutr Biochem. 2008;19:448–58.
228. Ma KY, Zhang ZS, Zhao SX, Chang Q, Wong YM, Yeung SY, et al. Red yeast increases excretion of bile acids in hamsters. Biomed Environ Sci. 2009;22:269–77.
229. Li JJ, Hu SS, Fang CH, Hui RT, Miao LF, Yang YJ, et al. Effects of xuezhikang, an extract of cholestin, on lipid profile and C-reactive protein: a short-term time course study in patients with stable angina. Clin Chim Acta. 2005;352:217–24.
230. Zhao SP, Liu L, Cheng YC, Shishehbor MH, Liu MH, Peng DQ, et al. Xuezhikang, an extract of cholestin, protects endothelial function through antiinflammatory and lipid-lowering mechanisms in patients with coronary heart disease. Circulation. 2004;110:915–20.
231. Liu L, Zhao SP, Cheng YC, Li YL. Xuezhikang decreases serum lipoprotein(a) and C-reactive protein concentrations in patients with coronary heart disease. Clin Chem. 2003;49:1347–52.
232. Lehrer S, Diamond EJ, Mamkine B, Droller MJ, Stone NN, Stock RG. C-reactive protein is significantly associated with prostate-specific antigen and metastatic disease in prostate cancer. BJU Int. 2005;95:961–2.
233. Solomon KR, Pelton K, Boucher K, Joo J, Tully C, Zurakowski D, et al. Ezetimibe is an inhibitor if tumor angiogenesis. Am J Pathol. 2009;174:1017–26.
234. Moyad MA, Merrick GS. Statins and cholesterol lowering after a cancer diagnosis: why not? Urol Oncol. 2005;23:49–55.
235. Klotz L. Active surveillance versus radical treatment for favorable-risk localized prostate cancer. Curr Treat Options Oncol. 2006;7:355–62.
236. Gotto Jr AM, Whitney E, Stein EA, Shapiro SR, Clearfield M, Weis S, et al. Relation between baseline and on treatment lipid parameters and first major acute major coronary events in the Air Force/Texas Coronary Atherosclerosis Prevention Study (AFCAPS/TexCAPS). Circulation. 2000;101:477–84.
237. Nakamura H, for the MEGA Study Group. Primary prevention of cardiovascular diseases among hypercholesterolemic Japanese with a low dose of pravastatin. Atheroscler Suppl. 2007;8:13–7.
238. Gordon RY, Cooperman T, Obermeyer W, Becker DJ. Marked variability of monacolin levels in commercial red yeast rice products: buyer beware. Arch Intern Med. 2010;170:1722–7.

239. Heber D, Lembertas A, Lu QY, Bowerman S, Go VL. An analysis of nine proprietary Chinese red yeast rice dietary supplements: implications of variability in chemical profile and contents. J Altern Complement Med. 2001;7:133–9.
240. Garnett WR. Interactions with hydroxymethylglutaryl-coenzyme A reductase inhibitors. Am J Health Syst Pharm. 1995;52:1639–45.
241. Schacter M. Chemical, pharmacokinetic and pharmacodynamic properties of statins: an update. Fundam Clin Pharmacol. 2005;19:117–25.
242. Moghadasian MH. Clinical pharmacology of 3-hydroxy-3-methylglutaryl coenzyme A reductase inhibitors. Life Sci. 1999;65:1329–37.
243. Hoffer LJ, Levine M, Assouline S, Melnychuk D, Padayatty SJ, Rosadiuk K, et al. Phase I clinical trial of I.V. ascorbic acid in advanced malignancy. Ann Oncol. 2008;19:1969–74.
244. Robitalle L, Mamer OA, Miller Jr WH, Levine M, Assouline S, Melnychuk D, et al. Oxalic acid excretion after intravenous ascorbic acid administration. Metabolism. 2009;58:263–9.
245. Thomas LD, Elinder CG, Tiselius HG, Wolk A, Akesson A. Ascorbic acid supplements and kidney stone incidence among men: a prospective study. JAMA Intern Med. 2013;173:386–8.
246. Ohno S, Ohno Y, Suzuki N, Soma G, Inoue M. High-dose vitamin C (ascorbic acid) therapy in the treatment of patients with advanced cancer. Anticancer Res. 2009;29:809–15.
247. Barnett CM, Nielson CM, Shannon J, Chan JM, Shikany JM, Bauer DC, et al. Serum 25-OH vitamin D levels and risk of developing prostate cancer in older men. Cancer Causes Control. 2010;21:1297–303.
248. Michaelsson K, Baron JA, Snellman G, Gedeborg R, Byberg L, Sundstrom J, et al. Plasma vitamin D and mortality in older men: a community-based prospective cohort study. Am J Clin Nutr. 2010;92:841–8.
249. Sanders KM, Stuart AL, Williamson EJ, et al. Annual high-dose oral vitamin D and falls and fractures in older women. JAMA. 2010;303:1815–22.
250. Bischoff-Ferrari HA, Giovannucci E, Willett WC, Dietrich T, Dawson-Hughes B. Estimation of optimal serum concentrations of 25-hydroxyvitamin D for multiple health outcomes. Am J Clin Nutr. 2006;84:18–28.
251. Zerwekh JE. Blood biomarkers of vitamin D status. Am J Clin Nutr. 2008;87(Suppl):1087S–91.
252. Isenor JE, Ensom MH. Is there a role for therapeutic drug monitoring of vitamin D level as a surrogate marker for fracture risk. Pharmacotherapy. 2010;30:254–64.
253. Kopes-Kerr C. Should family physicians routinely screen for vitamin d deficiency? No: screening is unnecessary, and routine supplementation makes more sense. Am Fam Physician. 2013;87(8):Online.
254. Murdoch DR, Slow S, Chambers ST, Jennings LC, Stewart AW, Priest PC, et al. Effects of vitamin D3 supplementation on upper respiratory tract infections in healthy adults: the VIDARIS randomized controlled trial. JAMA. 2012;308:1333–9.
255. Moyad MA. Dr Moyad's no bogus science health advice. Ann Arbor, MI: Ann Arbor Media Group; 2009.
256. Wolpowitz D, Gilchrest BA. The vitamin D questions: how much do you need and how should you get it? J Am Acad Dermatol. 2006;54:301–17.
257. Giovannucci E, Liu Y, Rimm EB, Hollis BW, Fuchs CS, Stampfer MJ, et al. Prospective study of predictors of vitamin D status and cancer incidence and mortality in men. J Natl Cancer Inst. 2006;98:451–9.
258. Aasheim ET, Hofso D, Hjelmesaeth J, Birkeland KI, Bohmer T. Vitamin status in morbidly obese patients: a cross-sectional study. Am J Clin Nutr. 2008;87:362–9.
259. Perez-Castrillon JL, Abad L, Vega G, Sanz-Cantalapiedra A, Garcia-Porrero M, Pinacho F, et al. Effect of atorvastatin on bone mineral density in patients with acute coronary syndrome. Eur Rev Med Pharmacol Sci. 2008;12:83–8.
260. Chen TC, Chimeh F, Lu Z, Mathieu J, Person KS, Zhang A, et al. Factors that influence the cutaneous synthesis and dietary sources of vitamin D. Arch Biochem Biophys. 2007;460:213–7.
261. Mozaffarian D, Rimm EB. Fish intake, contaminants, and human health: evaluating the risks and benefits. JAMA. 2006;296:1885–99.
262. Levis S, Gomez A, Jimenez C, Veras L, Ma F, Lai S, et al. Vitamin D deficiency and seasonal variation in an adult South Florida population. J Clin Endocrinol Metab. 2005;90:1557–62.
263. Jacobs ET, Alberts DS, Foote JA, Green SB, Hollis BW, Yu Z, et al. Vitamin D insufficiency in southern Arizona. Am J Clin Nutr. 2008;87:608–13.
264. Chel V, Wijnhoven HAH, Smit JH, Ooms M, Lips P. Efficacy of different doses and time intervals of oral vitamin D supplementation with or without calcium in elderly nursing home residents. Osteoporos Int. 2008;19:663–71.
265. Houghton LA, Vieth R. The case against ergocalciferol (vitamin D2) as a vitamin supplement. Am J Clin Nutr. 2006;84:694–7.
266. Welch TR, Bergstrom WH, Tsang RC. Vitamin D-deficient rickets: the reemergence of a once-conquered disease. J Pediatr. 2000;137:143–5.
267. Rajakumar K, Thomas SB. Reemerging nutritional rickets: a historical perspective. Arch Pediatr Adolesc Med. 2005;159:335–41.
268. Institute of Medicine. Dietary reference intakes for calcium and vitamin D. 2010. http://www.iom.edu/vitamind. Accessed 1 May 2013.
269. Slomski A. IOM endorses vitamin D, calcium only for bone health, dispels deficiency claims. JAMA. 2011;305:453–4.
270. Tangpricha V, Pearce EN, Chen TC, Holick MF. Vitamin D insufficiency among free-living healthy young adults. Am J Med. 2002;112:659–62.
271. Barger-Lux MJ, Heaney RP, Dowell S, Chen TC, Holick MF. Vitamin D and its major metabolites: serum levels after graded oral dosing in healthy men. Osteoporos Int. 1998;8:222–30.

272. Harris SS, Dawson-Hughes B, Perrone GA. Plasma 25-hydroxyvitamin D responses of younger and older men to three weeks of supplementation with 1800 IU/day of vitamin D. J Am Coll Nutr. 1999;18:470–4.
273. Harris SS, Dawson-Hughes B. Plasma vitamin D and 25OHD responses of young and old men to supplementation with vitamin D3. J Am Coll Nutr. 2002;21:357–62.
274. Heaney RP. Vitamin D: criteria for safety and efficacy. Nutr Rev. 2008;66(10 Suppl 2):S178–81.
275. Tuohimaa P, Tenkanen L, Ahonen M, Lumme S, Jellum E, Hallmans G, et al. Both high and low levels of blood vitamin D are associated with a higher prostate cancer risk: a longitudinal, nested case-control study in the Nordic countries. Int J Cancer. 2004;108:104–8.
276. Ahn J, Peters U, Albanes D, Purdue MP, Abnet CC, Chatterjee N, et al. Serum vitamin D concentration and prostate cancer risk: a nested case-control study. J Natl Cancer Inst. 2008;100:796–804.
277. Travis RC, Crowe FL, Allen NE, Appleby PN, Roddam AW, Tjonneland A, et al. Serum vitamin D and risk of prostate cancer in a case-control analysis nested within the European Prospective Investigation into Cancer and Nutrition (EPIC). Am J Epidemiol. 2009;169:1223–32.
278. Meyer HE, Robsahm TE, Bjorge T, Brustad M, Blomhoff R. Vitamin D, season, and risk of prostate cancer: a nested case-control study within Norwegian health studies. Am J Clin Nutr. 2013;97:147–54.
279. Brandstedt J, Almquist M, Manjer J, Maim J. Vitamin D, PTH, and calcium and the risk of prostate cancer: a prospective nested case-control study. Cancer Causes Control. 2012;23:1377–85.
280. Barnett CM, Beer TM. Prostate cancer and vitamin D: what does the evidence really suggest? Urol Clin N Am. 2011;38:333–42.
281. Vieth R. Why the optimal requirement for vitamin D3 is probably much higher than what is officially recommended for adults. J Steroid Biochem Mol Biol. 2004;89–90:575–9.
282. Pfeifer M, Begerow B, Minne HW. Vitamin D and muscle function. Osteoporos Int. 2002;13:187–94.
283. Glerup H, Mikkelsen K, Poulsen L, Hass E, Overbeck S, Andersen H, et al. Hypovitaminosis D myopathy without biochemical signs of osteomalacia bone involvement. Calcif Tissue Int. 2000;66: 419–24.
284. Bischoff-Ferrari HA, Dawson-Hughes B, Willett WC, Staehelin HB, Bazemore MG, Zee RY, et al. Effect of vitamin D on falls: a meta-analysis. JAMA. 2004;291:1999–2006.
285. Galvao DA, Nosaka K, Taaffe DR, Spry N, Kristjanson LJ, McGuigan MR, et al. Resistance training and reduction of treatment side effects in prostate cancer patients. Med Sci Sports Exerc. 2006;38:2045–52.
286. Kukuijan S, Nowson CA, Sanders K, Daly RM. Effects of resistance exercise and fortified milk on skeletal muscle mass, muscle size, and functional performance in middle-aged and older men: an 18-mo randomized trial. J Appl Physiol. 2009;107: 1864–73.
287. Kukuijan S, Nowson CA, Sanders KM, Nicholson GC, Seibel MJ, Salmon J, et al. Independent and combined effects of calcium-vitamin D3 and exercise on bone structure and strength in older men: an 18-month factorial design randomized trial. J Clin Endocrinol Metab. 2011;96:955–63.
288. Li K, Kaaks R, Linseisen J, Rohrmann S. Associations of dietary calcium intake and calcium supplementation with myocardial infarction and stroke risk and overall cardiovascular mortality in the Heidelberg cohort of the European Prospective Investigation into Cancer and Nutrition study (EPIC-Heidelberg). Heart. 2012;98:920–5.
289. Rodriguez C, McCullough ML, Mondul AM, Jacobs EJ, Fakhrabadi-Shokoohi D, Giovannucci EL, et al. Calcium, dairy products, and risk of prostate cancer in a prospective cohort of United States men. Cancer Epidemiol Biomarkers Prev. 2003;12:597–603.
290. Giovannucci E, Liu Y, Stampfer MJ, Willett WC. A prospective study of calcium intake and incident and fatal prostate cancer. Cancer Epidemiol Biomarkers Prev. 2006;15:203–10.
291. Baron JA, Beach M, Wallace K, Grau MV, Sandler RS, Mandel JS, et al. Risk of prostate cancer in a randomized clinical trial of calcium supplementation. Cancer Epidemiol Biomarkers Prev. 2005;14:586–9.
292. Kristal AR, Chi C, Tangen CM, Etzioni R, Thompson IM. Associations of demographic and lifestyle characteristics with prostate-specific antigen (PSA) concentration and rate of PSA increase. Cancer. 2006;106:320–8.
293. Planas J, Morote J, Orsola A, Salvador C, Trilla E, Cecchini L, et al. The relationship between daily calcium intake and bone mineral density in men with prostate cancer. BJU Int. 2007;99:812–6.
294. Wadhwa VK, Weston R, Mistry R, Parr NJ. Long-term changes in bone mineral density and predicted fracture risk in patients receiving androgen deprivation therapy for prostate cancer, with stratification of treatment based on presenting values. BJU Int. 2009;104:800–5.
295. Panju AH, Breunis H, Cheung AM, Leach M, Fleshner N, Warde P, et al. Management of decreased bone mineral density in men starting androgen-deprivation therapy for prostate cancer. BJU Int. 2009;103:753–7.
296. Baron JA, Beach M, Mandel JS, van Stolk RU, Haile RW, Sandler RS, et al. Calcium supplements for the prevention of colorectal adenomas. Calcium Polyp Prevention Study Group. N Engl J Med. 1999;340: 101–7.
297. Bonithon-Kopp C, Kronborg O, Giacosa A, Rath U, Faivre J. Calcium and fibre supplementation in prevention of colorectal adenoma recurrence: a randomized intervention trial. European Cancer Prevention Organization Study Group. Lancet. 2005;356:1300–6.

298. Borghi L, Schianchi T, Meschi T, Guerra A, Allegri F, Maggiore U, et al. Comparison of two diets for the prevention of recurrent stones in idiopathic hypercalciuria. N Engl J Med. 2002;346:77–84.
299. Saper RB, Rash R. Zinc: an essential micronutrient. Am Fam Physician. 2009;79:768.
300. Leitzmann MF, Stampfer MJ, Wu K, Colditz GA, Willett WC, Giovannucci EL. Zinc supplement use and risk of prostate cancer. J Am Cancer Inst. 2002;95:1004–7.
301. Age-Related Eye Disease Study Research Group. A randomized, placebo-controlled, clinical trial of high-dose supplementation with vitamins C and E, beta-carotene, and zinc for age-related macular degeneration and vision loss: AREDS Report Number 8. Arch Ophthalmol. 2001;119:1417–36.
302. Johnson AR, Munoz A, Gottlieb JL, Jarrard DF. High dose zinc increases hospital admissions due to genitourinary complications. J Urol. 2007;177:639–43.
303. Sanchez C, Lopez-Jurado M, Planells E, Llopis J, Aranda P. Assessment of iron and zinc intake and related biochemical parameters in an adult Mediterranean population from southern Spain: influence of lifestyle factors. J Nutr Biochem. 2009;20:125–31.
304. Fashner J, Ericson K, Werner S. Treatment of the common cold in children and adults. Am Fam Physician. 2012;86:153–9.
305. Pantuck AJ, Leppert JT, Zomorodian N, Aronson W, Hong J, Barnard RJ, et al. Phase II study of pomegranate juice for men with rising prostate-specific antigen following surgery or radiation for prostate cancer. Clin Cancer Res. 2006;12(13):4018–26.
306. Bell C, Hawthrone S. Ellagic acid, pomegranate and prostate cancer—a mini review. J Pharm Pharmacol. 2008;60:139–44.
307. Nelson JB, Sleep DJ, Isaacson JD, Carducci MA. Limitation of prostate-specific antigen doubling time as a predictor of outcome in hormone-naïve prostate cancer. J Clin Oncol. 2006;25(18S):233S-abstract 4566.
308. Freedland SJ, Humphreys EB, Mangold LA, Eisenberger M, Dorey FJ, Walsh PC, et al. Death in patients with recurrent prostate cancer after radical prostatectomy: time subgroups and their associated contributions to all-cause mortality. J Clin Oncol. 2007;25:1765–71.
309. Paller CJ, Ye X, Wozniak PJ, Gillespie BK, Sieber PR, Greengold RH, et al. A randomized phase II study of pomegranate extract for men with rising PSA following initial therapy for localized prostate cancer. Prostate Cancer Prostatic Dis. 2013;16:50–5.
310. Leitzmann MF, Platz EA, Stampfer MJ, Willett WC, Giovannucci E. Ejaculation frequency and subsequent risk of prostate cancer. JAMA. 2004;291:1578–86.
311. Zhou J, Smith S, Giovannucci E, Michaud DS. Reexamination of total fluid intake and bladder cancer in the Health Professionals Follow-up Study Cohort. Am J Epidemiol. 2012;175:696–705.
312. Sharifi N, Gulley JL, Dahut WL. An update on androgen therapy for prostate cancer. Endocr Relat Cancer. 2010;17:R305–15.
313. Wilson AC, Meethal SV, Bowen RL, Atwood CS. Leuprolide acetate: a drug of diverse clinical applications. Expert Opin Investig Drugs. 2007;16:1851–63.
314. Mottet N, Bellmunt J, Bolla M, Joniau S, Mason M, Mateev V, et al. EAU guidelines on prostate cancer. Part II: treatment of advanced, relapsing, and castration-resistant prostate cancer. Eur Urol. 2011;59:572–83.
315. Adler RA. Management of osteoporosis in men on androgen deprivation therapy. Maturitas. 2011;68:143–7.
316. Beebe-Dimmer J, Morgenstern H, Cetin K, Yee C, Bartoces M, Shahinian V, et al. Androgen deprivation therapy and cataract incidence among elderly prostate cancer patients in the United States. Ann Epidemiol. 2011;21:156–63.
317. Kim HS, Freedland SJ. Androgen deprivation therapy in prostate cancer: anticipated side-effects and their management. Curr Opin Support Palliat Care. 2010;4:147–52.
318. Saylor PJ, Keating NL, Smith MR. Prostate cancer survivorship: prevention and treatment of the adverse effects of androgen deprivation therapy. J Gen Intern Med. 2009;24 Suppl 2:S389–94.
319. Moyad MA. Promoting general health during androgen deprivation therapy (ADT): a rapid 10-step review for your patients. Urol Oncol. 2005;23:56–64.
320. Strum SB, McDermed JE, Scholz MC, Johnson H, Tisman G. Anaemia associated with androgen deprivation in patients with prostate cancer receiving combined hormone blockade. Br J Urol. 1997;79:933–41.
321. Malone S, Perry G, Segal R, Dahrouge S, Crook J. Long-term side-effects of intermittent androgen suppression therapy in prostate cancer: results of a phase II study. BJU Int. 2005;96:514–20.
322. Nilsson-Ehle H, Jagenburg R, Landahl S, Svanborg A. Blood hemoglobin declines in the elderly: implications for reference intervals from age 70 to 88. Eur J Haematol. 2000;65:297–305.
323. Ferrucci L, Maggio M, Bandinelli S, Basaria S, Lauretani F, Ble A, et al. Low testosterone levels and the risk of anemia in older men and women. Arch Intern Med. 2006;166:1380–8.
324. Hara N, Nishiyama T, Takizawa I, Saito T, Kitamura Y, Takahashi K. Decline of the red blood cell count in patients receiving androgen deprivation therapy for localized prostate cancer: impact of ADT on insulin-like growth factor-1 and erythropoiesis. Urology. 2010;75:1441–5.
325. Diamond TH, Higan CS, Smith MR, Guise TA, Singer FR. Osteoporosis in men with prostate carcinoma receiving androgen-deprivation therapy: recommendations for diagnosis and therapies. Cancer. 2004;100:892–9.
326. Wang W, Yussa T, Tsuchiya N, et al. Bone mineral density in Japanese prostate cancer patients under androgen-deprivation therapy. Endocr Relat Cancer. 2008;15:943–52.

327. Yuasa T, Maita S, Tsuchiya N, Ma Z, Narita S, Horikawa Y, et al. Relationship between bone mineral density and androgen-deprivation therapy in Japanese prostate cancer patients. Urology. 2010;75:1131–7.
328. Iso H. Lifestyle and cardiovascular disease in Japan. J Atheroscler Thromb. 2011;18:83–8.
329. Ryan CW, Huo D, Stallings JW, Davis RL, Beer TM, McWhorter LT. Lifestyle factors and duration of androgen deprivation affect bone mineral density of patients with prostate cancer during first year of therapy. Urology. 2007;70:122–6.
330. Planas J, Morote J, Orsola A, Salvador C, Trilla E, Cecchini L, et al. The relationship between daily calcium intake and bone mineral density in men with prostate cancer. BJU Int. 2007;99:812–5.
331. Wilcox A, Carnes ML, Moon TD, Tobias R, Baade H, Stamos E, et al. Androgen deprivation in veterans with prostate cancer: implications for skeletal health. Ann Pharmacother. 2006;40:2107–14.
332. Yee EF, White RE, Murata GH, Handanos C, Hoffman RM. Osteoporosis management in prostate cancer patients treated with androgen deprivation therapy. J Gen Intern Med. 2007;22:1305–10.
333. Smith MR, Egerdie B, Harnandez Toriz N, Feldman R, Tammela TL, Saad F, et al. Denosumab in men receiving androgen-deprivation therapy for prostate cancer. N Engl J Med. 2009;361:745–55.
334. Galvao DA, Taaffe DR, Spry N, Joseph D, Newton RU. Combined resistance and aerobic exercise program reverses muscle loss in men undergoing androgen suppression therapy for prostate cancer without bone metastases: a randomized controlled trial. J Clin Oncol. 2010;28:340–7.
335. Borsheim E, Bui QU, Tissier S, Kobayashi H, Ferrando AA, Wolfe RR, et al. Effect of amino acid supplementation on muscle mass, strength and physical function in the elderly. Clin Nutr. 2008;27:189–95.
336. Scognamiglio R, Avogaro A, Negut C, Piccolotto R, de Kreutzenberg SV, Tiengo A. The effects of oral amino acid intake on ambulatory capacity in elderly subjects. Aging Clin Exp Res. 2004;16:443–7.
337. Dillon EL, Sheffield-Moore M, Paddon-Jones D, Gilkison C, Sanford AP, Casperson SL, et al. Amino acid supplementation increases lean body mass, basal muscle protein synthesis, and insulin-like growth factor-I expression in older women. J Clin Endocrinol Metab. 2009;94:1630–7.
338. Pennings B, Boirie Y, Senden JM, Gijsen AP, Kuipers H, van Loon LJ. Whey protein stimulates postprandial muscle protein accretion more effectively than do casein and casein hydrolysate in older men. Am J Clin Nutr. 2011;93:997–1005.
339. Schmitz KH, Ahmed RL, Troxel AB, Cheville A, Lewis-Grant L, Smith R, et al. Weight lifting for women at risk for breast cancer-related lymphedema: a randomized trial. JAMA. 2010;304: 2699–705.
340. Nair KS, Rizza RA, O'Brien P, Dhatariya K, Short KR, Nehra A, et al. DHEA in elderly women and DHEA or testosterone in elderly men. N Engl J Med. 2006;355:1647–59.
341. Blackman MR, Sorkin JD, Munzer T, Bellantoni MF, Busby-Whitehead J, Stevens TE, et al. Growth hormone and sex steroid administration in healthy aged women and men: a randomized controlled trial. JAMA. 2002;288:2282–92.
342. Taaffe DR, Pruitt L, Reim J, Hintz RL, Butterfield G, Hoffman AR, et al. Effect of recombinant growth hormone on the muscle strength response to resistance exercise in elderly men. J Clin Endocrinol Metab. 1994;79:1361–6.
343. Levine GN, D'Amico AV, Berger P, Clark PE, Eckel RH, Keating NL, et al. Androgen-deprivation therapy in prostate cancer and cardiovascular risk: a science advisory from the American Heart Association, American Cancer Society, and American Urological Association: endorsed by the American Society for Radiation Oncology. Circulation. 2010;121:833–40.
344. Nguyen PL, Je Y, Schutz FA, Hoffman KE, Hu JC, Parekh A, et al. Association of androgen deprivation therapy with cardiovascular death in patients with prostate cancer: a meta-analysis of randomized trials. JAMA. 2011;306:2359–66.
345. Yannucci J, Manola J, Garnick MB, Bhat G, Bubley GJ. The effect of androgen deprivation therapy on fasting serum lipid and glucose parameters. J Urol. 2006;176:520–5.
346. Fetterman Jr JW, Zdanowicz MM. Therapeutic potential of n-3 polyunsaturated fatty acids in disease. Am J Health Syst Pharm. 2009;66:1169–79.
347. Taouis M, Dagou C, Ster C, Durand G, Pinault M, Delarue J. N-3 polyunsaturated fatty acids prevent the defect of insulin receptor signaling in muscle. Am J Physiol Endocrinol Metab. 2002;282: E664–71.
348. Lombardo YB, Chicco AG. Effects of dietary polyunsaturated n-3 fatty acids on dyslipidemia and insulin resistance in rodents and humans. A review. J Nutr Biochem. 2006;17:1–13.
349. Fedor D, Kelley DS. Prevention of insulin resistance by n-3 polyunsaturated fatty acids. Curr Opin Clin Nutr Metab Care. 2009;12:138–46.
350. Carpenter YA, Portois L, Malaisse WJ. N-3 fatty acids and the metabolic syndrome. Am J Clin Nutr. 2006;83(Suppl):1499S–504.
351. Rudkowska I. Fish oil for cardiovascular disease: impact on diabetes. Maturitas. 2010;67:25–8.
352. Derweesh IH, Diblasio CJ, Kincade MC, Malcolm JB, Lamar KD, Patterson AL, et al. Risk of new-onset diabetes mellitus and worsening glycaemic variables for established diabetes in men undergoing androgen-deprivation therapy for prostate cancer. BJU Int. 2007;100:1060–5.
353. Kris-Etherton PM, Harris WS, Appel LJ, AHA Nutrition Committee, American Heart Association. Omega-3 fatty acids and cardiovascular disease: new recommendations from the American Heart Association. Arterioscler Thromb Vasc Biol. 2003;23:151–2.
354. Braith RW, Stewart KJ. Resistance exercise training: its role in the prevention of cardiovascular disease. Circulation. 2006;113:2642–50.

355. Barton DL, Soori GS, Bauer BA, Sloan JA, Johnson PA, Figueras C, et al. Pilot study of Panax quinquefolius (American ginseng) to improve cancer-related fatigue: a randomized, double-blind, dose-finding evaluation: NCCTG trial N03CA. Support Care Cancer. 2010;18:179–87.
356. Cormie P, Newton RU, Taaffe DR, Spry N, Joseph D, Akhill Hamid M, et al. Exercise maintains sexual activity in men undergoing androgen suppression for prostate cancer: a randomized controlled trial. Prostate Cancer Prostatic Dis. 2013;16:170–5.
357. Kontos M, Agbaje OF, Rymer J, Fentiman IS. What can be done about hot flushes after treatment for breast cancer? Climacteric. 2010;13:4–21.
358. Moyad MA. Complementary therapies for reducing the risk of osteoporosis in patients receiving luteinizing hormone-releasing hormone treatment/orchiectomy for prostate cancer: a review and assessment of the need for more research. Urology. 2002;59(4 Suppl 1):34–40.
359. Irani J, Salomon L, Oba R, Bouchard P, Mottet N. Efficacy of venlafaxine, medroxyprogesterone acetate, and cyproterone acetate for the treatment of vasomotor hot flushes in men taking gonadotropin-releasing hormone analogues for prostate cancer: a double-blind, randomized trial. Lancet. 2010;11: 147–54.
360. Langenstroer P, Kramer B, Cutting B, Amling C, Poultan T, Lance R, et al. Parenteral medroxyprogesterone for the management of luteinizing hormone releasing hormone induced hot flashes in men with advanced prostate cancer. J Urol. 2005;174: 642–5.
361. Lucas M, Asselin G, Merette C, Poulin MJ, Dodin S. Effects of ethyl-eicosapentaenoic acid omega-3 fatty acid supplementation on hot flashes and quality of life among middle-aged women: a double-blind, placebo-controlled, randomized clinical trial. Menopause. 2009;16:357–66.
362. Freeman MP. Omega-3 fatty acids in major depressive disorder. J Clin Psychiatry. 2009;70 Suppl 5:7–11.
363. Martins JG. EPA but not DHA appears to be responsible for the efficacy of omega-3 long chain polyunsaturated fatty acid supplementation in depression: evidence from a meta-analysis of randomized controlled trials. J Am Coll Nutr. 2009;28:525–42.
364. Ryan JL, Heckler CE, Roscoe JA, Dakhll SR, Kirshner J, Flynn PJ, et al. Ginger (Zingiber officinale) reduces acute chemotherapy-induced nausea: a URCC CCOP study of 576 patients. Support Care Cancer. 2012;20:1479–89.
365. Mijnhout GS, Kollen BJ, Alkhalaf A, Kleefstra N, Bilo HJ. Alpha lipoic acid for symptomatic peripheral neuropathy in patients with diabetes: a meta-analysis of randomized controlled trials. Int J Endocrinol. 2012;2012:456279.
366. Koh EH, Lee WJ, Lee SA, Kim EH, Cho EH, Jeong E, et al. Effects of alpha-lipoic acid on body weight in obese subjects. Am J Med. 2011;124:85e1–8.
367. Marshall JR, Tangen CM, Sakr WA, Wood Jr DP, Berry DL, Klein EA, et al. Phase III trial of selenium to prevent prostate cancer in men with high-grade prostatic intraepithelial neoplasia: SWOG S9917. Cancer Prev Res. 2011;4:1761–9.
368. Fleshner NE, Kapusta L, Donnelly B, Tanguay S, Chin J, Hersey K, et al. Progression from high-grade prostatic intraepithelial neoplasia to cancer: a randomized trial of combination vitamin-E, soy and selenium. J Clin Oncol. 2011;29: 2386–90.
369. Algotar AM, Stratton MS, Ahmann FR, Ranger-Moore J, Nagle RB, Thompson PA, et al. Phase 3 clinical trial investigating the effect of selenium supplementation in men at high-risk for prostate cancer. Prostate. 2013;73:328–35.
370. Stratton MS, Algotar AM, Ranger-Moore J, Stratton SP, Slate EH, Hsu CH, et al. Oral selenium supplementation has no effect on prostate-specific antigen velocity in men undergoing active surveillance for localized prostate cancer. Cancer Prev Res (Phila). 2010;3:1035–43.
371. Bauer CM, Ishak MB, Johnson EK, Beebe-Dimmer JL, Cooney KA. Prevalence and correlates of vitamin and supplement usage among men with a family history of prostate cancer. Integr Cancer Ther. 2012;11:83–9.
372. McCullough MK, Patel AV, Kushi LH, Patel R, Willet WC, Doyle C, et al. Following cancer prevention guidelines reduces risk of cancer, cardiovascular disease, and all-cause mortality. Cancer Epidemiol Biomarkers Prev. 2011;20:1089–97.
373. Thomas RJ, Holm M, Williams M, Bowman E, Bellamy P, Andreyev J, et al. Lifestyle factors correlate with the risk of late pelvic symptoms after prostatic radiotherapy. Clin Oncol (R Coll Radiol). 2013;25:246–51.
374. Park SW, Kim TN, Nam JK, Ha HK, Shin DG, Lee W, et al. Recovery of overall exercise ability, quality of life, and continence after 12-week combined exercise intervention in elderly patients who underwent radical prostatectomy: a randomized controlled trial. Urology. 2012;80:299–305.

8 Lifestyle Changes, CAM, and Kidney Stones: Heart Health = Kidney Health

Introduction: Heart Health and Kidney Health

Is heart health tantamount to kidney health? I believe this is the case, although it does not appear to be perceived in this fashion because the research still needs to mature. For example, no previous study before the CARDIA (Coronary Adult Risk Development in Young Adults) study had examined subclinical arterial disease and stones [1]. CARDIA was a population-based observational study of 5,115 Caucasian and African-American men and women that were between the ages of 18 and 30 years at recruitment and then followed for 20 years. Researchers found there were 3.9 %, or 200, participants that reported a history of kidney stones during this time, and those with symptomatic stones were correlated with higher carotid wall thickness after 20 years, especially of the internal carotid/bulb region. A significant ($p=0.01$) 1.6 times a higher risk of kidney stone participants had carotid disease, even after looking at all confounding atherosclerotic risk factors. Interestingly, the participants were an average age of 25 years when this study started, and after 20 years the majority of them went from normal weight to being overweight and obese. The average glucose and triglycerides also increased dramatically. Again, even after controlling for these risk factors, there was still a significant correlation between stones and cardiovascular disease. Perhaps physicians should inquire about the cardiovascular health of patients with a history of kidney stones. Also, it appears to be time to convince individuals to follow a heart-healthy lifestyle program to reduce the risk of kidney stones. The conclusion of this study was more profound compared to any words this author could utilize in this book: "The association between a history of kidney stones and subclinical carotid atherosclerosis in young adults adds further support to the notion that nephrolithiasis and atherosclerosis share common systemic risk factors and/or pathophysiology."

A Mayo Clinic or Olmstead County, Minnesota, study of 4,564 stones formers matched with 10,680 controls during a mean follow of 9 years found a 38 % increased risk for myocardial infarction (MI), which was reduced to 31 % after adjusting for other comorbidities and chronic kidney disease (CKD) [2]. Kidney stones have been correlated with a higher risk of MI (OR-1.3, $p<0.05$) and stroke (OR = 1.3; $p<0.05$) in other studies including a cohort of 23,349 questionnaires collected from individuals 15 years or older in the IV Portuguese National Health Survey [3]. A cross-sectional study of 13,418 Japanese men 30–69 years of age found 404 stone formers on ultrasound (3 %) and 1,231 with a past history of stones. Multivariate-adjusted OR for overweight/obesity, hypertension, gout/hyperuricemia, and chronic kidney disease were significantly increased in past and current stone formers versus controls. This led the authors to suggest an association with kidney stones and traditional risk factors for heart disease [4].

M.A. Moyad, *Complementary & Alternative Medicine for Prostate and Urologic Health*,
DOI 10.1007/978-1-4614-8492-9_8, © Springer Science+Business Media New York 2014

It is also possible that associations of cardiovascular disease with kidney stones are not as strong when adjusting for multiple confounding variables [2], and when larger samples with stronger analytical methods are utilized, cardiovascular associations will be attenuated and at times eliminated because stone disease is complex and has multiple etiologies. For example, in the National Health and Nutrition Examination Survey III of 14,879 men and women with a reported 683 participants reporting a history of stones (median follow-up 14.9 years), the correlation between cardiovascular mortality and all-cause mortality was no longer significant in the adjusted analysis for age, gender, race, and poverty. Yet, in the unadjusted analysis, it was highly significant with hazard ratios or risk of approximately 2.0 and $p<0.0001$ [5]. Therefore, the evidence suggests an association with cardiovascular health but not necessarily a consistent independent predictor or cardiovascular events. Still, if patients are made aware that reducing cardiovascular disease (CVD) risk lowers the risk of kidney stones and vice versa, the potential to reduce the burden of both conditions seems plausible and at least a "first do no harm" approach.

Comprehensive Lifestyle Changes, Stones, and Heart Health

If CVD increases the risk of kidney stones, then what would occur if multiple healthy lifestyle changes were incorporated into a clinical study to prevent kidney stones? A historic 5-year randomized trial from Parma, Italy, was published in the New England Journal of Medicine [6]. This trial demonstrated that a lower intake of animal protein and sodium and a normal intake of calcium reduced the risk for a kidney stone formation in individuals with a previous kidney stone compared to a low-calcium diet group. This was arguably one of the longest clinical trials ever published to address this issue. A total of 120 men (mean age 45 years) were included who had been diagnosed with idiopathic hypercalciuria (urinary calcium excretion >300 mg/day) on an unrestricted diet, experiencing recurrent formation of calcium oxalate stones (at least two documented events), and on no current treatments. A total of 60 men were placed on a normal-calcium diet (1,200 mg/day of calcium from food and not supplements) and low-animal protein (52 g per day or less) and low-sodium chloride (2,925 mg/day or 40 %, as sodium is equivalent to 1,170 mg/day of sodium) intervention diet. Another group of 60 men were placed in the low-calcium diet (400 mg/day) and instructed to avoid milk, yogurt, and cheese so that calcium ingestion would be reduced to just several hundred milligrams per day. Both groups were recommended to avoid large quantities of oxalate-rich foods (walnuts, spinach, chocolate, etc.) and to drink 2–3 L of water per day. The primary outcome of the study was time to a symptomatic kidney stone or the presence of an identified stone on an imaging test. Over 5 years, men that received the intervention diet (normal calcium, low protein, and salt) reduced their risk of a recurrent stone by 50 % (relapse rate of 40 vs. 20 %, $p=0.04$) versus the control group (low-calcium diet). Urinary calcium was reduced significantly in both groups (−170 mg/day), but urinary oxalate excretion increased by a mean of 5.4 mg per day in the low-calcium group and was reduced in the normal-calcium group (−7.2 mg per day). This was a groundbreaking trial because it demonstrated the real importance of comprehensive lifestyle changes on kidney stone risk. The only problem was the fact that determining what had the largest impact or even an impact on kidney stone recurrence (protein, salt, and/or calcium) could not be determined.

The comprehensive DASH (Dietary Approaches to Stop Hypertension) study demonstrated an ability to dramatically lower blood pressure (−7.1 mm Hg systolic in non-hypertensive and −11.5 mm Hg systolic in hypertensive) similar to what is accomplished with medication using a comprehensive diet and lifestyle program along with reducing sodium below 1,200 mg (1/2 teaspoon) or 2,300 mg per day (1 teaspoon) compared to approximately 3,500 mg per day (1.5 teaspoons) [7, 8]. Diastolic blood pressure reductions of over 5 mm Hg in hypertensives was an average finding with some dietary changes alone.

The recommendations from DASH have been applied to other studies to determine if these comprehensive lifestyle changes could reduce the risk of kidney stones and the preliminary results are dramatic. For example, in the Health Care Professionals Follow-up Study of 45,821 men with 18 years of follow-up and the Nurses' Health Study I and II of approximately 195,000 women with 14–18 years of follow-up each, researchers constructed a DASH diet score and evaluated incident kidney stone risk [9]. A total of 5,645 kidney stones were documented over a combined 50-year follow-up period, and those with higher DASH scores also had greater intakes of potassium, magnesium, oxalate, calcium, and vitamin C and lower sodium intake, and this group experienced a 40–45 % reduction in the risk of a kidney stone. Again, this suggests that the sum of personal lifestyle behaviors and parameters are far more powerful on cardiovascular and kidney health compared to one or just a few changes. The eight general recommendations from the original DASH diet and from this cohort were the following [7–9]:

1. Higher intake of grains (7–8 daily servings)
2. Higher intake of vegetables (4–5 servings a day)
3. Higher intake of fruits (4–5 servings a day)
4. Low-fat or no-fat dairy products (2–3 servings a day)
5. Low to moderate intake of red and processed meat, poultry, or fish (2 or fewer servings a day) and low fats and oils (2–3 servings a day, the DASH diet had 27 % of total calories as fat, which is moderate)
6. Higher intake of nuts, seeds, and dry beans (4–5 servings a week)
7. Low intake of sweets (5 servings a week, also low in fat) and sweetened beverages
8. 1,500 mg or less of sodium per day or 2,400 mg a day, depending on the individual situation, and keep in mind that most sodium reduction comes from eating healthier such as reducing intake of processed foods—not from the salt shaker

Higher DASH diet scores reduced kidney stone risk even in those with reduced calcium intakes and excluding hypertensive participants did not change these results [9]. In other words, men and women of all ages appear to be able to reduce the risk of stones utilizing a comprehensive DASH diet and lifestyle program. A closer analysis into this diet in 3,426 participants with and without a history of stones found higher DASH scores (better compliance) compared to lower scores to have significantly higher urinary calcium excretion (10–12 %), higher urinary oxalate (4–18 %) and citrate (11–16 %), and urinary volume (16–32 %) [10]. Higher DASH scores were also correlated with greater urine potassium, magnesium, phosphate, and pH. The authors theorized it is the increase in citrate and urine volume along with other stone inhibitors in dairy and plants that were beneficial. The normalization of calcium and reduced animal protein and salt should have also provided some benefit. Calcium oxalate stone formers are often instructed to reduce the intake of oxalate from some foods, but these studies suggest this is not needed in some cases because it could also result in a lower intake of vegetables, fruits, and whole grains.

Hypertension

Older and preliminary observational studies have found a fairly consistent relationship between hypertension and kidney stones or vice versa [11–16]. The mechanism of action has not been elucidated, but could be due to higher urinary calcium excretion, increased urinary uric acid, and decreased urinary citrate, especially in the setting of obesity, but again this needs more attention. It appears the current strongest theory is the increase in calcium excretion, which was found to 12 % higher (25.6 mg per day more) in one well-controlled statistical retrospective series of 462 stone-forming patients [16]. Arguably one of the biggest factors for cardiovascular disease risk now has a correlation with stone risk.

Dyslipidemia, High LDL, High Triglycerides, Inflammatory Markers, and Treatment (Statins?)

High cholesterol/dyslipidemia may be an emerging risk factor for calcium oxalate and uric acid stones [17]. Yet few large observational studies have ever been conducted in this area of urology to determine if cholesterol-lowering agents via inflammation reduction or simply protecting kidney tissue from damage could cause risk reduction. Preliminary laboratory studies suggest a potential risk reduction with statins via inhibition of renal crystal retention [18]. Arguably the first human study of statin use was derived from outpatient electronic military health records from the Southwestern USA, which identified adult patients with dyslipidemia and stones [19]. The cohort consisted of 57,232 subjects with dyslipidemia and 1,904 subjects with stones. Patients on statins had a significantly lower risk of kidney stones (3.1 vs. 3.7 %; OR = 0.83, $p < 0.001$) on univariate analysis. Statin patients were significantly older, more likely to be female, and have comorbidities. Interestingly, multivariate analysis (adjusted for age, sex, and comorbidity) showed a stronger significant reduction (OR = 0.51, $p < 0.001$) in stone risk with statin use. More prospective studies are needed, but again the ability of statins to reduce inflammatory markers could be one primary mechanism of action [20]. It is of interest that not just higher LDL cholesterol but abnormally high triglycerides may increase the risk of kidney stones [17, 21]. It is also of interest that triglycerides are one of the five potential traits found in those patients with metabolic syndrome and fish oil or marine-derived omega-3 fatty acids (EPA and DHA) reduce triglycerides and may reduce some risk factors for kidney stones [22].

Obesity/Bariatric Surgery/Weight-Loss Diets and Drugs and/or Pre- and Diabetes (Glucose Intolerance)

An analysis of three large prospective cohorts involving almost a quarter of a million participants found higher body weight in men and women to be a risk factor for stones, with a RR of 1.44 in men to 1.89–1.92 in older and younger women [23]. An increased risk with increasing BMI appears to be a consistent finding from other observational series. Overall, higher BMI and waist circumference are risk factors for kidney stones [24, 25]. Whether the risk exists because of lower urinary citrate, higher uric acid, and oxalate has been well discussed. Regardless, it is known that obesity appears to cause a shift in primary kidney stone risk from a reduction in calcium oxalate stones to more prevalent uric acid stone disease [26, 27].

Diabetes is also a well-studied and consistent risk factor for a variety of stone disease [28–34]. Similar to obesity, especially for type 2 diabetics, there may be an increase in the risk of uric acid stones. Insulin resistance creates a lower urine pH via deficient ammonia production and thus an increase in risk [32]. There is also the potential for inhibitory ureteral peristalsis, which can increase the risk of stones via urinary stasis [33]. Although more oxalate excretion occurs in diabetics, the reduced urinary pH has been a consistent observation [34].

Some older obesity medications, such as orlistat, and bariatric surgery are correlated with hyperoxaluria, stone formation, and oxalate nephropathy [31]. Other weight-loss medications more recent to the marketplace such as the combination of phentermine and topiramate (Qsymia) also appear to slightly raise the risk of kidney stones at higher (92 vs. 46 mg) topiramate dosages [35]. Roux-en-Y surgery appears to cause hyperoxaluria, low urine volume, and hypocitraturia, whereas gastric binding may cause less risk due to low urine volumes and higher calcium excretion [36], but actual weight loss with banding is significantly less compared to other surgical bariatric procedures [37]. Weight gain utilizing carbohydrates and rapid weight-loss diets adhering to low-carbohydrate intake could increase the risk of calcium oxalate and uric acid stones [32, 38]. Although, whether or not one type of diet, low fat or low carbohydrate, increases the risk of stone disease more than another is controversial. For example, a 2-year comparative trial of 307 obese individuals found no impact of low-carbohydrate diets on bone density, GFR, albuminuria, or fluid and electrolytes compared to a low-fat diet [39]. Arguably, it is best to lose weight over time to improve cardiovascular health and reduce the risk of stones rather than focus specifically on the type of weight-reduction program utilized. Short-term studies of low-carbohydrate diets have suggested an increase in stone risk based on acid load [40], but again over a long-period of time, the increase in risk of stone disease is questionable compared to other popular diets [39].

Metabolic Syndrome (More Is Not Better)

After the discussion on obesity and glucose intolerance, it should not be surprising that preliminary research is beginning to demonstrate an increased risk of stone disease with an increasing number of metabolic syndrome traits, for example, from 3 % with 0 traits to almost 10 % with all five traits (abnormal glucose, blood pressure, central obesity, high triglycerides, and low HDL) [41]. Perhaps one of the strongest contributors to this risk is hypertension [42], although obesity also increases risk and metabolic syndrome patients also have an increased risk for uric acid stones [43].

Exercise and/or Water/Hydration and Fluid Types

Surprisingly few studies have addressed the impact of exercise on stone disease. Two studies have found a suggested increase risk of stone disease, but this was in the setting of reduced hydration during and after activity [44, 45]. Immobility or bed rest is associated with an increased risk [46, 47], and exercise aids in weight loss [48]. Perhaps the message to patients should be to increase physical activity in the setting of increased hydration until their urine appears clear when voiding. And exercise might operate via other pathways to reduce kidney stone risk apart from weight loss in the setting of adequate hydration; for example, inflammatory markers such as C-reactive protein (CRP) and fibrinogen appear to be consistently reduced in studies of heart disease patients [49].

Water intake is an accepted risk-reducing strategy against stone disease, especially to prevent calcium stone recurrence [50, 51]. This strategy is commonly mentioned in some guidelines, along with pharmacologic interventions such as allopurinol, citrate, and thiazides [50]. Water intake greater than 2 L per day to produce a urine output of greater than 2.5 L per day reduced stone recurrence as much as 61 % [51]. This would again suggest water intake is a conventional medical recommendation to prevent relapse and, arguably, reduce the risk of first time stone disease, but this has not been adequately addressed. Still, fruits and vegetables utilized in comprehensive lifestyle programs to reduce the risk of incident stone disease are not just high in electrolytes (potassium and magnesium) but also water content [9]. High-moisture foods such as fruits and vegetables could account for 20–25 % of human daily water intake [52].

A variety of noncaloric and some caloric fluids from water to caffeinated and decaffeinated coffee and alcoholic beverages may reduce risk, but higher sugar or soda and fruit juice beverages may increase risk [53]. Alcohol consumption can also be dehydrating, so patients should be told to drink water right before, during, and after alcohol consumption to maintain hydration and discourage increased caloric consumption from alcoholic beverages.

Citrate is a known inhibitor of calcium kidney stone formation. Lemonade from real lemons (homemade) or lemon juice has become the paradigm of a targeted ideal beverage for increased urinary citrate [54]. Increased alkali intake can increase urine pH, which could help prevent kidney stones. Multiple sodas that appear to contain a concentration of citrate equal to or greater than alkali or total alkali of lemonade used to treat low urine citrate calcium kidney stones (6.30 mEq/L citrate as alkali and 6.30 as total alkali) include Diet Sunkist Orange, Diet 7UP, Sprite Zero, Diet Canada Dry Ginger Ale, Sierra Mist Free, Diet Orange Crush, Fresca, and Diet Mountain Dew. It is also of interest that colas, including those that are caffeine free, have the lowest total alkali or less than 1.0 mEq/L [55].

Other citrate-based fruit juices (apart from lemon juice and lemonade from real lemons) such as Ruby Red grapefruit juice, orange, pineapple, cranberry, lemon/lime Gatorade, and Crystal Light lemonade sugar-free drink mix are also excellent sources of citrate [54]. Yet, in the age of a global obesity epidemic, which can raise stone risk, I am concerned about the caloric content of these products, which in many cases equals a serving of high caloric alcohol [48]. Therefore, lower caloric options such as Crystal Light or sugar-free drink mixes or reduced caloric or no-calorie citrate-based beverages are more ideal. Still, lemon and lime juice containing 1.44 and 1.38 g of citric acid per ounce and lemon and lime juice concentrates containing 1.10 and 1.06 g per ounce are still the paradigm of comparison [56]. Again, clinicians and patients need to be sensitive to the caloric content of all citrate sources, the need to dilute these sources, or simply advocate for low- or no-calorie sources in those with weight and waist issues.

Dietary Fiber

Minimal research has been conducted on the impact of higher fiber intakes with stone risk. Several small studies suggest no advantage, the potential for an increase, and even a reduction in the risk of stone disease [57–62]. The problem with many of these protocols is that water intake is controlled, and with increased fiber ingestion, fluid intake needs to be dramatically increased; compliance issues abound when attempting to increase fiber intake. It is arguable that if water intake was allowed to increase by upwards of 1 L for every 10–15 g of fiber, there would be no impact or a potential advantage of dietary fiber intake. Phytate (multiple negative charges as an ion) in fibers can also bind with calcium to form complexes and potentially reduce the risk of hypercalciuria and stones [60, 61], and may complement conventional treatment [62]. Fiber in fruits and vegetables along with nutrients (magnesium, potassium, low in sodium) and water content could reduce the risk of stones. Regardless, fiber intake is a healthy overall and cardiovascular disease risk-reducing strategy [63]. Still, it cannot be claimed that it has any definitive beneficial impact on stone risk at this time, despite the author's belief that the benefit outweighs the risk.

Dietary Oxalate Content Controversies (Bioavailable? Soluble Versus Insoluble?)

Some educational sources provide a long and comprehensive list of high-oxalate foods and their dosages which should be avoided by some previous calcium oxalate stone formers. This tradition will not occur in this chapter perhaps due to the iconoclastic thought or purpose to instead focus more on the larger issue. Vegetarians consume and excrete more oxalate in the diet compared to those that eat meat, but vegetarians appear to have a lower risk of recurrent kidney stone risk [64, 65]. Encouraging the consumption of a predominantly plant-based diet appears to offer more of a benefit compared to counting the milligrams of oxalate from foods. For example, drinking tea usually has zero calories and helps for weight-loss programs and fluid intake that could also reduce stone risk, but can be high in dietary oxalate, but it is low in bioavailable oxalate (percentage of the total appearing in the urine) [66, 67]. A test of seven high-oxalate foods (spinach, chocolate, tea, vegetable juice, cranberry juice, pecans, and orange) found only spinach to cause hyperoxaluria in normal subjects (increase of 29.3 mg in 8 h) [67]. The real issue is the amount of soluble compared to insoluble oxalates occurring in a product [68], which impacts the bioavailability.

Plant oxalate exists in two forms: the water-soluble (absorbable) salts attached to potassium, sodium, and ammonium ions and the insoluble salts attached to calcium, magnesium, and iron that are not absorbed and become part of fecal material [68–70]. A soluble or water-soluble oxalate from plants can bind to intestinal material (e.g., calcium) and not be absorbed, or it can get absorbed and appear in the urine. Plants high in soluble oxalates are more concerning and may or may not have a greater chance of increasing urinary oxalate, especially when consumed with other food and beverage items. For example, when spices were tested, green cardamom (99 %) had the highest concentration of soluble oxalate followed by turmeric powder (91–95 %), ginger

(87 %), malabathrum leaf (59 %), and black cardamom (59 %) [71, 72]. Cinnamon (6 % soluble) was the only spice that contained primarily insoluble oxalate only. Also, oxalate excretion amounts are measured as single ingested food source, but when other foods or even calcium or magnesium is ingested with dietary oxalate, it can potentially and significantly reduce absorption (magnesium as much as calcium, but have +2 charge and oxalate has a −2 charge) [73].

Additionally, there is evidence to suggest that individuals ingesting healthy food sources of oxalate might also increase the probability of housing intestinal oxalate-degrading flora such as *Oxalobacter formigenes*, a gram-negative and anaerobic bacterium whose primary energy source is oxalate itself [74]. The American Dietetic Association (ADA) recommends a dietary oxalate intake of 40–50 mg per day or less for those at risk of oxalate stones [75], but I do believe caution should be emphasized in cases where eliminating any food providing ample nutrients or low caloric intake as part of a weight-loss program is a primary goal. High food sources of oxalate, which are usually discouraged in high-risk oxalate stone formers, include the following [76, 77]:

- Beets
- Black teas
- Bran concentrates and cereals
- Chocolate
- Legumes (beans, peanuts, soybeans)
- Nuts (some tree nuts)
- Rhubarb
- Spinach

Still, there are nuances to these recommendations, which should be emphasized. For example, these foods are healthy and could be a part of a heart-healthy weight-loss program, or, for example, soy products are high in phytate binding calcium compounds, and tofu, for example, contains minimal soluble oxalate [77, 78]. Again, until there is more definitive proof that some of these foods incorporated into a comprehensive lifestyle program such as DASH [9] to prevent stones actually increase the risk of stone disease, there should be ample room for debate on what to restrict and not to restrict when in a kidney stone prevention program.

Table 8.1 Some basic cardiovascular risk factors associated with a higher risk of kidney stones[a]

Dyslipidemia (high LDL and/or triglycerides)
Glucose intolerance/diabetes
Hypertension
Metabolic syndrome
Obesity
Physical inactivity
Unhealthy diet

[a]Note: Chronic tobacco usage and higher dosages of tobacco, although not a consistent independent risk factor for stone disease, increase the risk of hypertension, which could also eventually increase stone risk. Additionally, tobacco users are less likely to follow heart-healthy lifestyle changes, and smoking is a major risk factor for bladder cancer and worse outcomes from urologic treatments

Another compromising option is to prevent a viable alternative to patients concerned about removing some healthy foods from diet. For example, kale is a low-calorie and low-oxalate vegetable, which has greater calcium absorbability versus spinach and could also bind intestinal oxalate [79]. This allows some patients to maintain normal calcium dietary intake and remain less concerned with high-oxalate food sources. Low-calorie teas such as green or herbal tea instead of black tea are an option [77], and some commercial chocolates contain added calcium, and these should be tested for oxalate bioavailability. This is just a short list of alternative thoughts and ideas to patients concerned about oxalate ingestion. Now, before beginning the discussion on dietary supplements and other factors and stone risk, the reader should be reminded of the various cardiovascular risk factors associated with stone disease mentioned in the first half of this chapter, and these are listed in Table 8.1.

Calcium and Vitamin D Supplements

The Women's Health Initiative (WHI) randomized 36,282 postmenopausal women to 1,000 mg of calcium carbonate and 400 IU of vitamin D_3 daily or placebo [80]. Calcium and vitamin D increased the risk of self-reported kidney stones (HR = 1.17; 95 % CI, 1.02–1.34), and the Number

Needed to Harm (NNH) was 272 over 7 years. Participants were already ingesting high intakes of dietary calcium at baseline (1,150 mg/day) [80].

A total of 449 women in the calcium and vitamin D group and 381 in the placebo group reported a kidney stone during the clinical trial. Rates of kidney stones did not differ between the various demographic, dietary, and other hypothesized risk factors. Neither total calcium intake nor the use of supplements at the beginning of the study was associated with the risk of stones. Even those individuals that did not ingest their calcium supplements on a regular basis also experienced a slight increased risk of a kidney stone.

Idiopathic hypercalciuria (IH) in this population of participants might explain the potential increase in stone risk in the supplement users [48]. IH is found in 5–7 % of the adult population, and such a large randomized trial of calcium and vitamin D (arguably the largest ever done in medicine) should balance the number of IH individuals fairly equally among the two arms of the trial. What is also interesting again is that the average person in the study was again already receiving 1,150 mg of dietary calcium and 365 IU of dietary vitamin D before the study was initiated.

Although some systematic reviews suggest no overall risk of stones, it is difficult to ignore the findings of excessive amounts of calcium not providing only the potential for harm and minimal benefit [81]. A large prospective cohort of over 91,700 women with 12-year follow-up found dietary supplements of calcium associated with an increased risk of kidney stones (RR = 1.2), but dietary calcium intake was correlated with a lower risk. It is also if interest that increased sucrose and sodium also increased stone risk and increased fluid and potassium reduced stone risk [82]. There has also been some concern over clinical trials suggesting higher rates of myocardial infarction with excess calcium supplementation [83]. It would be prudent to follow the conservative and evidence-based Institute of Medicine (IOM) guidelines suggesting daily total calcium intakes of 1,000 mg per day in 19- to 50-year-old males and females, 1,000 mg per day also in 51- to 70-year-old males, and 1,200 mg in 51± year-old females and 70± year-old males [84]. Calcium citrate dietary supplements may not increase the risk of kidney stones and should be the preferred calcium supplement for those needing supplementation at a higher risk of calcium oxalate nephrolithiasis [48]. They can be utilized with and without food but are not as concentrated as lower-cost calcium carbonate supplements that need to be ingested with food. Still, calcium supplements, including calcium citrate, increase the risk of constipation, especially in the elderly.

Vitamin D is a controversial supplement because in higher dosages it has the potential to cause hypercalcemia [84]. The IOM recommendations appear to be conservative and accurate in recommending 600 IU per day for adults (men and women) up to the age of 70 years and 800 IU for 70+ individuals. Yet, there is no strong and consistent evidence to suggest higher urinary calcium levels on higher vitamin D levels right now [85, 86]. Regardless, bolus dosing should be discouraged until these questions are further answered and higher intakes have not been shown to consistently benefit individuals more than moderate dose intakes.

Cranberry and Cranberry Dietary Supplements and Oxalate

One research group noticed that an individual utilizing cranberry supplements for urinary health was diagnosed with a kidney stone soon after initiating these supplements and decided to further investigate this question, which had not been previously answered [87]. A total of five subjects utilized cranberry supplements at the recommended daily dosage on the label for 7 days, and then urinary oxalate levels increased significantly (p=0.01) by an average of over 43 %. If over 10 % consistent increases as noted by these authors can cause calcium and oxalate to bind and crystallize or form a stone, then this is concerning. The average normal intake of oxalate from the diet is about 150 mg/day, but two cranberry tablets from this study could be expected to contain over 350 mg of oxalate per day. Another problem with many cranberry concentrate supplements is that they can contain a good amount or at least some plain vitamin C (known oxalate-increasing compound). Sodium levels also increased from this study and so did the ability of calcium and oxalate to bind together. Yet, magnesium and potassium also increased in the volunteers, which could slightly reduce risk of kidney stones. What this study showed is that most supplements do not report their potential oxalate content or ability to increase oxalate, and this needs more research. In the meantime, most individuals that have a high risk for kidney stones do not need to be on cranberry supplements unless a company can report their oxalate amount in a pill.

Cranberry juice is fraught with mixed issues and messages. Some studies reported a low bioavailability of oxalate from cranberry juice [67] and a reduction in oxalate excretion and increases in citrate in individuals with no stone risk [88]. Still, it provides an acid load and can increase urinary calcium and oxalate in other individuals [89]. It is interesting when cranberry juice (19.87 mmol/L) is analyzed for citrate content, it has been greater in some cases compared to homemade lemonade (17.42 mmol/L) [54]. In other words, cranberry concentrate supplements appear to be high in oxalate in some cases, cranberry juice is high in calories in some cases and has a mixed stone risk, and this is objective information that should be passed on to the patient. Personally, I favor the use of cranberry supplements over cranberry juice for those with UTIs, because intuitively the pills do not appear to add to the obesity epidemic in terms of caloric contribution (100–150 cal per 8 oz vs. little to no calories with pills) [48] and have worked as well thus far for the prevention of UTIs [90]. Also, the impact of cranberry juice for UTIs is being questioned, and the compliance rates of drinking cranberry juice daily for months in some trials have been poor. In children the juice may also have some efficacy, but the acidity and long-term commitment to daily use also can contribute to compliance issues [91]. If someone has a high risk for oxalate stone and UTI recurrence, then again some idea of the contribution of the amount of oxalate from the supplement would be of assistance in deciding if the benefit was worth the risk.

Inosine (Nucleoside Supplements) or D-Ribose Dietary Supplements

Inosine is not just a nucleoside produced when hypoxanthine is connected to a ribose ring (ribofuranose) via a glycosidic bond [92, 93], but it is also sold as a dietary supplement. Inosine is produced in the body, where it assists with energy production (precursor to adenosine used for the production of ATP) and increasing red blood cell concentrations of 2,3-diphosphoglycerate (2,3-DPG), which is why there was always interest in determining if supplementing with this compound could boost athletic performance. Inosine has other roles in the body; it is found in organ meats, and there is some found in brewer's yeast, but the supplements appear to provide the largest quantities. Inosine has not been impressive as an athletic enhancement product at large dosage (up to 10,000 mg per day) [94, 95]. Also, individuals with gout or others with uric acid concerns should not take this supplement because it can significantly raise uric acid levels.

Interestingly, this supplement has and will continue to be tested in dosages of 500–3,000 mg per day in clinical trials to raise the uric acid level to anywhere from 6 to 9 mg/dL (no more or less) in neurological inflammatory disorders such as in multiple sclerosis (MS) and Parkinson's patients to determine if there could be a clinical benefit [96–99]. Uric acid is a natural inhibitor or scavenger of certain compounds such as peroxynitrite, which could otherwise promote inflammation and axon degeneration [97]. Some MS and Parkinson's patients have been known to harbor lower uric acid levels compared to those without MS and Parkinson's, and those with higher uric acid appear in some cases to have a slower progression of their disease. Some preliminary 1-year testing suggests dosages of 2,000–3,000 mg per day might provide a benefit, but 4 out of 16 patients were also diagnosed with kidney stones during the study [98]. Other adverse effects did not occur; for example, inosine supplementation did not raise blood pressure, but uric acid significant increases of 4.2 at baseline to 7.1 mg per 100 mL occurred with these supplements [100]. Other somewhat related nucleoside (hypoxanthine attached to ribose = nucleoside inosine, found in tRNA) dietary supplements such as D-ribose have not been shown to increase uric acid at dosages as high as 5,000–10,000 mg per day [101, 102].

Magnesium (Dietary and Supplements)

Higher dietary magnesium intake appears to reduce the risk of hyperoxaluria in those with nephrolithiasis [103]. The conundrum of magnesium from foods is that higher sources are found in whole grains, spinach, nuts, and legumes, which have been also considered higher oxalate sources [104]. Dietary magnesium supplements many have some efficacy [103, 105], especially when combined with other kidney stone inhibitors, but dosages of magnesium are not simple to increase because of bowel toxicity (loose stools and diarrhea), which can occur [106]. Magnesium is also excreted renally, so it needs to be utilized with caution in those with renal disease. It appears dietary sources are generally healthy and more sensible at the moment for many patients and could reduce stone risk. Magnesium has a +2 charge (like calcium) as a cation and oxalate has a −2 charge, which should maintain the interest in this compound potentially lowering oxalate levels.

Omega-3 Dietary Supplements from Marine Sources (EPA and DHA) and Omega-6 Supplementation

Fish oil supplements (1,200 mg /day of the active ingredients EPA and DHA) were analyzed in a retrospective study of 29 patients (followed for a mean of 9–10 months) along with dietary changes (fluid, sodium, protein, citric juices) in patients with hypercalciuria (urinary calcium >250 mg/day in males or >200 mg/day for females) and demonstrated a significant potential to lower urinary calcium (349–247 mg/day) and oxalate (45–32 mg/day) and increase citrate (737–940 mg/day) [107]. The authors theorized that by affecting what is known as prostaglandin metabolism, which causes a reduction in compounds like PGE2 that normally can increase the risk of stones by increasing calcium in the urine, omega-3 compounds may have efficacy. Specifically, the dietary changes added to fish oil in their study included 2 L/day of urine, reduced sodium (less than 2,400 mg), protein reduction, normal calcium intake, and citric juices (4 oz concentrated lemon/lime juice per day). Overall, there was a 52 % response rate to the dietary change and fish oil supplement over an average period of 10 months, and 24 % of the patients were normocalciuric by study end, and there was an average of approximately 30 % reduction in urinary calcium after 6 months, and urine oxalate reduced in about a third of patients.

Older clinical research has suggested the ability of fish oil (e.g., EPA) to lower urinary calcium and oxalate levels in recurrent stone formers and the potential for benefit in the notable studies of Greenland Eskimos that demonstrated a lower risk of heart disease with a greater omega-3 intake from fish [22]. EPA has more research against kidney stones compared to DHA in fish oil, but both can be anti-inflammatory, which also may reduce the ability of calcium to bind to other components. Fish oil omega-3 fatty acids may impact the transport of oxalate so lower amounts are absorbed and appear in the urine. Another study of 18 months that used 1,800 mg of EPA found high baseline calcium levels in the urine were significantly reduced, but those with already normal calcium levels experienced no change [108]. This same research group followed 29 patients over a mean of 36 months on 1,800 mg of EPA preventive treatment and found reductions in stone formation during treatment, which were significant when compared to off treatment over a total observational period of 8 years [108]. Another small clinical study of 15 healthy subjects ingesting 900 mg of EPA and 600 mg of DHA over 30 days reduced significantly urinary oxalate excretion and the risk of calcium oxalate crystallization.

The problem with this exciting initial data is preliminary prospective observational research from three large cohorts (Health Professionals Follow-Up Study and Nurses' Health Study I and II) documented 3,956 incident kidney stones over a combined 36 years of follow-up including 234,000 individuals, and no relationship was found for fatty acid intake including fish oil supplements and incident kidney stones [109]. Older women in one cohort (NHS1) actually had a significant increase in risk in the highest quintile of EPA and DHA intake with a multivariate risk of 1.28 ($p=0.04$). Overall, there was no association in risk of stones and fatty acids in the other two cohorts. Another issue needs consideration before endorsing fish oil in urology, and this is the ongoing recent unimpressive data outside of urology where far more data existed initially for enthusiasm. Phase 3-like clinical trials on the recent effect of fish oil have been similar to placebo. For example, no impact of fish oil was found in a large trial on macular degeneration progression (AREDS2) [110], as well as a more definitive primary prevention cardiovascular health clinical trial in high-risk patients [111], or for prevention of postoperative atrial fibrillation [112], and from a comprehensive meta-analysis of cardiovascular events and disease [113].

Another issue is whether or not omega-3 dietary supplements function any better against kidney stone risk compared to omega-6 supplementation. For example, a significant increase in citrate and/or reduced calcium in the urine utilizing 1,000 mg of evening primrose oil (EPO) per day was found in a small preliminary study, along with decreases in oxalate [114]. EPO is a high source of the omega-6 anti-inflammatory compound known as "GLA" or "gamma-linolenic acid" and linoleic acid, which can then convert to DGLA and then PGE1, which is an anti-inflammatory compound. This needs further research; similar to omega-3 supplements, they have not received enough rigorous or placebo-controlled investigations. Still, similar anti-inflammatory effects of omega-3 and omega-6 compounds preliminarily occur outside of the field of urology (e.g., for conjunctival inflammation in patients with dry eye syndrome) [115].

Probiotic (Natural)-*Oxalobacter formigenes* and Lactic Acid Bacteria

Oxalobacter formigenes (*O. formigenes*), mentioned earlier, is a gram-negative and anaerobic bacterium whose primary metabolic energy source is oxalate itself [74, 116]. It is a natural gut probiotic, and other probiotics known as lactic acid bacteria, despite ample attention on the Internet and from other sources, have yet to prove they consistently lower oxalate levels to normal (less than 40–45 mg per day in the urine). This area of research just needs time to evolve because someone or some commercial entity should be able to offer a version of this bacterium in the future. Either *O. formigenes* will be offered as a probiotic or we will find a supplement or probiotics that can significantly and consistently increase the amount of this bacterium in the colon. *O. formigenes* utilization (solution delivered via a gastrostomy tube) twice a day for 4 weeks in select patients with primary hyperoxaluria type I (infantile oxalosis) has demonstrated the potential for plasma oxalate reduction [117]. However, a randomized trial of 43 patients observed no significant differences with placebo in urinary oxalate levels in those with primary hyperoxaluria [118]. Research may soon identify other strains of bacteria or better or more diverse deliver systems for *O. formigenes* and in the ideal patient populations (genetic predisposition, dietary, recurrent oxalate stone formers, etc.). Other species of bacteria may simply be isolated based on geographic location of individuals [119].

The human gut can be colonized by *O. formigenes* during infancy, and by age 8 almost all children test positive for it, compared to only 60–80 % of adults, and this is explained partially by the use of antibiotics [120–123] and, partially, in my opinion, unhealthy lifestyle and dietary changes and other supplements, drugs, and other scenarios that have not been fully tested against this bacterium as of yet. For example, morbidly obese patients appeared to have had a low colonization rate (8 %) with *O. formigenes* before bariatric surgery, which suggests that the hyperoxaluria observed after surgery is not due to the loss of colonization from this bacterium [124].

Other bacterial species ("lactic acid bacteria") could have a role in oxalate breakdown [125], such as *Lactobacillus acidophilus*, and other strain combinations over 4 weeks on one older study provided a potential 40 % oxalate reduction [126], but a bacterium that can be consistently relied on commercially has not occurred. There have been dramatic reductions in the risk of calcium oxalate stone recurrence (as high as 70 %) in some studies [127] and other studies suggesting minimal benefit [118]. However, these data need to mature, because it is possible that there is just a correlation between colonization and improved lifestyle changes that simultaneously reduce kidney stone risk dramatically by themselves. In addition, just because a probiotic has the ability to reduce oxalate levels does not necessarily translate to a lower risk of recurrent stone disease, and based on cost and delivery system, it needs to show some advantage over what could be accomplished with some minimal to moderate lifestyle changes. A final issue is the intrastool and interstool variability of the amount of *O. formigenes* detected by certain methods such as real-time polymerase chain reaction (PCR) [128]. Thus, there is great excitement but great detail to still be investigated and elucidated.

Vitamin B_6 Supplements (Pyridoxine HCL): An Effective Endogenous Oxalate Reducer in Some Conditions

Primary hyperoxaluria type 1 is the most common form of this genetic condition, which due to an enzymatic defect, and large concentrations of oxalate can be so damaging that in the advanced stages the primary effective form of treatment is kidney-liver transplantation [129]. Some treatment guidelines for this condition now recommend not only a higher fluid intake but a starting dose of 5 mg/kg per day not to exceed 20 mg/kg per day of vitamin B_6 with the goal of reducing urine oxalate excretion by less than 30 %. Other special dietary interventions are not generally recommended other than those for "concurrent diseases in the absence of CKD."

Vitamin B_6 (pyridoxine) is a cofactor in the alanine-glyoxylate-transaminase (AGT, an aminotransferase) pathway and could reduce the synthesis of oxalate through the induction of enzymatic activity [129–135]. For this reason, it has been a partial success story in decreasing oxalate production in some patients with primary hyperoxaluria type 1 because it simply causes a shift in the breakdown of glyoxylic acid toward glycine as opposed to oxalic itself. In other words, more glycine is produced from glyoxylic acid because of vitamin B_6, instead of oxalate, which is also an end product of glyoxylic acid. Lactate dehydrogenase (LDH) is the enzyme that normally converts glyoxylic acid into oxalate, and it competes with the B_6 AGT pathway. Less glyoxylic acid (glyoxylate) becomes available as a substrate for LDH when more B_6 is available. Interestingly, ethylene glycol-induced hyperoxaluria treatment in the laboratory appears beneficial when a vitamin B_6 compound is utilized [133]. Ethylene glycol tastes sweet and some animals and children are attracted to it. Veterinarians deal with this issue often because some dogs and cats consume radiator fluid. Vitamin B_6 involvement as a cofactor in multiple enzymatic pathways involving amino acid metabolism has drawn interest in multiple medical areas and not just for ethylene glycol poisoning but acute isoniazid overdose, certain mushroom poisonings such as Gyromitra mushroom or false morel [134].

There have been case studies of recurrent calcium oxalate stone formers taking 100 mg of vitamin B_6 daily with some long-term success [132]. The general recommended daily dietary intake of B_6 is approximately 1.2–1.7 mg per day in adults, but to reduce high oxalate levels, the most common dosage used thus far is 50–100 mg per day or slightly higher (up to 200 mg) of pyridoxine HCL based on oxalate levels from a 24-h urine composition test [135]. For example, a retrospective study of over 300 patients with 95 being diagnosed with idiopathic hypercalciuria also given dietary advice, and utilizing 50–100 mg a day of vitamin B_6 with some eventually utilizing a maximum of 200 mg per day based on the amount of oxalate in the urine (50–60 mg oxalate per day, B6 of 50 mg, but over 60 mg oxalate per day then 100 mg B6 or higher), was published [135]. A total of 39 % of these patients normalized the amount of oxalate in their urine (55–33, $p = 0.0004$), but 75 % of them significantly benefitted in term of improved urinary parameters (oxalate from 58–40, $p < 0.0001$) with diet and vitamin B_6 supplements, and researchers reported no serious side effects, such as sensory peripheral neuropathy, that can occur when ingesting too much vitamin B_6. Mean follow-up was 18.4 months and mean age of 50 years.

Pyridoxine in 250- to 500-mg daily doses provided a potential benefit to 8 (no stones occurred) of 12 patients with a history of recurrent calcium oxalate stones and idiopathic hypercalciuria. It significantly reduced urinary oxalate excretion ($p<0.025$) up to 18 months of treatment [136]. Another small study of two groups of stone formers, idiopathic and enteric, found it appeared effective for idiopathic but not enteric at dosages of 300 mg per day. This study suggested patients with intestinal hyperabsorption of oxalate may not benefit from B_6 [137]. A study published in 1967 followed calcium oxalate kidney stone patients on 10 mg of vitamin B_6 and 200 mg of magnesium oxide, and 30 of the 36 patients on this program over 5 years did not have another stone or reduced their risk [138]. Oxalate levels did not decrease but citrate levels increased significantly. Thus, there has been a long-term interest in using B_6 for stone reduction, and yet no definitive trial has been published since this time.

Some companies sell a more active form or the type of B6 that is detected in the blood known as "pyridoxal-5-phosphate" (P-5-P or P5P), but it appears the majority of the past studies have utilized pyridoxine HCL or the lower cost version of B_6 [139]. There is one past study of pyridoxal phosphate at 60 mg for 3 months, and it significantly reduced urinary oxalate excretion in patients with idiopathic hypercalciuria alone. These patients were also placed on a regular calcium diet. This is of enormous interest, but again the issue with vitamin B_6 supplements is the lack of ample individual or comparative data against some control or placebo.

One notable large prospective epidemiologic study of over 85,500 women with no history of stones reported 1,078 incident stone cases during 14 years of follow-up [140]. A higher consumption of B_6 was associated with a 34 % lower multivariate-adjusted risk in the group consuming 40 mg or more per day versus the lowest intake (less than 3 mg per day) occurred. Fish, chickpeas, chicken breast, and fortified cereals are high in vitamin B_6, but can only contribute about 0.5–1 mg per serving, which is not realistic in terms of competing with clinical studies to reduce abnormally high levels of oxalate. More observational work is obviously needed.

Some companies sell tablets over the counter as high as 500 mg per tablet, but this is too high and can again increase the risk of a sensory peripheral neuropathy at dosages of 300–500 mg per day [134, 141]. Some publications refer to recommending 1–10 mg per kg based on oxalate levels, but before this can be determined in patients with stone disease, it appears that 50–200 mg of B_6 usually in the form of pyridoxine hydrochloride is a cost-effective and safe dietary supplement from past studies [135]. Vitamin B_6 can be ingested with and without meals, but I always recommend with meals when given a choice because it can reduce gastrointestinal side effects. It is arguably time for more rigorous testing of B_6 in patients other than those with primary hyperoxaluria I to determine its overall use in stone disease.

Vitamin C Versus Buffered Vitamin C (Calcium Ascorbate or Other Sources) and the Metabolic Paradox of Increased Oxalate, but Reduced Serum Uric Acid (SUA) and Increased Urinary Uric Acid

Vitamin C has consistently been one of most utilized dietary supplements in the USA [142] and around the world [143]. The overall popularity of vitamin C supplements with the public among all age groups [142, 144, 145], and even among healthcare professionals themselves [144, 146], is notable, and it would be prudent to further elucidate the impact on stone disease. This is a controversial area because it is well known that high intakes of vitamin C supplements can increase oxalate levels [147, 148], but whether or not they significantly increase the risk of kidney stones is an area of debate. What is not controversial is the observation that increases in oxalate concentration are an abnormal metabolic consequence that should be generally discouraged and prevented.

Regardless of the etiology, hyperoxaluria can contribute to kidney injury and damage [149, 150].

Past clinical trials have consistently demonstrated large increases in oxalate with increased vitamin C from dietary supplements [151–153]. This occurred in previous stone formers and in individuals with no history of kidney stones. Healthy men and women can produce large quantities of urinary oxalate, regardless of stone risk status, when ingesting larger doses of concentrated ascorbic acid from dietary supplements. For example, a previous clinical trial of calcium oxalate stone formers ingesting 1,000 (group 1) or 2,000 mg (group 2) per day of vitamin C and non-stone formers ingesting 1,000 mg (group 3) for a total of only 3 days found that all three groups experienced significant increases in oxalate excretion: 61 % increase in oxalate in group 1, 41 % in group 2, and 56 % in group [151]. Significant increases in calcium oxalate urinary supersaturation also occurred in all three groups. Urinary pH did not change after vitamin C was ingested in any of the groups. A separate crossover clinical trial (two 6-day intervals) where participants were given 1,000 mg of vitamin C and then a placebo found a significant increase in urinary oxalate occurred in stone formers (33 %) and non-stone formers (20 %) [152]. Again, no change in urinary pH occurred. A third crossover trial of 29 stone and 19 non-stone formers consuming 2,000 mg of ascorbic acid compared to no intake for 6-day intervals found similar results to the other trials [153]. A total of 40 % of both the stone and non-stone formers experienced increases in the 24-h urinary oxalate concentrations of ≥10 % and in the Tiselius index (potential measure of stone risk). No change in oxalate concentrations occurred in the other 60 %. The authors suggested caution in ingesting high doses of ascorbic acid in individuals with or without a history of stones, because an individual's versus a population's response to vitamin C supplements in regard to potential oxalate changes is not consistently predictable from this and previous trials. Thus, it is accepted currently that high urine levels of oxalate occur with higher doses of ascorbic acid (1,000–2,000+ mg/day), but some individuals, for an unknown intrinsic or extrinsic reason and regardless of previous stone history, do not experience a change in oxalate.

Past observational studies have found mixed results in terms of stone risk. The large (n = 45,619 males) prospective epidemiologic Health Professionals Follow-up Study (HPFS) found a 41 % increase in the 14-year incidence of stones (1,473 cases with no previous history) in men with 1,000 mg or greater of daily supplemental vitamin C intake compared to those ingesting less than 90 mg [154]. Interestingly, magnesium, potassium, and/or fluid intake all appeared to reduce risk in this study (similar to what was mentioned earlier in this chapter). An earlier report from the Nurses' Health Study (NHS, n = 85,557) found no relationship between vitamin C and stone risk (1,078 cases, 14-year follow-up) in women even when comparing 1,500 mg or more per day versus less than 250 mg per day [140]. This was the same study observing the potential for vitamin B6 to reduce the risk of kidney stones (40 or more mg/day vs. <3 mg/day).

Perhaps one of the largest and most comprehensive studies on 24-h urinary oxalate places part of the vitamin C argument in perspective. A cross-sectional investigation of 3,348 stone and non-stone formers from the men in the HPFS, and women in the NHS, and the Nurses' Health Study II (NHS II) was published [155]. Median urinary oxalate levels were below 40 mg, and the association between dietary and urinary oxalate levels was similar regardless of nephrolithiasis history. Individuals consuming 1,000 mg/day or more of vitamin C compared to <90 mg/day excreted significantly (p < 0.001) more (6.8 mg/day) urinary oxalate. Body mass index (BMI), total fructose intake, and 24-h urinary magnesium, potassium, and phosphorus levels were also positively correlated with urinary oxalate levels, and age and calcium intake were inversely correlated with urinary oxalate. Participants with diabetes excreted 2.0 mg/day greater urinary oxalate (p < 0.01) compared to those without diabetes. The authors concluded dietary oxalate from most foods minimally contributes to urinary oxalate, but vitamin C supplementation has a more direct correlation, and increased calcium supplementation a more inverse correlation, so both of these supplements are potentially more significant contributors to oxalate concentrations.

A more recent population-based, prospective cohort of Swedish men recruited 48,850 participants, aged 45–79 years at baseline [156]. Using a self-administered questionnaire ascorbic acid usage and 20 other supplement types were recorded. Excluded from analysis were men with previous stone disease and users of supplements other than vitamin C because of potential confounding. A total of 11 years of follow-up identified 436 first incident cases of kidney stones, and vitamin C was correlated with a dose-dependent twofold significant increased risk. Vitamin C ingestion of fewer than 7 (median) and 7 or more tablets per week demonstrated significant increased relative risk of 1.66 and 2.23 versus supplement nonusers in multivariate analysis (P for trend = 0.001). No specific dosages were recorded (just tablet number), but the authors believe the majority of patients in this study ingested 1,000 mg per day. A commentary following the article estimated 1 kidney stone per 680 high-dose vitamin C users per year if this data is accurate [157].

Since ascorbic acid itself increases oxalate levels, and calcium discourages oxalate absorption, there was a curiosity of whether or not a more buffered (pH neutral) vitamin C such as calcium ascorbate (Ester-C) could discourage increased oxalate when compared to plain vitamin C. This comparative study in urology was urgently needed in my opinion because of potential safety, educational, and preventive implications and because of the popularity of vitamin C supplements. Our team used a randomized, double-blind, crossover study (1,000 mg/day for 5 days and then 2,000 mg/day for 5 additional days and then crossover with a 7-day washout) and found an overall reduction in oxalate with calcium ascorbate and an increase in the vitamin C group. This finding became significant when comparing the percentage of subjects experiencing these changes ($p = 0.04$) or reductions in 24-h urine oxalate levels and oxalate concentration compared to vitamin C [158, 159]. A total of 25 % more subjects experienced a reduction in 24-h oxalate (59 vs. 34 %) and oxalate concentration (72 vs. 46 %) over the 10-day treatment period when utilizing calcium ascorbate. This clinical study was conducted in individuals without a history of stone disease, and a total of 43 individuals had competed 24-h urinary oxalate data when utilizing ascorbic acid and 41 after using calcium ascorbate. A 10 % increase (subjective benchmark of risk) or greater in 24-h oxalate was observed for 28 % on calcium ascorbate compared to 51 % on plain ascorbic acid. There were no significant differences in creatinine or 24-h urine volumes between treatment phases. It is of interest that older and other studies of a similar or another vitamin C formulation found the potential for similar reductions or no adverse changes in oxalate [160, 161]. Personally, this research should be of enormous interest and will hopefully continue on a larger scale to determine if buffered vitamin C has a less pronounced effect on oxalate increases in individuals with and without a history of stone disease. This preliminary evidence is arguably of more interest now based on the belief that vitamin C raises oxalate significantly and the potential for oxalate kidney stones at higher dosages. Similar to the question left open with vitamin B_6 and oxalate in non-stone and stone formers, the issue of lowering oxalate with a pH neutral or buffered vitamin C needs to be answered. Calcium ascorbate is a low-cost and generic option now for those high-risk or non-risk kidney stone patients that want to continue high-dose vitamin C despite concerns over oxalate increases.

Plain vitamin C, however, is currently in somewhat of a perceived metabolic or serum versus urine paradox or conundrum. In preliminary research vitamin C (ascorbic acid) supplements have shown the ability to slightly to moderately reduce serum uric acid levels (SUA), which arguably could prevent gout [162], but the impact on uric acid stone disease is unknown and could theoretically be increased. A meta-analysis of vitamin C on serum uric acid identified 13 randomized controlled trials with a total of 556 participants, median dose of 500 mg per day, and median study duration of 30 days [163]. Pretreatment serum uric acid (SUA) levels were in the range of 2.9–7.0 mg/dL. The combined impact of these trials resulted in a significant ($p = 0.03$) reduction in SUA of −0.35 mg/dL

(–20.8 μmols/L), but the heterogeneity of the trials were also significant ($p < 0.01$). Larger reductions in uric acid were found in placebo-controlled trials. This suggests the potential for vitamin C to prevent incident gout and potentially recurrence, although none of the studies included in this meta-analysis utilized patients with gout.

One clinical trial of 500 mg of vitamin C versus placebo for 2 months found that vitamin C reduced their uric acid levels on average by –0.5 mg/dL and there was no change in the placebo group ($p < 0.0001$) [164]. Changes in SUA were inversely correlated with changes in serum ascorbic acid ($p = 0.0002$). In those individuals with abnormally higher uric acid levels to start with (>7.0 mg/dL), vitamin C reduced uric acid by as much as –1.5 mg/dL on average ($p = 0.0008$). These observations were consistent across subgroups defined by age, sex, race, BMI, chronic illness, diuretic use, and quartiles of baseline SUA and serum ascorbic acid. A potential mechanism of action was observed from this trial and other sources [164–166], which included an increased estimated glomerular filtration rate (GFR) in the current study [164], and/or the potential for reduced or competitive reabsorption is plausible because vitamin C and uric acid are both reabsorbed at the proximal tubule by anion-exchange transport [165, 166]. Vitamin C also appears to reduce SUA via sustained uricosuria (which is reversed by acetylsalicylic acid) without acidification of urine [165]. Thus, it is still theoretically plausible based on the quantity of uric acid appearing in the urine that it could induce or increase the probability of gouty arthritis or uric acid stones in higher risk individuals [165]. There is also some past preliminary research to partially contest some of the negative and positive past findings when large doses (4 or 12 g) of ascorbic acid were given to nongouty subjects (no change in uric acid occurred) [167], and a clinical trial of 500 mg of vitamin C demonstrated significant inferiority to allopurinol in those with a history of gout [168]. The authors of one study suggested that patients with hyperuricosuria or gout are at higher risk of exacerbation with vitamin C and not normal subjects [167]. And, the potential exists that there is more excitement for gout prevention instead of recurrence or "established gout," and beneficial results (–0.3 mg/dL) are not generally and clinically significant and could be due to uric acid assay variability [168]. Regardless, the authors of the latter study acknowledge that the uric acid effects could be weak on a lower dosage of vitamin C (500 mg) and due to medication interactions, especially low-dose aspirin (less than 325 mg reduces uric acid clearance, but >3 g has uricosuric effects), and diuretics could further minimize the effects of vitamin C [168]. Still, the potential for harm exists, and it should be discussed with patients that higher doses of vitamin C could theoretically increase the risk of oxalate or uric acid stone disease, especially in those patients with ongoing issues of urine oxalate or uric acid levels. Calcium ascorbate, discussed earlier in this section, can raise serum vitamin C levels similarly to plain vitamin C [158, 159], but its impact on SUA or urinary uric acid is not well known and needs to be further studied. In the meantime, similar effects on uric acid should first be assumed before research is completed with ascorbic acid and any other form of ascorbic acid (first do no harm).

Interestingly, observational studies point to even greater gout preventive abilities with vitamin C supplements at 1,000 or 1,500 mg per day via SUA reductions, but again this is preliminary [169, 170]. A prospective 20-year follow-up study of 46,994 males with no history of gout found compared to men receiving less than 250 mg/day of vitamin C, the multivariate relative risk of gout was 17 % lower for a total vitamin C intake of 500–999 mg/day, 34 % lower for 1,000–1,499 mg/day, and 45 % lower for 1,500 mg/day or larger ($p < 0.001$ for trend). A similar multivariate significant reduction in risk (p for trend <0.001) was found when comparing supplemental vitamin C users versus nonusers. Another similar analysis of males in this cohort found significant inverse association of vitamin C intake with SUA.

It should also be noted that cherries, tart cherry juice, cherry juice concentrate, and cherry extract supplements could reduce SUA via anthocyanin compounds reducing inflammation and/or because of their high vitamin C content, but they also could increase urinary uric acid [171]. Cherries (bing sweet, etc.) and other cherry derivatives have some preliminary data to reduce the risk of gout and gout attacks [171–176]. The largest observational study utilized 633 individuals with gout, and cherry intake over a 2-day time period was correlated with a 35 % lower risk of gout attacks versus no intake, and cherry extract demonstrated a similar correlation [172]. Cherry in combination with allopurinol use reduced the risk of gout attacks by 75 % compared to time periods without either exposure. In a pilot presented but unpublished prospective randomized control of using cherry juice concentrate, patients ingesting cherry juice concentrate had a significant reduction in the number of gout attacks within 4 months ($p<0.05$) [173, 174]. An impact is not observed in the control group consuming pomegranate juice. A total of 55 % of patients ingesting cherry juice were attack free and discontinued their intake of NSAIDs within 60 days of consuming this juice. Retrospective studies by the same group showed a potential for the reductions of attacks regardless of whether or not patients were on uric acid lowering therapy [174]. These researchers suggest IL-1 (a mediator of gouty inflammation) inhibition from monocytes normally activated by urate crystals to be more of primary action based on their research compared to vitamin C [175]. It is plausible tart cherry juice, for example, or cherry products reduce inflammatory markers and even uric acid ($p<0.05$) as observed in a preliminary study of marathon runners [176]. And, there is the suggestion juice has an advantage over non-processed cherries because it is more widely available throughout the year [174]. Still, the caloric contribution of some of these juices could be high, and since weight gain also increases the risk of stones, it would seem logical to also test low-calorie options such as dietary supplement extracts [48]. The issue of increasing urinary uric acid or not needs clarity, as does primary mechanism of action (vitamin C or another anti-inflammatory compounds).

Again some argue against the vitamin C theory in cherries [174], but cherries/extracts may contain an unusually large amount of dehydroascorbic acid that has a greater absorption rate by the body compared to regular ascorbic acid or vitamin C [171], and once cellular uptake occurs, conversion back to ascorbic acid results [158]. This mechanism of dehydroascorbic acid conversion to ascorbic acid is arguably one main mechanism, whereby far greater concentrations (10–20 times or more) of vitamin C in certain body tissues and organ systems compared to blood vitamin C levels occur [158]. Regardless, the entire topic of cherry and vitamin C is of notable interest and is another point of discussion with patients, along with the positives and negatives associated with CAM (just like conventional medicine).

Vitamin E? No Thank you?

It is imperative that clinicians always consider the broader implications of a recommendation for one entity (forest over the tree). Vitamin E is the paradigm of this, whereby in most medical disciplines, especially urology, there is concerning data over a significant increased risk of prostate cancer at a dosage of 400 IU [177, 178]. And, the plethora of concerns over high-dose vitamin E has existed for some time in multiple areas of medicine [179–182]. This does not imply that vitamin E has no role in medicine at all in high dosages because in rare cases where benefit may outweigh the harm it is still utilized such as for steatohepatitis [183, 184] or as part of a macular degeneration supplement for those with moderate to advanced disease [185]. Thus, the role of vitamin E in stone prevention should be nonexistent because so many other safer and more effective methods are available. Still, there are some kidney protective properties of vitamin E [186, 187], but it is difficult to ever visualize where the benefit against stones will ever outweigh the harm for high-dose supplementation.

Zinc and an Increased Stone Risk?

Zinc is found in higher concentration compared to any other heavy metal in calcium-based kidney stones (found in nucleus and crust) [188]. Significantly higher urinary zinc excretion has been found in calcium stone formers compared to non-stone-forming controls [189]. This would suggest that zinc could promote calcium-based stone aggregation. A post hoc analytical study of

343 patients from the notable Age-Related Eye Disease Study 1 (AREDS1) [185] using the dosage of 80 mg zinc found an increased risk of hospital admission due to genitourinary complications [190]. This included a nonsignificant increased risk of urinary lithiasis in men compared to placebo (RR = 4.08, or 2.0 vs. 0.5 %). Higher dietary zinc intake (>15 mg/day vs. <7.0 mg) may be associated with a higher risk of kidney stones from a large US-based cross-sectional study. It was noted by the authors that the largest source of dietary zinc intake is derived from animal sources, which could indicate an increased animal protein intake. Yet, when correcting for protein intake, there was no association found [191]. In fact, several large prospective studies and some clinical studies have not found an association of increased protein intake alone with calcium-based kidney stones [82, 192, 193]. Zinc could be a confounding factor in this relationship or concern with animal protein, but overall, the primary message with zinc should currently be similar to that of vitamin E. There is the potential for more harm than good with zinc in the area of stone disease [194], and the potential for an increased risk of prostate conditions and an increased risk of prostate cancer does exist from past epidemiologic data [195, 196]. Until more data are acquired, it would be prudent to be safe rather than sorry and suggest no separate zinc supplementation apart from a low-dose multivitamin or temporary usage, for example, the common cold [197].

Miscellaneous (Acupuncture, Artificial Sweeteners and Potassium Citrate Palatability, and Other Juices)

Some CAM options are surprising in terms of their potential role in urology and kidney stones. For example, good preliminary clinical data exists for acupressure or acupuncture to reduce anxiety before undergoing an emergent kidney stone procedure such as ESWL [198–200]. It also has the ability to provide an analgesic effect, which could hopefully reduce the need or desire for sedative prescription medications.

Several other CAM factors could be discussed, but they are at their infancy in terms of research. Raspberry appears to be utilized in some areas of the Middle East for stones, and there is some laboratory evidence to suggest a potential for benefit [201]. A separate clinical study of 12 healthy males consuming 330 mL of different juices and 24-h urine collections found some diverse observations [202]. Cranberry juice acidifies urine and increases urinary oxalate and uric acid excretion, but it could be used for brushite and struvite stones and UTI prevention. Black currant juice increases urine pH, excretion of citric and oxalic acid, but there was no impact of plum juice. Again, the benefit-to-risk ratio needs to be carefully evaluated before a recommendation is advocated.

Encouraging caloric excess from certain juices, as mentioned earlier, may reduce stone risk in the acute setting but due to weight and waist gain could increase the risk of stones in the future and other health issues. It appears simple to recommend a caloric juice as a solution or preventive aid, but in the setting of a true obesity epidemic, the patient and clinician need to evaluate these CAM options carefully. It is also of interest that some artificial sweeteners, which are calorie free, might improve the compliance of oral potassium citrate supplementation, so the ability of low caloric dietary options to enhance conventional medicine is also another benefit of CAM [203].

Conclusion

The prevention of a first kidney stone or the recurrence of stones appears complicated with so many potential recommendations, but in reality it can be simplified for patients and some healthcare professionals. There are even some genetic factors clearly involved in the risk and recurrence of stone disease [204], but the ability to alter this risk has to be exemplified by the numerous beneficial lifestyle changes discussed in this chapter. Heart health is tantamount to kidney health. Table 8.2 is a comprehensive listing of diverse lifestyle changes, supplements, and other factors

Table 8.2 A comprehensive list for health care professionals and patients of primarily CAM, along with some conventional options, which impact the risk of kidney stones

Intervention/parameter	Impact on stone disease/other commentary
Acupuncture/acupressure and other CAM relaxation or stress-reducing interventions	May reduce stress and anxiety before conventional medical kidney stone procedures, such as ESWL, and could reduce some of the need for sedative or pain medications for renal colic
Antibiotics	The indiscriminate and chronic use of antibiotics for potentially viral conditions such as sore throat or mild to moderate sinusitis could result in the partial or complete elimination of bacteria such as *Oxalobacter formigenes*, which normally utilizes dietary oxalate in the gut
Calcium (dietary and supplements)	Approximately 1,000–1,200 mg of dietary calcium per day may reduce the risk of kidney stone recurrence and stone disease (binds oxalate in gut calcium has 2 positive charges vs. the 2 negative charges of oxalate), but lower and higher intakes, especially from calcium carbonate supplements, can increase the risk of stones. Calcium citrate supplements may reduce or have no effect on kidney stone risk and can be taken with or without meals (unlike calcium carbonate) but are more costly in general, require more pills, and can increase the risk of constipation over time. Total daily dietary calcium should be calculated with a nutritionist, and then any deficit should be increased with more food sources (kale, low-calorie dairy/yogurt, etc.) or if unsuccessful adding dietary supplements (calcium citrate in previous oxalate stone formers)
Cardiovascular disease	Higher risk of cardiovascular disease (CVD) appears to be associated with a higher risk of stone disease and vice versa
Citrate/citrate beverage sources/supplements	Multiple non-cola diet soda and other beverages are high in citrate and could compete with real lemonade or lemons added to water in terms of adequate citrate intake to reduce stone risk. Citrate is a good buffer and can help keep urine at a higher pH, and as an ion it has three negative charges that can bind to complexes of positive charges in calcium, for example, to further eliminate its precipitation capacity. Potassium citrate dietary supplements can only be sold in 99-mg tablets in the USA so prescription potassium citrate sources are ideal for those that need assistance in increasing citrate from a pill. There are compliance and taste issues with prescription citrate sources, but adding artificial sweetener (Splenda®, etc.) helps, and nothing matches the efficacy of the prescription when needed. For example, drinking large quantities of real lemonade is not the answer and would add another estimated 1,700 cal. per week to equate the effects of potassium citrate prescription medicine (add 10–20 lb per year)
Cranberry concentrate dietary supplements/juice	May contain significantly higher quantities of oxalate, but it depends on the brand. Whether or not it is enough to cause kidney stones has not been adequately studied. It is my hope that companies producing cranberry supplements would voluntarily test oxalate levels and report them to the public
DASH (Dietary Approaches to Stop Hypertension) diet	Eight healthy lifestyle changes/components appear to profoundly reduce the risk of a first kidney stone and is heart healthy (increase in fruits, veggies, nuts and legumes, low-fat dairy products, and whole grains and reduce red and processed meat, sodium, and sweetened beverages)
Diabetes/prediabetes/glucose intolerance/insulin resistance	Consistent increase risk of kidney stones especially uric acid stones. More severe disease is associated with even higher risks of stones
Dyslipidemia/high LDL cholesterol/high triglycerides/ statins and other treatments	Preliminary research to suggest an increased risk of kidney stones with dyslipidemia. Cholesterol-lowering medication (e.g., statins) may reduce the risk of stone disease via multiple pathways including a reduction in inflammatory markers. High triglycerides could increase risk and is also a part of metabolic syndrome. Marine omega-3 fatty acids (EPA and DHA) lower triglycerides and may reduce stone risk
Exercise/immobility	Exercise without adequate hydration can increase the risk of stones (e.g., increased calciuria), but weight loss and hydration with exercise lowers the risk of stones. Hydrate until urine is clear in color and exercise also stimulates weight loss and reduces inflammatory markers (CRP, fibrinogen, etc.), which could aid in kidney stone risk reduction
Fad dieting (low carbohydrate, low fat, etc.)	The concern over low-carbohydrate dieting, for example, and stone disease is somewhat exaggerated because sustained weight loss over time is more heart and kidney healthy compared to a focus on the dieting method used. Preliminary 2-year research of low-carbohydrate versus low-fat diet suggests similar weight loss and stone risk. Rapid weight loss and in large amounts can increase the risk of calcium oxalate and uric acid stones

(continued)

Table 8.2 (continued)

Intervention/parameter	Impact on stone disease/other commentary
Fluid intake/hydration/ water and other beverages (lemon/lime and other juices and soda)	>2–2.5 L of fluid intake per day (ideally water) appears to be associated with a lower risk of kidney stones via a urine output of at least 2.5 L per day. Low or noncaloric soda is preferred over higher caloric soda and fruit juices. Citrate-based diluted drinks such as lemon/lime juice and low-calorie Crystal Light lemonade drink mixes are also beneficial to increase citrate levels. Real lemons and lemon juice and limes, diluted in water, may reduce the risk of a kidney stone. Multiple low caloric and non-cola products appear to improve fluid status and lower the risk of stones. Dehydration increases the risk of stone disease. Enough water should be consumed to at least create a light or clear colored urine
Fruits and veggies	Good source of potassium, magnesium, fiber, and water can raise urine pH or just provide more citric acid, which all contribute to lowering the risk of stone disease. Citrus fruits (and juices) have more citric acid, which also has the ability to simply discourage stone formation
Hypertension	Consistent increase risk of kidney stones via an increased risk of calcium excretion. Kidney stones could also cause an increase risk of hypertension
Idiopathic hypercalciuria (IH)	Common and perhaps part of the reason a slight change in urinary calcium from over supplementation of calcium or from other sources could increase the risk of a kidney stone
Inflammation/ inflammatory markers	IL-6, hs-CRP and other inflammatory markers increase in some patients with higher stone risk (dyslipidemia, hypertension, obesity, diabetes, etc.)
Inosine or ribose dietary supplementation (nucleoside-based supplements)	Inosine supplements are used for athletic enhancement (not been effective) or in testing to slow the progression of neurologic inflammatory diseases especially Parkinson's and multiple sclerosis (MS), but significantly raises uric acid and kidney stone risk from preliminary clinical trials. Inosine may function as a scavenger or peroxynitrite at dosages of 2,000+ mg per day or other damaging compounds, but its potential to raise uric acid and kidney stone risk should also be given more attention. D-Ribose supplements used in dosages as high as 10,000 mg per day for increasing energy and reducing fatigue have had no impact on uric acid levels thus far
Magnesium (dietary and supplements)	Recommend daily allowance from food sources is 310–420 mg based on age and situation. Higher intakes of dietary magnesium have been associated with lower stone risk (bind oxalate in gut, magnesium has two positive charges and oxalate has two negative charges), especially when higher concentrations of magnesium are found in the urine. Magnesium dietary supplements should be tested at lower dosages (100–200 mg/day) with other stone inhibitors, but have not been thoroughly studied, and high dosages of magnesium supplements can increase the risk of soft stools and diarrhea
Metabolic syndrome (abnormal glucose, high blood pressure, central obesity, low HDL, and high triglycerides)	A potential increased risk of stone disease with an increased number of metabolic syndrome traits
Obesity/overweight/ bariatric surgery	Consistent increase risk with a higher BMI and/or waist circumference, especially for uric acid stones, but also calcium oxalate stones. Bariatric surgery results in the potential for increased intestinal oxalate absorption and excretion and calcium oxalate stones and also uric acid stones. Rapid weight gain and weight loss increases the risk for stones (calcium and uric acid)
Omega-3 fatty acids (marine source or EPA and DHA) and omega-6 fatty acids	Omega-3 fatty acids (EPA and DHA) are FDA approved to reduce triglycerides and may also reduce urinary calcium and/or oxalate excretion and kidney stone risk. In combination with dietary counseling dosages as low as 1,200–1,800 mg/day could assist in lowering urinary calcium or oxalate (preliminary research). Omega-6 supplements (e.g., evening primrose oil) also contain anti-inflammatory effects and may also reduce calcium and/or oxalate excretion. Both omega-3 and omega-6 need more rigorous studies against placebo control before they can be advocated

(continued)

Table 8.2 (continued)

Intervention/parameter	Impact on stone disease/other commentary
Oxalate (compound with two negative charges) from endogenous or exogenous-food and beverage sources (soluble vs. insoluble)	Primary hyperoxaluria I, for example, is a rare autosomal recessive condition, which demonstrates the potential serious toxicity of excessive oxalate production without the ability for degradation. In the advanced stages, liver-kidney transplantation is needed. Other causes of increased oxalate also occur, which can lead to recurrent stone disease. Normally, about one-third of oxalate is derived from food/supplements (vitamin C for example) and two-thirds are derived/produced by the liver (endogenous), and in some cases excessive intestinal absorption also occurs (e.g., post-bariatric surgery). Increased absorption of oxalate is a concern in up to 50 % of patients with calcium oxalate stone disease. A rare vitamin B_6 deficiency may also contribute to increased oxalate level, and inflammatory bowel disease or short bowel syndrome can lead to increased oxalate absorption. Oxalate ion is a compound with two negative charges—thus, calcium with two positive charges can bind to dietary oxalate in gut and it can be eliminated in the feces. Soluble (absorbable/bioavailable) versus insoluble (nonabsorbable) oxalate amounts are added together to give a total oxalate content. Soluble oxalate amounts help to determine the amount of oxalate that could occur in the urine. Foods and beverages high in soluble oxalate are more concerning. Regardless, many foods considered high-oxalate foods are overall healthy and should not be discouraged in some patients (normal to low oxalate in urine on average) and are also low in bioavailable oxalate. For example, tea has no calories, high in nutrients, and is low in bioavailable oxalate. Spinach has a high soluble oxalate content and high bioavailability but is also nutrient dense and low caloric and could be a part of some weight-loss programs. Turmeric and ginger have high soluble oxalates compared to cinnamon (mostly insoluble), which has a low soluble oxalate content
Phytate	May be associated with a lower risk of kidney stones. It is the most abundant type of phosphate (main storage form, also known as IP6 or inositol-hexaphosphate) in plants and forms insoluble complexes with calcium in the gastrointestinal tract (has multiple negative charges), which can reduce excessive calcium absorption and urinary excretion. There is some concern that oxalate absorption could then be increased because of lower free gut calcium, but this does not appear to be the case and phytate also appears to inhibit crystal formation in the urine. Phytate is found in many foods (bran cereal, dark bread, beans, seeds, nuts) and is especially a component of foods with fiber. As fiber intake increases so does phytate intake
Potassium and potassium dietary supplements/potassium citrate prescription sources	Recommend daily allowance from food sources for adults is generally 4,700 mg per day. So, it is not easy to achieve potassium (or magnesium) from diet unless someone has a moderately healthy diet. Increased potassium to sodium ratio in the diet may lower the risk of stone disease more than isolated sodium restriction. Potassium dietary supplements can only be sold in the USA at a dosage of 99 mg maximum, which is why extreme potassium citrate needs are best derived from prescription sources (adding sucralose, the artificial sweetener, to some liquid solutions could improve taste, and sucralose has no calories and is not generally absorbed by the GI tract)
Prescription medications commonly used for stone disease	Thiazides are standard treatment for calcium stone formers with idiopathic hypercalciuria. Potassium alkali/citrate is used for those with hypocitraturia, but in some cases calcium phosphate stones can occur with this treatment. Allopurinol has been used for calcium oxalate stone formers with hyperuricosuria. Antibiotics are used for struvite stones (along with complete removal)
Probiotic-*Oxalobacter formigenes* and other potential oxalic acid utilizing bacteria (lactic acid bacteria)	A gram-negative anaerobic bacterium in flora of some individuals that uses oxalate as a primary energy source. Interestingly, some oxalate dietary consumption increases the probability of containing this intestinal bacterium. If a probiotic dietary supplement could be discovered that utilizes this bacterium or increases the chances of some colonization of this bacterium, it would be ideal. Research is still mixed on whether or not such an effective probiotic can be effective in reducing stone recurrence in the near future. It is also plausible that more discriminating use of antibiotics and mild to moderate lifestyle changes to reduce stone risk could increase colonization probability of this bacterium or work synergistically or even better. Other bacteria can degrade oxalate in the intestines (e.g., *L. acidophilus*) but have not been as thoroughly studied
Protein (animal)/red and processed meat	Inconsistent or weak relationships that suggest higher intakes of animal protein increase the risk of stones, but a high plant and/or animal protein and low glycemic/reduced–caloric intake diet may cause weight loss and diabetes risk reduction, which could lower the risk of kidney stones in the long term. Reducing red and processed or non-lean meat is healthy and may also reduce stone disease. Animal proteins do have the ability to increase the acid load

(continued)

Table 8.2 (continued)

Intervention/parameter	Impact on stone disease/other commentary
Smoking and tobacco	Not an overt risk factor for stone disease but chronic tobacco exposure could increase the risk of cardiovascular disease including high blood pressure, which could increase the risk of stones
Sodium (or potassium to sodium ratio)	Processed food should be reduced because it is the primary source of high sodium intake in the diet (not the salt shaker), and identifying foods high in potassium and low in sodium (fruits, veggies, nuts, etc.) may be more important compared to just isolated sodium reduction (high potassium to sodium ratio in foods is healthy). Some studies suggest that some sodium intake is needed to trigger voluntary increased fluid intake. Excessive sodium increases urinary calcium by increasing the fluid volume of the body and reducing the ability of the kidney to reabsorb calcium from the urine, and it can also cause calcium to leech from bones, further increasing the risk of having too much calcium in the urinary tract, and it reduces citrate and it increases the chance that calcium and oxalate will crystallize forming a stone
Sucrose/sugar/refined carbohydrates/fruit juices/ fructose	Temporary or chronic insulin increases may mimic diabetic disease, and these inflammatory changes from refined carbohydrates or sugars can increase the amount of calcium excreted in the urine (independent of calcium intake) and reduce the pH of urine. Fructose (component of sugar found in many beverage/fruit juices) may also contribute to a higher risk
Topiramate and weight-loss drugs that contain this compound (Qsymia)	Qsymia is an FDA weight-loss drug with topiramate and phentermine, and it has slightly increased the risk of stones in some clinical trials at higher dosages. Orlistat and other medications used to cause moderate to rapid and large amounts of weight loss could increase the risk of stone disease
Uric acid	Excessive amounts in the urine could lead to a uric acid stone, which can be found in those with gout but is also becoming more common in obesity and diabetes. A reduction in urine pH favors precipitation of a uric acid stone. Inosine dietary supplements increase urinary uric acid and stone risk. Ascorbic acid supplements may also increase uric acid excretion and stone risk (oxalate and uric acid stone risk)
Vitamin B_6 (pyridoxine)	Vitamin B_6 dietary supplements (pyridoxine hydrochloride) appear to reduce endogenous oxalate production by shifting metabolism in the body to produce glycine instead of oxalate, especially in those with primary hyperoxaluria type 1. Other hyperoxaluric conditions (endogenous and exogenous) may or may not benefit with vitamin B_6 supplementation but needs more research compared to a control group. Dosages of 50–100 mg/day of pyridoxine hydrochloride may be helpful in reducing urinary oxalate. Higher dosages (>200–300) are problematic because it can cause a sensory neuropathy. The other more active form of vitamin B_6 (P5P, pyridoxal-5-phosphate) needs more research, but has some preliminary research for those with idiopathic hypercalciuria at 60 mg/day
Vitamin C (ascorbic acid) and calcium ascorbate (buffered or less acidic vitamin C) and cherries/ extract/concentrates	Plain vitamin C increases oxalate levels at dosages of 1,000–1,500+ that could increase the risk of oxalate stone disease. Preliminary evidence suggests buffered/pH neutral vitamin C (calcium ascorbate) might not increase oxalate levels as significantly compared to plain vitamin C and could also cause less GI upset and could be an alternative to plain vitamin C. However, plain vitamin C (1,000–1,500+) may significantly lower serum uric acid (SUA) levels, and it being studied to prevent gout with early interesting results. It does not appear to be as effective for those with gout. It is being studied with standard gout prophylaxis. Vitamin C may operate by increasing filtration and blocking reabsorption of proximal tubule uric acid, which means there is a theoretical risk of an increased risk of a uric acid stones if this is the case. Some good dietary sources of vitamin C (tart cherry, cherries, cherry juice concentrate) are also being studied to prevent gout and gout recurrence and may have an effect via their vitamin C level and/or anti-inflammatory mechanism. They may also increase urinary uric acid levels
Vitamin D	Serum vitamin D levels have not been associated thus far with an increase in urinary calcium in those with and without a history of kidney stones. Although a bolus dosage could be concerning, small increases (500–1,000 IU at a time) in supplement dose should be encouraged until more safety data is collected. Vitamin D also helps to suppress parathyroid hormone in moderation (600–1,000 IU per day), which could arguably discourage calcium stone formation in some individuals
Vitamin E supplements	Some minor data suggest protective kidney effects, but overall their notorious history in urology at 400 IU per day (increases the risk of prostate cancer) and from other areas of medicine suggests that this supplement will have no role in stone prevention in the future

that impact stone risk, and this should be shared with healthcare professionals and patients.

Kidney stone risk and recurrence symbolize an outstanding opportunity in urology to demonstrate the importance of lifestyle and the ability to be the impetus not only for kidney health but overall mental and physical health. On the mental health side, the stress precipitated by stone disease or the ability of stress to increase the risk of stone disease is of interest [205, 206]. What if healthcare professionals in urology could also have some role in helping patients lose weight/waist; reduce their cholesterol, blood pressure, and glucose; improve their diet; increase the commitment to exercise; or even eliminate tobacco (an indirect contributor to stones via hypertensive risk) [207, 208]? This would not only improve a patient's chance of living longer and better, but an ancillary benefit could be a life free of stone disease.

References

1. Reiner AP, Kahn A, Eisner BH, Pletcher MJ, Sadetsky N, Williams OD, et al. Kidney stones and subclinical atherosclerosis in young adults: the CARDIA study. J Urol. 2011;185:920–5.
2. Rule AD, Roger VL, Melton LJ, Bergstraih EJ, Li X, Peyser PA, et al. Kidney stones associate with increased risk for myocardial infarction. J Am Soc Nephrol. 2010;21:1641–4.
3. Domingos F, Serra A. Nephrolithiasis is associated with an increased prevalence of cardiovascular disease. Nephrol Dial Transplant. 2011;26:864–8.
4. Ando R, Nagaya T, Suzuki S, Takahashi H, Kawai M, Okada A, et al. Kidney stone formation is positively associated with conventional risk factors for coronary heart disease in Japanese men. J Urol. 2013;189:1340–6.
5. Tang J, Mettler P, McFann K, Chonchoi M. The association of prevalent kidney stone disease with mortality in US adults: The National Health and Nutrition Examination Survey III, 1988–1994. Am J Nephrol. 2013;37:501–6.
6. Borghi L, Schianchi T, Meschi T, Guerra A, Allegri F, Maggiore U, et al. Comparison of two diets for the prevention of recurrent stones in idiopathic hypercalciuria. N Engl J Med. 2002;346:77–84.
7. Appel LJ, Moore TJ, Obarzanek E, Vollmer WM, Svetkey LP, Sacks FM, DASH Collaborative Research Group, et al. A clinical trial of the effects of dietary patterns on blood pressure. N Engl J Med. 1997;336:1117–24.
8. Sacks FM, Svetkey LP, Vollmer WM, Appel LJ, Bray GA, Harsha D, DASH-Sodium Collaborative Research Group, et al. Effects on blood pressure of reduced dietary sodium and the Dietary Approaches to Stop Hypertension (DASH) diet. N Engl J Med. 2001;344:3–10.
9. Taylor EN, Fung TT, Curhan GC. DASH-style diet associates with reduced risk for kidney stones. J Am Soc Nephrol. 2009;20:2253–9.
10. Taylor EN, Stampfer MJ, Mount DB, Curhan GC. DASH-style diet and 24-hour urine composition. Clin J Am Soc Nephrol. 2010;5:2315–22.
11. Cappuccio FP, Siani A, Barba G, Mellone MC, Russo L, Farinaro E, et al. A prospective study of hypertension and the incidence of kidney stones in men. J Hypertens. 1999;17:1017–22.
12. Cappuccio FP, Strazzullo P, Mancini M. Kidney stones and hypertension: population based study of an independent clinical association. BMJ. 1990;300:1234–6.
13. Borghi L, Meschi T, Guerra A, Briganti A, Schlanchi T, Allegri F, et al. Essential arterial hypertension and stone disease. Kidney Int. 1999;55:2397–406.
14. Madore F, Stampfer MJ, Rimm EB, Curhan GC. Nephrolithiasis and risk of hypertension. Am J Hypertens. 1998;11:46–53.
15. Madore F, Stampfer MJ, Willett WC, Speizer FE. Nephrolithiasis and risk of hypertension in women. Am J Kidney Dis. 1998;32:802–7.
16. Eisner BH, Porten SP, Bechis SK, Stoller ML. Hypertension is associated with increased urinary calcium excretion in patients with nephrolithiasis. J Urol. 2010;183:576–9.
17. Inci M, Demirtas A, Sarli B, Akinsai E, Baydilli N. Association between body mass index, lipid profiles, and types of urinary stones. Ren Fail. 2012;34:1140–3.
18. Tsujihata M, Yoshioka I, Tsujimura A, Nonomura N, Okuyama A. Why does atorvastatin inhibit renal crystal retention? Urol Res. 2011;39:379–83.
19. Sur RL, Masterson JH, Palazzi KL, L'esperance JO, Auge BK, Change DC, et al. Impact of statins on nephrolithiasis in hyperlipidemic patients: a 10-year review of an equal access health care system. Clin Nephrol. 2013;79:351–5.
20. Bonnet J, McPherson R, Tedgul A, Simoneau D, Nozza A, Martineau P, et al. Comparative effects of 10-mg versus 80-mg atorvastatin on high-sensitivity C-reactive protein in patients with stable coronary artery disease: results of the CAP (Comparative Atorvastatin Pleiotropic effects) study. Clin Ther. 2008;30:2298–313.
21. Akoudad S, Szkio M, McAdams MA, Fulop T, Anderson CA, Coresh J, et al. Correlates of kidney stone disease differ by race in a multi-ethnic middle-aged population: the ARIC study. Prev Med. 2010;51:416–20.
22. Buck AC, Davies RL, Harrison T. The protective role of eicosapentaenoic acid [EPA] in the pathogenesis of nephrolithiasis. J Urol. 1991;146:188–94.

23. Taylor EN, Stampfer MJ, Curhan GC. Obesity, weight gain, and the risk of kidney stones. JAMA. 2005;293:455–62.
24. Del Valle EE, Negri AL, Spivacow FR, Rosende G, Forrester M, Pinduli I. Metabolic diagnosis in stone formers in relation to body mass index. Urol Res. 2012;40:47–52.
25. Taylor EN, Curhan GC. Body size and 24-hour urine composition. Am J Kidney Dis. 2006;48:905–15.
26. Lee SC, Kim YJ, Kim TH. Impact of obesity in patients with urolithiasis and its prognostic usefulness in stone recurrence. J Urol. 2008;179:570–4.
27. Ekeruo WO, Tan YH, Young MD, Dahm P, Maloney ME, Mathias BJ, et al. Metabolic risk factors and the impact of medical therapy on the management of nephrolithiasis in obese patients. J Urol. 2004;172:159–63.
28. Taylor EN, Stampfer MJ, Curhan GC. Diabetes mellitus and the risk of nephrolithiasis. Kidney Int. 2005;68:1230–5.
29. Chung SD, Chen YK, Lin HC. Increased risk of diabetes in patients with urinary calculi: a 5-year followup study. J Urol. 2011;186:1888–93.
30. Tasca A. Metabolic syndrome and bariatric surgery in stone disease etiology. Curr Opin Urol. 2011;21:129–33.
31. Ahmed MH, Ahmed HT, Khalil AA. Renal stone disease and obesity: what is important for urologists and nephrologists? Ren Fail. 2012;34:1348–54.
32. Asplin JR. Obesity and urolithiasis. Adv Chronic Kidney Dis. 2009;16:11–20.
33. Canada AE, Isgoren AE. Re: Increased risk of diabetes in patients with urinary calculi: a 5-year followup study: S-D Chung, Y-K Chen and H-C lin J Urol 2011;186:1888–1893. J Urol. 2012;187:2279–80.
34. Eisner BH, Porten SP, Bechis SK, Stoller ML. Diabetic kidney stone formers excrete more oxalate and have lower urine pH than nondiabetic stone formers. J Urol. 2010;183:2244–8.
35. Gadde KM, Allison DB, Ryan DH, Peterson CA, Troupin B, Schwlers ML, et al. Effects of low-dose, controlled release, phentermine plus topiramate combination on weight and associated comorbidities in overweight and obese adults (CONQUER): a randomized, placebo-controlled, phase 3 trial. Lancet. 2011;16(377):1341–52.
36. Penniston KL, Kaplon DM, Gould JC, Nakada SY. Gastric band placement for obesity is not associated with increased urinary risk of urolithiasis compared to bypass. J Urol. 2009;182:2340–6.
37. Tice JA, Karliner L, Walsh J, Petersen AJ, Feldman MD. Gastric banding or bypass? A systematic review comparing the two most popular bariatric procedures. Am J Med. 2008;121:885–93.
38. Lemann J, Piering WF, Lennon EJ. Possible role of carbohydrate-induced calciuria in calcium oxalate kidney-stone formation. N Engl J Med. 1969;280:232–7.
39. Friedman AN, Ogden LG, Foster GD, Klein S, Stein R, Miller B, et al. Comparative effects of low-carbohydrate high-protein versus low-fat diets on the kidney. Clin J Am Soc Nephrol. 2012;7:1103–11.
40. Reddy ST, Wang CY, Sakhaee K, Brinkley L, Pak CY. Effect of low-carbohydrate high-protein diets on acid–base balance, stone-forming propensity, and calcium metabolism. Am J Kidney Dis. 2002;40:265–74.
41. West B, Luke A, Durazo-Arvizu RA, Cao G, Shoham D, Kramer H. Metabolic syndrome and self-reported history of kidney stones: the National Health and Nutrition Examination Survey (NHANES III) 1988–1994. Am J Kidney Dis. 2008;51:741–7.
42. Jeong IG, Kang T, Bang JK, Park J, Kim W, Hwang SS, et al. Association between metabolic syndrome and the presence of kidney stones in a screened population. Am J Kidney Dis. 2011;58:383–8.
43. Kadlec AO, Greco K, Fridirici ZC, Hart ST, Vellos T, Turk TM. Metabolic syndrome and urinary stone composition: what factors matter most? Urology. 2012;80:805–10.
44. Sakhaee K, Nigam S, Snell P, Hsu MC, Pak CY. Assessment of the pathogenetic role of physical exercise in renal stone formation. J Clin Endocrinol Metab. 1987;65:974–9.
45. Sriboonlue P, Prasongwatana V, Tosukhowong P, Tungsanga K, Bovornpadoongkitti S. Increased risk of urinary stone disease by physical exercise. Southeast Asian J Trop Med Public Health. 1996;27:172–7.
46. Okada A, Ohshima H, Itoh Y, Yasui T, Tozawa K, Kohri K. Risk of renal stone formation induced by long-term bed rest could be decreased by premedication with bisphosphonate and increased by resistive exercise. Int J Urol. 2008;15:630–5.
47. Monga M, Macias B, Groppo E, Kostelec M, Hargens A. Renal stone risk in a simulated microgravity environment: impact of treadmill exercise with lower body negative pressure. J Urol. 2006;176:127–31.
48. Moyad MA. Dr. Moyad's no bogus science health advice. Ann Arbor, MI: Spry; 2010.
49. Swardfager W, Herrmann N, Cornish S, Mazereeuw G, Marzolini S, Sham L, et al. Exercise intervention and inflammatory markers in coronary artery disease: a meta-analysis. Am Heart J. 2012;163:666–76.
50. Fink HA, Wilt TJ, Eldman KE, Garimella PS, MacDonald R, Rutks IR, et al. Medical management to prevent recurrent nephrolithiasis in adults: a systematic review for an American College of Physicians Clinical Guideline. Ann Intern Med. 2013;158:535–43.
51. Fink HA, Akornor JW, Garimella PS, MacDonald R, Cutting A, Rutks IR, et al. Diet, fluid, or supplements for secondary prevention of nephrolithiasis: a systematic review and meta-analysis of randomized trials. Eur Urol. 2009;56:72–80.
52. Sharp RL. Role of whole foods in promoting hydration after exercise in humans. J Am Coll Nutr. 2007;26(5 Suppl):592S–6.
53. Curhan GC, Willett WC, Speizer FE, Stampfer MJ. Beverage use and risk for kidney stones in women. Ann Intern Med. 1998;128:534–40.

54. Haleblian GE, Leitao VA, Pierre SA, Robinson MR, Albala DM, Ribeiro AA, et al. Assessment of citrate concentration in citrus fruit-based juices and beverages: implications for management of hypocitraturic nephrolithiasis. J Endourol. 2008;22:1359–66.
55. Eisner BH, Asplin JR, Goldfarb DS, Ahmad A, Stoller ML. Citrate, malate and alkali content in commonly consumed diet sodas: implications for nephrolithiasis treatment. J Urol. 2010;183:2419–23.
56. Penniston KL, Nakada SY, Holmes RP, Assimos DG. Quantitative assessment of citric acid in lemon juice, lime juice, and commercially-available fruit juice products. J Endourol. 2008;22:567–70.
57. Hiatt RA, Ettinger B, Caan B, Quesenberry Jr CP, Duncan D, Citron JT. Randomized controlled trial of a low animal protein, high fiber diet in the prevention of recurrent calcium oxalate kidney stones. Am J Epidemiol. 1996;144:25–33.
58. Rotily M, Leonetti F, Iovanna C, Berthezene P, Dupuy P, Vazi A, et al. Effects of low animal protein or high-fiber diets on urine composition in calcium nephrolithiasis. Kidney Int. 2000;57:1115–23.
59. Dussol B, Iovanna C, Rotily M, Morange S, Leonetti F, Dupuy P, et al. A randomized trial of low-animal-protein or high-fiber diets for secondary prevention of calcium nephrolithiasis. Nephron Clin Pract. 2008;110:185–94.
60. Ebisuno S, Morimoto S, Yasukawa S, Ohkawa T. Results of long-term rice bran treatment on stone recurrence in hypercalciuric patients. Br J Urol. 1991;67:237–40.
61. Shah PJ, Green NA, Williams G. Unprocessed bran and its effect on urinary calcium excretion in idiopathic hypercalciuria. Br Med J. 1980;281:426–9.
62. Ala-Opas M, Elomaa I, Porkka L, Alfthan O. Unprocessed bran and intermittent thiazide therapy in prevention of recurrent urinary calcium stones. Scand J Urol Nephrol. 1987;21:311–4.
63. Kaczmarczyk MM, Miller MJ, Freund GG. The health benefits of dietary fiber: beyond the usual suspects of type 2 diabetes mellitus, cardiovascular disease and colon cancer. Metabolism. 2012;61:1058–66.
64. Marangella M, Bianco O, Martini C, Petrarulo M, Vitale C, Linari F. Effect of animal and vegetable protein intake on oxalate excretion in idiopathic calcium stone disease. Br J Urol. 1989;63:348–51.
65. Robertson WG, Peacock M, Heyburn PJ, Hanes FA, Rutherford A, Clementson E, et al. Should recurrent calcium oxalate stone formers become vegetarians? Br J Urol. 1979;51:427–31.
66. Brinkley LJ, Gregory J, Pak CY. A further study of oxalate bioavailability in foods. J Urol. 1990;144:94–6.
67. Brinkley L, McGuire J, Gregory J, Pak CY. Bioavailability of oxalate in foods. Urology. 1981;17:534–8.
68. Brogren M, Savage GP. Bioavailability of soluble oxalate from spinach eaten with and without milk products. Asia Pac J Clin Nutr. 2003;12:219–24.
69. Radek M, Savage GP. Oxalates in some Indian green leafy vegetables. Int J Food Sci Nutr. 2008;59:246–60.
70. Noonan SC, Savage GP. Oxalate content of foods and its effect on humans. Asia Pac J Clin Nutr. 1999;8:64–74.
71. Ghosh Das S, Savage GP. Total and soluble oxalate content of some Indian spices. Plant Foods Hum Nutr. 2012;67:186–90.
72. Tang M, Larson-Meyer DE, Liebman M. Effect of cinnamon and turmeric on urinary oxalate excretion, plasma lipids, and plasma glucose in healthy subjects. Am J Clin Nutr. 2008;87:1262–7.
73. Liebman M, Costa G. Effects of calcium and magnesium on urinary oxalate excretion after oxalate loads. J Urol. 2000;163:1565–9.
74. Jiang J, Knight J, Easter LH, Neiberg R, Holmes RP, Assimos DG. Impact of dietary calcium and oxalate, and Oxalobacter formigenes colonization on urinary on urinary oxalate excretion. J Urol. 2011;186:135–9.
75. American Dietetic Association. Urolithiasis/urinary stones. In: ADA Nutrition Care Manual. Chicago, IL: American Dietetic Association; 2005. p. 483–6.
76. Massey LK. Food oxalate: factors affecting measurement, biological variation, and bioavailability. J Am Diet Assoc. 2007;107:1191–4.
77. Massey LK, Sutton RAL. Modification of dietary oxalate and calcium reduces urinary oxalate in hyperoxaluric patients with kidney stones. J Am Diet Assoc. 1993;93:1305–7.
78. Al-Wahsh IA, Horner HT, Palmer RG, Reddy MB, Massey LK. Oxalate and phytate of soy foods. J Agric Food Chem. 2005;53:5670–4.
79. Heaney RP, Weaver CM. Calcium absorption from kale. Am J Clin Nutr. 1990;51:656–7.
80. Jackson RD, LaCroix AZ, Gass M, Wallace RB, Robbins J, Lewis CE, Women's Health Initiative Investigators, et al. Calcium plus vitamin D supplementation and the risk of fractures. N Engl J Med. 2006;354:669–83.
81. Candelas G, Martinez-Lopez JA, Rosario MP, Carmona L, Loza E. Calcium supplementation and kidney stone risk in osteoporosis: a systematic literature review. Clin Exp Rheumatol. 2012;30:954–61.
82. Curhan GC, Willett WC, Speizer FE, Spiegelman D, Stampfer MJ. Comparison of dietary calcium with supplemental calcium and other nutrients as factors affecting the risk for kidney stones in women. Ann Intern Med. 1997;126:497–504.
83. Shaker HK, Stigleman S. Clinical inquiry: can calcium supplements cause serious adverse effects in healthy people? J Fam Pract. 2012;61:620–1.
84. Institute of Medicine. Dietary reference intakes for calcium and vitamin D. Report brief, November 2010. Washington, DC: Institute of Medicine; 2001. Available at: http://www.iom.edu/~/media/Files/Report%20Files/2010/Dietary-Reference-Intakes-for-Calcium-and-Vitamin-D/Vitamin%20D%20and%20Calcium%202010%20Report%20Brief.pdf. Accessed on 14 May 2012.

85. Eisner BH, Thavaseelan S, Sheth S, Halebilian G, Pareek G. Relationship between serum vitamin D and 24-hour urine calcium in patients with nephrolithiasis. Urology. 2012;80:1007–10.
86. Leaf DE, Korets R, Taylor EN, Tang J, Asplin JR, Goldfarb DS, et al. Effect of vitamin D repletion on urinary calcium excretion among kidney stone formers. Clin J Am Soc Nephrol. 2012;7:829–34.
87. Terris MK, Issa MM, Tacker JR. Dietary supplementation with cranberry concentrate tablets may increase the risk of nephrolithiasis. Urology. 2001;57:26–9.
88. McHarg T, Rodgers A, Charlton K. Influence of cranberry juice on the urinary risk factors for calcium oxalate kidney stone formation. BJU Int. 2003;92:765–8.
89. Gettman MT, Ogan K, Brinkley LJ, Adams-Huet B, Pak CY, Pearle MS. Effect of cranberry juice consumption on urinary stone risk factors. J Urol. 2005;174:590–4.
90. Jepson RG, Williams G, Craig JC. Cranberries for preventing urinary tract infections. Cochrane Database Syst Rev. 2012;10, CD001321.
91. Goldman RD. Cranberry juice for urinary tract infection in children. Can Fam Physician. 2012;58: 398–401.
92. Harmsen E, de Tombe PP, de Jong J, Achterberg PW. Enhanced ATP and GTP synthesis from hypoxanthine or inosine after myocardial ischemia. Am J Physiol. 1984;246:H37–43.
93. Currell K, Derave W, Everaert I, McNaughton L, Slater G, Burke LM, et al. A–Z of nutritional supplements: dietary supplements, sports nutrition foods and ergogenic aids for health and performance-Part 20. Br J Sports Med. 2011;45:530–2.
94. McNaughton L, Dalton B, Tarr J. Inosine supplementation has no effect on aerobic or anaerobic cycling performance. Int J Sports Nutr. 1999;9:333–44.
95. Starling RD, Trappe TA, Short KR, Sheffield-Moore M, Jozsi AC, Fink WJ, et al. Effect of inosine supplementation on aerobic and anaerobic cycling performance. Med Sci Sports Exerc. 1996;28:1193–8.
96. Kovacs Z, Juhasz G, Palkovits M, Dobolyi A, Kekesi KA. Area, age, and gender dependence of the nucleoside system in the brain: a review of current literature. Curr Top Med Chem. 2011;11:1012–33.
97. McCarty MF, Barroso-Aranda J, Contreras F. High-dose folate and dietary purines promote scavenging of peroxynitrite-derived radicals-clinical potential in inflammatory disorders. Med Hypotheses. 2009;73: 824–34.
98. Markowitz CE, Spitsin S, Zimmerman V, Jacobs D, Udupa JK, Hooper DC, et al. The treatment of multiple sclerosis with inosine. J Altern Complement Med. 2009;15:619–25.
99. Liu B, Shen Y, Xiao K, Tang Y, Cen L, Wei J. Serum uric acid levels in patients with multiple sclerosis: a meta-analysis. Neurol Res. 2012;34:163–71.
100. Spitsin S, Markowitz CE, Zimmerman V, Koprowski H, Hooper DC. Modulation of serum uric acid levels by inosine in patients with multiple sclerosis does not affect blood pressure. J Hum Hypertens. 2010;24:359–62.
101. Kreider RB, Melton C, Greenwood M, Rasmussen C, Lundberg J, Earnest C, et al. Effects of oral D-ribose supplementation on anaerobic capacity and selected metabolic markers in healthy males. Int J Sports Nutr Exerc Metab. 2003;13:76–86.
102. Seifert JG, Subudhi AW, Fu MX, Riska KL, John JC, Shecterle LM, et al. The role of ribose on oxidative stress during hypoxic exercise: a pilot study. J Med Food. 2009;12:690–3.
103. Eisner BH, Sheth S, Dretler SP, Herrick B, Pais Jr VM. High dietary magnesium intake decreases hyperoxaluria in patients with nephrolithiasis. Urology. 2012;80:780–3.
104. Volpe SL. Magnesium in disease prevention and overall health. Adv Nutr. 2013;4:378S–83.
105. Jaipakdee S, Prasongwatana V, Premgamone A, Reungjui S, Tosukhowong P, Tungsanga K, et al. The effects of potassium and magnesium supplementations on urinary risk factors of renal stone patients. J Med Assoc Thai. 2004;87:255–63.
106. Guerrera MP, Volpe SL, Mao JJ. Therapeutic uses of magnesium. Am Fam Physician. 2009;80:157–62.
107. Ortiz-Alvarado O, Miyaoka R, Kriedberg C, Leavitt DA, Moeding A, Stessman M, et al. Urology. 2012;79:282–6.
108. Yasui T, Suzuki S, Itoh Y, Tozawa K, Tokudome S, Kohri K. Eicosapentaenoic acid has a preventive effect on the recurrence of nephrolithiasis. Urol Int. 2008;81:135–8.
109. Taylor EN, Stampfer MJ, Curhan GC. Fatty acid intake and incident nephrolithiasis. Am J Kidney Dis. 2005;45:267–74.
110. The Age-Related Eye Disease Study 2 (AREDS2) Research Group. Lutein + zeaxanthin and omega-3 fatty acids for age-related macular degeneration: the age-related eye disease study 2 (AREDS2) randomized clinical trial. JAMA. 2013;309:2005–15.
111. Risk and Prevention Study Collaborative Group. N-3 fatty acids in patients with multiple cardiovascular risk factors. N Engl J Med. 2013;368:1800–8.
112. Mozaffarian D, Marchioli R, Macchia A, Silleta MG, Ferrazzi P, Gardner TJ, OPERA Investigators, et al. Fish oil and postoperative atrial fibrillation: the Omega-3 fatty acids for prevention of post-operative atrial fibrillation (OPERA) randomized trial. JAMA. 2012;308:2001–11.
113. Rizos EC, Ntzani EE, Bika E, Kostapanos MS, Elisaf MS. Association between omega-3 fatty acid supplementation and risk of major cardiovascular disease events: a systematic review and meta-analysis. JAMA. 2012;308:1024–33.
114. Rodgers A, Lewandowski S, Allie-Hamdulay S, Pinnock D, Baretta G, Gambaro G. Evening primrose oil supplementation increases citraturia and decreases other urinary risk factors for calcium oxalate urolithiasis. J Urol. 2009;182:2957–63.
115. Brignole-Baudoulin F, Baudoulin C, Aragona P, Rolando M, Labetoulle M, Pisella PJ, et al. A multicentre, double-masked, randomized, controlled trial assessing the effect of oral supplementation of omega-3 and omega-6 fatty acids on a conjunctival

inflammatory marker in dry eye patients. Acta Opthalmol. 2011;89:e591–7.

116. Allison MJ, Dawson KA, Mayberry WR, Foss JG. Oxalobacter formigenes gen. nov., sp. Nov: oxalate degrading anaerobes that inhabit the gastrointestinal tract. Arch Microbiol. 1985;141:1–7.
117. Hoppe B, Dittlich K, Fehrenbach H, Plum G, Beck BB. Reduction of plasma oxalate levels by oral application of Oxalobacter formigenes in 2 patients with infantile oxalosis. Am J Kidney Dis. 2011;58:453–5.
118. Hoppe B, Groothoff JW, Hulton SA, Cochat P, Niaudet P, Kemper MJ, et al. Efficacy and safety of Oxalobacter formigenes to reduce urinary oxalate in primary oxaluria. Nephrol Dial Transplant. 2011;26:3609–15.
119. Assimos D. Re: Sensitivity of human strains of Oxalobacter formigenes to commonly prescribed antibiotics. J Urol. 2013;189:171–2.
120. Kelly JP, Curhan GC, Cave DR, Anderson TE, Kaufman DW. Factors related to colonization with Oxalobacter formigenes in U.S. adults. J Endourol. 2011;25:673–9.
121. Duncan SH, Richardson AJ, Kaul P, Holmes RP, Allison MJ, Stewart CS. Oxalobacter formigenes and its potential role in human health. Appl Environ Microbiol. 2002;68:3841–7.
122. Kharlamb V, Schelker J, Francois F, Jiang J, Holmes RP, Goldfarb DS. Oral antibiotic treatment of Helicobacter pylori leads to persistently reduced intestinal colonization rates with Oxalobacter formigenes. J Endourol. 2011;25:1781–5.
123. Lange JN, Wood KD, Wong H, Otto R, Mufarrij PW, Knight J, et al. Sensitivity of human strains of Oxalobacter formigenes to commonly prescribed antibiotics. Urology. 2012;79:1286–9.
124. Duffey BG, Miyaoka R, Holmes R, Assimos D, Hinck B, Korman E, et al. Oxalobacter colonization in the morbidly obese and correlation with urinary stone risk. Urology. 2011;78:531–4.
125. Federici F, Vitali B, Gotti R, Pasca MR, Gobbi S, Peck AB, et al. Characterization and heterologous expression of the oxalyl coenzyme A decarboxylase gene from Bifidobacterium lactis. Appl Environ Microbiol. 2004;70:5066–73.
126. Campieri C, Campieri M, Bertuzzi V, Swennen E, Matteuzzi D, Stefoni S, et al. Reduction of oxaluria after an oral course of lactic acid bacteria at high concentration. Kidney Int. 2001;60:1097–105.
127. Kaufman DW, Kelly JP, Curhan GC, Anderson TE, Dretler SP, Preminger GM, et al. Oxalobacter formigenes may reduce the risk of calcium oxalate kidney stones. J Am Soc Nephrol. 2008;19:1197–203.
128. Prokopovich S, Knight J, Assimos DG, Holmes RP. Variability of Oxalobacter formigenes and oxalate in stool samples. J Urol. 2007;178:2186–90.
129. Cochat P, Hulton SA, Acquaviva C, Danpure CJ, Daudon M, De Marchi M, OxalEurope, et al. Primary hyperoxaluria type 1: indications for screening and guidance for diagnosis and treatment. Nephrol Dial Transplant. 2012;27:1729–36.
130. Milliner DS, Eickholt JT, Bergstrahl EJ, Wilson DM, Smith LH. Results of long-term treatment with orthophosphates and pyridoxine in patients with primary hyperoxaluria. N Engl J Med. 1994;331:1553–8.
131. Williams HE, Smith Jr RH. Primary hyperoxaluria. In: Stansbury JB, Wyngaarden JB, Fredrickson PS, Goldstein SL, Brown MS, editors. The metabolic basis of inherited disease. 5th ed. New York: McGraw-Hill; 1983. p. 204–10.
132. Goldenberg RM, Girone JAC. Oral pyridoxine in the prevention of oxalate kidney stones. Am J Nephrol. 1996;16:552–3.
133. Scheinman JI, Voziyan PA, Belmont JM, et al. Pyridoxamine lowers oxalate excretion and kidney crystals in experimental hyperoxaluria: a potential therapy for primary hyperoxaluria. Urol Res. 2005;33:368–71.
134. Lheureux P, Penaloza A, Gris M. Pyridoxine in clinical toxicology: a review. Eur J Emerg Med. 2005;12:78–85.
135. Ortiz-Alvarado O, Miyaoka R, Kriedberg C, Moeding A, Stessman M, Monga M. Pyridoxine and dietary counseling for the management of idiopathic hyperoxaluria in stone-forming patients. Urology. 2011;77:1054–8.
136. Mitwalli A, Aylomamitis A, Grass L, Oreopoulos DG. Control of hyperoxaluria with large doses of pyridoxine in patients with kidney stones. Int Urol Nephrol. 1988;20:353–9.
137. Jaeger P, Portmann L, Jacquet AF, Burckhardt P. Pyridoxine can normalize oxaluria in idiopathic renal lithiasis. Schweiz Med Wochenschr. 1986;116:1783–6.
138. Gershoff SN, Prien EL. Effect of daily MgO and vitamin B6 administration to patients with recurring calcium oxalate kidney stones. Am J Clin Nutr. 1967;20:393–9.
139. Nakada T, Sasagawa I, Furuta H, Katayama T, Shimazaki J. Effect of high calcium diet on urinary oxalate excretion in urinary stone-forming patients. Eur Urol. 1988;15:264–70.
140. Curhan GC, Willett WC, Speizer FE, et al. Intake of vitamin B6 and C and the risk of kidney stones in women. J Am Soc Nephrol. 1999;10:840–5.
141. Berger A, Schaumberg HH. More on neuropathy from pyridoxine abuse. N Engl J Med. 1984;311:986–7.
142. Radimer K, Bindewald B, Hughes J, Ervin B, Swanson C, Picciano MF. Dietary supplement use by US adults: data from the National Health and Nutrition Examination Survey, 1999–2000. Am J Epidemiol. 2004;160:339–49.
143. Hirayama F, Lee AH, Binns CW, Watanabe F, Ogawa T. Dietary supplementation by older adults in Japan. Asia Pac J Clin Nutr. 2008;17:280–4.
144. Gardiner P, Woods C, Kemper KJ. Dietary supplement use among health care professionals enrolled in an online curriculum on herbs and dietary supplements. BMC Complement Altern Med. 2006;6:21.

145. Picciano MF, Dwyer JT, Radimer KL, Wilson DH, Fisher KD, Thomas PR, et al. Dietary supplement use among infants, children, and adolescents in the United States, 1999–2002. Arch Pediatr Adolesc Med. 2007;161:978–85.
146. Frank E, Bendich A, Denniston M. Use of vitamin-mineral supplements by female physicians in the United States. Am J Clin Nutr. 2000;72:969–75.
147. Hall PM. Preventing kidney stones: calcium restriction not warranted. Cleve Clin J Med. 2002;69:885–8.
148. Moe OW. Kidney stones: pathophysiology and medical management. Lancet. 2006;367:333–44.
149. Khan SR. Animal models of kidney stone formation: an analysis. World J Urol. 1997;15:236–43.
150. Robijn S, Hoppe B, Vervaet BA, D'Haese PC, Verhulst A. Hyperoxaluria: a gut-kidney axis? Kidney Int. 2011;80:1146–58.
151. Baxmann AC, De OG, Mendonca C, Heilberg IP. Effect of vitamin C supplements on urinary oxalate and pH in calcium stone-forming patients. Kidney Int. 2003;63:1066–71.
152. Traxer O, Huet B, Poindexter J, Pak CY, Pearle MS. Effect of ascorbic acid consumption on urinary stone risk factors. J Urol. 2003;170(2 Pt 1):397–401.
153. Massey LK, Liebman M, Kynast-Gales SA. Ascorbate increases human oxaluria and kidney stone risk. J Nutr. 2005;135:1673–7.
154. Taylor EN, Stampfer MJ, Curhan GC. Dietary factors and the risk of incident kidney stones in men: new insights after 14 years of follow-up. J Am Soc Nephrol. 2004;15:3225–32.
155. Taylor EN, Curhan GC. Determinants of 24-hour urinary oxalate excretion. Clin J Am Soc Nephrol. 2008;3:1453–60.
156. Thomas LD, Elinder CG, Tiselius HG, Wolk A, Akesson A. Ascorbic acid supplements and kidney stone incidence among men: a prospective study. JAMA Intern Med. 2013;173:386–8.
157. Fletcher RH. The risk of taking ascorbic acid. JAMA Intern Med. 2013;173:375–94.
158. Moyad MA, Combs MA, Crowley DC, Baisley JE, Sharma P, Vrablic AS, et al. Vitamin C with metabolites reduce oxalate levels compared to ascorbic acid: a preliminary and novel clinical urologic finding. Urol Nurs. 2009;29:95–102.
159. Moyad MA, Combs MA, Baisley JE, Evans M. Vitamin C with metabolites: additional analysis suggests favorable changes in oxalate. Urol Nurs. 2009;29:383–5.
160. Wright JV, Suen RM, Kirk FR. Comparative studies of "Ester-C" versus L-ascorbic acid. Int Clin Nutr Rev. 1990;10:7–10.
161. Pancorbo D, Vazquez C, Fletcher MA. Vitamin C-lipid metabolites: uptake and retention and effect on plasma C-reactive protein and oxidized LDL levels in healthy volunteers. Med Sci Monit. 2008;14:CR547–51.
162. Suresh E, Das P. Recent advances in management of gout. OJM. 2012;105:407–17.
163. Juraschek SP, Miller 3rd ER, Gelber AC. Effect of oral vitamin C supplementation on serum uric acid: a meta-analysis of randomized controlled trials. Arthritis Care Res (Hoboken). 2011;63:1295–306.
164. Huang HY, Appel LJ, Choi MJ, Gelber AC, Charleston J, Norkus EP, et al. The effects of vitamin C supplementation on serum concentrations of uric acid: results of a randomized controlled trial. Arthritis Rheum. 2005;52:1843–7.
165. Stein HB, Hasan A, Fox IH. Ascorbic acid-induced uricosuria: a consequence of megavitamin therapy. Ann Intern Med. 1976;84:355–8.
166. Berger L, Gerson CD, Yu TF. The effect of ascorbic acid on uric acid excretion with a commentary on the renal handling of ascorbic acid. Am J Med. 1977;62: 71–6.
167. Mitch WE, Johnson MW, Kirshenbaum JM, Lopez RE. Effect of large doses of ascorbic acid on uric acid excretion by normal subjects. Clin Pharmacol Ther. 1981;29:318–21.
168. Stamp LK, O'Donnell JL, Frampton C, Drake J, Zhang M, Chapman PT. Clinically insignificant effect of supplemental vitamin C on serum urate in patients with gout: a pilot randomized controlled trial. Arthritis Rheum. 2013;65:1636–42.
169. Choi HK, Gao X, Curhan G. Vitamin C intake and the risk of gout in men: a prospective study. Arch Intern Med. 2009;169:502–7.
170. Gao X, Curhan G, Forman JP, Ascherio A, Choi HK. Vitamin C intake and serum uric acid concentration in men. J Rheumatol. 2008;35:1853–8.
171. Jacob RA, Spinozzi GM, Simon VA, Kelley DS, Prior RL, Hess-Pierce B, et al. Consumption of cherries lowers plasma urate in healthy women. J Nutr. 2003;133:1826–9.
172. Zhang Y, Neogi T, Chen C, Chaisson C, Hunter DJ, Choi HK. Cherry consumption and decreased risk of recurrent gout attacks. Arthritis Rheum. 2012;64: 4004–11.
173. Schlesinger N, Ron Y, Chen CC. Do cherries reduce acute gouty attacks in patients with gouty arthritis? [abstract]. Ann Rheum Dis. 2007;67 Suppl 3:0742.
174. Schlesinger N, Schlesinger M. Previously reported prior studies of cherry juice concentrate for gout flare prophylaxis: comment on the article by Zhang et al. Arthritis Rheum. 2013;65:1135–6.
175. Schlesinger N, Rabinowitz R, Schlesinger M. Pilot studies of cherry juice concentrate for gout flare prophylaxis. J Arthritis. 2012;1:1–5.
176. Howatson G, McHugh MP, Hill JA, Brouner J, Jewell AP, van Someren KA, et al. Influence of tart cherry juice on indices of recovery following marathon running. Scand J Med Sci Sports. 2010;20: 843–52.
177. Lippman SM, Klein EA, Goodman PJ, Lucia MS, Thompson IM, Ford LG, et al. Effect of selenium and vitamin E on risk of prostate cancer and other cancers: the Selenium and Vitamin E Cancer Prevention Trial (SELECT). JAMA. 2009;301: 39–51.

178. Klein EA, Thompson Jr IM, Tangen CM, Crowley JJ, Lucia MS, Goodman PJ, et al. Vitamin E and the risk of prostate cancer: the Selenium and Vitamin E cancer prevention trial (SELECT). JAMA. 2011;306:1549–56.
179. Miller 3rd ER, Pastor-Barriuso R, Dalal D, Riemersma RA, Appel LJ, Guallar E. Meta-analysis: high-dosage vitamin E supplementation may increase all-cause mortality. Ann Intern Med. 2005;142:37–46.
180. Lonn E, Bosch J, Yusuf S, Sheridan P, Pogue J, Arnold JM, The HOPE and HOPE TOO Trial Investigators, et al. Effects of long-term vitamin E supplementation on cardiovascular events and cancer: a randomized controlled trial. JAMA. 2005;293:1338–47.
181. Sesso HD, Buring JE, Christen WG, Kurth T, Belanger C, MacFadyen J, et al. Vitamins E and C in the prevention of cardiovascular disease in men: the Physicians' Health Study II randomized controlled trial. JAMA. 2008;300:2123–33.
182. Moyad MA. Selenium and vitamin E supplements for prostate cancer: evidence or embellishment? Urology. 2002;59(4 Suppl 1):9–19.
183. Sanyal AJ, Chalasani N, Kowdley KV, McCullough A, Diehl AM, Bass NM, NASH CRN, et al. Pioglitazone, vitamin E, or placebo for nonalcoholic steatohepatitis. N Engl J Med. 2010;362:1675–85.
184. Pacana T, Sanyal AJ. Vitamin E and nonalcoholic fatty liver disease. Curr Opin Clin Nutr Metab Care. 2012;15:641–8.
185. Age-Related Eye Disease Study Research Group. A randomized, placebo-controlled, clinical trial of high-dose supplementation with vitamins C and E, beta carotene, and zinc for age-related macular degeneration and vision loss. ARED Report No. 8. Arch Ophthalmol. 2001;119:1417–36.
186. Thamilselvan S, Menon M. Vitamin E therapy prevent hyperoxaluria-induced calcium oxalate crystal deposition in the kidney by improving renal tissue antioxidant status. BJU Int. 2005;96:117–26.
187. Huang HS, Chen J, Chen CF, Ma MC. Vitamin E attenuates crystal formation in rat kidneys: role of renal tubular cell death and crystallization inhibitors. Kidney Int. 2006;70:699–710.
188. Bazin D, Chevallier P, Matzen G, Jungers P, Daudon M. Heavy elements in urinary stones. Urol Res. 2007;35:179–84.
189. Trinchieri A, Mandressi A, Luongo P, Longo G, Pisani E. The influence of diet on urinary risk factors for stones in healthy subjects and idiopathic renal calcium stone formers. Br J Urol. 1991;67:230–6.
190. Johnson AR, Munoz A, Gottlieb JL, Jarrard DF. High dose zinc increases hospital admissions due to genitourinary complications. J Urol. 2007;177:639–43.
191. Tang J, McFann K, Chonchol M. Dietary zinc intake and kidney stone formation: evaluation of NHANES III. Am J Nephrol. 2012;36:549–53.
192. Curhan GC, Willett WC, Knight EL, Stampfer MJ. Dietary factors and the risk of incident kidney stones in younger women: Nurses' Health Study II. Arch Intern Med. 2004;164:885–8891.
193. Breslau NA, Brinkley L, Hill KD, Pak CY. Relationship of animal protein-rich diet to kidney stone formation and calcium metabolism. J Clin Endocrinol Metab. 1988;66:140–6.
194. Trinchieri A, Mandressi A, Luongo P, Rovera F, Longo G. Urinary excretion of citrate, glycosaminoglycans, magnesium and zinc in relation to age and sex in normal subjects and in patients who form calcium stones. Scand J Urol Nephrol. 1992;26:379–86.
195. Lagiou P, Wuu J, Trichopoulou A, Hsieh C-C, Adami H-O, Trichopoulos D. Diet and benign prostatic hyperplasia: a study in Greece. Urology. 1999;54:284–90.
196. Leitzmann MF, Stampfer MJ, Wu K, Colditz GA, Willett WC, Giovannucci EL. Zinc supplement use and risk of prostate cancer. J Natl Cancer Inst. 2002;95:1004–7.
197. Fashner J, Ericson K, Werner S. Treatment of the common cold in children and adults. Am Fam Physician. 2012;86:153–9.
198. Mora B, Iannuzzi M, Lang T, Steinlechner B, Barker R, Dobrovits M, et al. Auricular acupressure as a treatment for anxiety before extracorporeal shock wave lithotripsy in the elderly. J Urol. 2007;178:160–4.
199. Wang SM, Punjala M, Weiss D, Anderson K, Kalin ZN. Acupuncture as an adjunct for sedation during lithotripsy. J Altern Complement Med. 2007;13: 241–6.
200. Miyaoka R, Monga M. Use of traditional Chinese medicine in the management of urinary stone disease. Int Braz J Urol. 2009;35:396–405.
201. Kessler T, Jansen B, Hesse A. Effect of blackcurrant-, cranberry- and plum juice consumption on risk factors associated with kidney stone formation. Eur J Clin Nutr. 2002;56:1020–3.
202. Ghalayini IF, Al-Ghazo MA, Harfell MN. Prophylaxis and therapeutic effects of raspberry (Rubus idaeus) on renal stone formation in Balb/c mice. Int Braz J Urol. 2011;37:259–66.
203. Mechlin C, Kalorin C, Asplin J, White M. Splenda® improves tolerance of oral potassium citrate supplementation for prevention of stone formation: results of a randomized double-blind trial. J Endourol. 2011;25:1541–5.
204. Vezzoli G, Terranegra A, Arcidiacono T, Soldati L. Genetics and calcium nephrolithiasis. Kidney Int. 2011;80:587–93.
205. Miyaoka R, Ortiz-Alvarado O, Kriedberg C, Alanee S, Chotikawanich E, Monga M. Correlation between stress and kidney stone disease. J Endourol. 2012;26:551–5.
206. Najem GR, Seebode JJ, Samady AJ, Feuerman M, Friedman L. Stressful life events and risk of symptomatic kidney stones. Int J Epidemiol. 1997;26: 1017–23.
207. Thuy AB, Blizzard L, Schmidt MD, Luc PH, Granger RH, Dwyer T. The association between smoking and hypertension. J Hypertens. 2010;28:245–50.
208. Virdis A, Giannarelli C, Neves MF, Taddei S, Ghiadoni L. Cigarette smoking and hypertension. Curr Pharm Des. 2010;16:2518–25.

9 Review of Lifestyle and CAM for Miscellaneous Urologic Topics (Bladder Cancer, CP/CPPS, IC/PBS, Kidney Cancer): Part One

I. Bladder Cancer (Lifestyle)

Arguably, one of the strongest correlations between smoking and cancer risk or progression is not just lung cancer, but bladder cancer [1–5]. Data now suggest equal risks for men and women, and smoking after bladder treatment may also increase the risk of cancer recurrence and heart disease. Smoking cessation programs need to be emphasized [4], but additionally, a simultaneous or follow-up weight-loss program should be suggested, in my opinion, because of the high risk for weight gain within 12 months of quitting (mean of 10 pounds or more in first 12 months) [6]. Other forms of tobacco exposure may also be associated with an increased risk, such as cigar and water pipes, smokeless tobacco, and environmental tobacco [5].

Bladder cancer is not associated with an increasing BMI or obesity [7], but this cancer is confounded by the ability of weight loss to be sustained while consistently using tobacco products. Regardless, evidence suggests the possibility of more complications and worse oncologic outcomes in obese patients receiving radical cystectomy, for example [8].

A higher intake of cruciferous vegetable consumption has been associated with a lower risk of bladder cancer from a variety of meta-analyses and some of the largest prospective epidemiologic studies [9, 10], and this beneficial consistent association is unusual for most cancers in terms of diet currently with the exception of another urologic cancer, kidney cancer (fruit and vegetables associated with a lower risk) [11]. Greater fluid intake has also been associated with the potential for a lower risk of bladder cancer, but over time and further analysis, this risk has been attenuated [12], and there has been no impact thus far on recurrence rates with greater fluid intake after superficial bladder cancer diagnosis and treatment [13]. This association of increased fluid consumption and the potential for a lower risk of bladder cancer and kidney stone risk [14] are unique among the cancers and among specialties. Other lifestyle and dietary changes have not been consistently associated with bladder cancer risk, except there is some preliminary weak evidence to suggest increased consumption of red meat and saturated fat may increase risk and higher intakes of plant omega-3 (alpha-linolenic acid) may reduce risk [15, 16]. A summary of the proper perspective on diet or lifestyle and bladder cancer suggests that heart-healthy changes (e.g., not smoking) are associated with lower bladder cancer risk, but outside of tobacco and cruciferous vegetable intake, the impacts of lifestyle changes are tenuous. Still, this observation needs to be put into perspective for patients. Up to half and arguably more bladder cancer cases are tied into

M.A. Moyad, *Complementary & Alternative Medicine for Prostate and Urologic Health*,
DOI 10.1007/978-1-4614-8492-9_9, © Springer Science+Business Media New York 2014

lifestyle changes such as smoking, and this in and out itself is an enormous and tragic public health story, which needs ongoing educational and urgent attention.

Cholesterol-lowering drugs (statins) have had a nebulous history with bladder cancer, but overall there is no relationship with risk or outcomes in patients treated with bladder cancer (neutral effect) [17, 18]. There is also a concern with the type 2 diabetic drug pioglitazone and an increased risk of bladder cancer [19], but the benefit-to-risk ratio needs to be reviewed along with other potential options, and ironically there is the potential for long-term diabetes to increase the risk of bladder and other cancers [20, 21]. Exposure to ionizing radiation, cyclophosphamide, and ifosfamide can also increase the risk of bladder cancer [15].

Exposure to excess arsenic (inorganic) in drinking water at concentrations above 300 μg/L is a strong risk factor for bladder cancer, but has at least favorably impacted municipal water supply standards around the world [5, 22]. Municipal and private well water systems should be checked yearly/regularly for arsenic, in my opinion. And perhaps the most well-known occupational risk for any cancer exists for bladder cancer. The strong correlation with aromatic amines such as 2-naphthylamine, 4-aminobiphenyl, benzidine, and even 4,4′-methylenebis(2-chloroaniline) is found in products from the rubber, dye, and industries, and also motor vehicle exhaust, paints, hair dyes (permanent dyes and regular exposure), cigarette smoke, fungicides, plastics, and metals are well known [5].

Interestingly, another method whereby water exposure (not consumption) increases bladder cancer risk is from schistosomiasis. Schistosoma haematobium is a parasitic infection more common in developing countries or areas in the Middle East and Africa [23]. An intense inflammatory reaction in the bladder caused by chronic infection with this parasite increases the risk of squamous cell carcinoma of bladder. This cancer is a classic example of the ongoing and increasing interest in a variety of tumors that may be caused by chronic inflammation (liver, esophageal, intestinal, etc.).

II. Bladder Cancer (CAM/Dietary Supplements)

Low-Dose Multivitamin for Prevention

Centrum Silver was utilized in the largest and most rigorous trial to date to determine if it could reduce the risk of total cancer and cardiovascular events [24, 25]. This study was known as the Physicians' Health Study II (PHS II), and it was a randomized, double-blind, placebo-controlled trial of over 14,000 male US physicians aged 50 years or older at baseline (mean age 64 years). A total of 1,312 of these men had a history of cancer at randomization. The study actually began in 1997, and follow-up was completed through June 1, 2011. The median follow-up was 11.2 years, and 2,669 men were diagnosed with cancer (approximately half were prostate cancer). Men ingesting a multivitamin had a significant 8 % reduction in the risk of cancer, but men with a baseline history of cancer experienced a significant 27 % decrease [24]. No significant impact was observed for individual cancers, but when combining all of the nonsignificant individual cancer reductions, the significant modest reduction occurred in total cancer risk (primary endpoint). There was a nonsignificant 12 % reduction in cancer deaths in the multivitamin group compared to placebo. One cancer that appeared to have a larger reduction (−28 %; $p=0.10$; 41 vs. 57 cases) in risk compared to others was bladder cancer, but no impact on bladder cancer deaths (−16 %; 15 vs. 18 cases; $p=0.62$). Side effects were similar to a placebo except for a higher number of rashes (2,125 vs. 2,002 men; 7 % increase risk; $p=0.03$) with the supplement, and there was also a 9 % significant reduced risk of hematuria (1,194 vs. 1,292 men; $p=0.02$) when taking the supplement compared to placebo. Only a limited number of current smokers were included in this trial (3–4 %), and smoking status subgroup analysis suggested a potentially more pronounced nonsignificant (28 %; HR=0.72) reduction in overall cancer risk (former smokers and nonsmokers had HR of 0.99 and 0.89) with the multivitamin. It was not mentioned with current smokers whether cancer risk was greater for one type of cancer or another, and the number of cancer cases in this group was small (53 vs. 70 events). Patients should also be told that in this study those with a parental history of cancer appeared to derive no benefit from the multivitamin, but again those with no history or a baseline history appeared to have a modest benefit.

There was no impact on cardiovascular events overall compared to placebo with the exception of a potential chance finding of a lower significant risk of fatal myocardial infarction in favor of Centrum Silver for those with no baseline history of cardiovascular disease (CVD), but a small number of events occurred (22 vs. 39 cases; adjusted HR = 0.56; $p = 0.03$) [25]. In men with a baseline history of CVD, there were nine fatal MI events (5 vs. 4). It seems safe to recommend Centrum Silver or children's multivitamin daily to men (and perhaps women) to potentially reduce the risk of cancer with either no impact or a potential for reduction in bladder cancer risk or perhaps hematuria. Why a children's multivitamin? The study began in 1997, and the Centrum utilized during this entire study consisted of lower dosages of most ingredients, similar to a children's multivitamin sold today in the USA. No impressive epidemiologic data for a multivitamin existed before this clinical trial to suggest a positive or negative impact on in bladder cancer risk [26], and perhaps this is still the case after the landmark Centrum trial, but at least the discussion of safety with a low-dose multivitamin can now be discussed with confidence.

Again, all of these data suggest that there is also no impressive data to suggest utilizing high-dose or megadose supplements to prevent bladder or any other cancer, and there is enough evidence to suggest significant harm when utilizing this high- or megadose approach [27–34]. This is similar to the evidence that has already existed in terms of cardiovascular risk increases with larger intakes of dietary supplements [35–37].

Megadose Vitamins and Minerals for Adjuvant Treatment of Superficial Bladder Cancer (Less Is More)

In a small and randomized study from the 1990s, there was a suggestion that megadoses of a supplement compared to a recommended daily allowance (RDA) supplement may reduce the risk of non-muscle-invasive bladder cancer recurrence after BCG treatment [38]. However, a larger follow-up study was needed to confirm these preliminary findings, which, to the researchers credit, occurred [39]. Patients were BCG-naïve with carcinoma in situ; Ta or T1 bladder cancer was randomized to receive intravesical BCG or BCG + interferon alpha-2b and then further randomized to receive an RDA (minimal intake) or megadose supplement. Each RDA tablet of vitamins contained 25 % of the recommended daily dose, and patients took two tablets twice daily of either the RDA or the megadose supplement. Each megadose tablet (again patient four tablets a day throughout the trial) contained:

- 9,000 IU of vitamin A
- 25 mg of B6
- 500 mg of vitamin C
- 400 IU of vitamin D_3
- 400 mcg of folate
- 100 IU of vitamin E
- 7.6 mg of zinc

Induction BCG was given weekly for 6 weeks and then at 4, 7, 13, 19, 25, and 37 months [39]. The primary endpoint was biopsy-confirmed recurrence or cytology that was positive. A total of 670 patients were randomized, and at 24-month median follow-up, there were no significant differences between the RDA and megadose supplements groups. The following recurrence-free survival numbers were BCG + RDA 63 %, BCG + megadose supplement 59 %, BCG + Interferon + RDA 55 %, and BCG + Interferon + megadose supplement 61 %. Megadose supplements and/or interferon alpha-2b added to BCG did not impact time to recurrence in patients with non-muscle-invasive bladder cancer. And there was a slight nonsignificant increased risk of recurrence with BCG and the megadose supplement.

When the first small megadose study published in the 1990s in the Journal of Urology [38], it was visionary and impressive and served as an inspiration to continue to pursue CAM in urology, from my perspective. Megadose vitamins probably did reduce the risk of recurrence, in my opinion, from the earlier study because researchers were arguably dealing with a population of individuals with some minor and perhaps overt deficiencies in a variety of vitamins and minerals. Decades later in the USA, for example, patients are not generally deficient, but they appear to be oversupplemented or sufficient in most cases with antioxidants from foods, beverages, and supplements [40]. As I have argued throughout this book, it makes it difficult to truly conduct a large clinical trial of a truly deficient healthy population over a long period of time, despite some authors requesting such studies [41]. When clinical trials are designed to supplement for nutritional deficiencies, the issue by the time the trial commences these deficiencies will no longer exist, which contaminates the ability of the trial to test the original hypothesis.

The megadose supplement itself in the later bladder cancer clinical trial was also controversial in my opinion. It contained newly added folic acid and vitamin D compared to the original formulation utilized in the preliminary successful study [38, 39]. Why was the formula altered from what was potentially successful in the preliminary study? Would this be allowed in a definitive phase 3 pharmaceutical study, where the phase 1 or 2 study had a successful outcome and safety with a specific dose and formulation, and it was altered in the phase 3 trial? Arguably these added nutrients, especially folic acid, also have data to suggest that they could also increase recurrence of certain cancers or other abnormalities when given at higher doses [27–30]. And it is interesting that lower doses of these supplements may be providing the benefits needed without adding the significant increased risks or overall concerns for most individuals [42, 43].

A large clinical trial called SELEBLAT (Selenium and Bladder Cancer Trial) is being conducted that is testing 200 μg of selenium (from yeast source) a day to determine if it can reduce the risk of bladder cancer recurrence after conventional treatment over 3 years compared to a placebo [44]. The study is multicenter, accruing subjects at 18 hospitals in Belgium. There will be many questions to be answered with this trial because even if there is some partial efficacy, the concern over using higher dosages of selenium and other antioxidants long-term abound from past clinical studies (see Chap. 7) [31–34, 45, 46]. Regardless, SELEBLAT will provide an answer to the value of high-dose selenium in urology outside of its lack of value for prostate prevention and treatment.

Probiotic: *Lactobacillus casei* (Prevention and Treatment)

Two older randomized controlled, double-blind investigational trials were conducted in patients with superficial transitional cell cancer (TCC) of the bladder to determine the effect of oral *L. casei* Shirota powder (biolactis powder-BLP, 3 g/day) on recurrence post-transurethral resection [47, 48]. Study 1 (BLP Study Group) randomized 23 subjects in the BLP arm and 25 on placebo [47], while study 2 (also from BLP Study Group) allocated 61 to BLP and 64 to placebo [48]. The two arms in study 1 had similar clinical qualities, but their 50 % recurrence-free interval after BLP treatment was 1.8 times longer ($p=0.03$) versus the placebo arm (350 days vs. 195 days) [47]. Study 2 referred patients to one of three subgroups according to their tumor status [48]. Subgroup A consisted of multiple primary tumors, B consisted of single recurrent tumors, and C consisted of multiple recurrent bladder tumors. The 50 % recurrence-free interval in subgroups A and B was longer, with BLP versus placebo (688 vs. 543 days). No significant difference was recognized in subgroup C. Multivariate analysis showed that the result with BLP was significantly greater than the placebo ($p=0.01$). Mild diarrhea was the primary side effect in 4.6 % of the individuals (three patients) taking BLP and did not require treatment. These preliminary observations suggest that BLP powder has a good safety profile short term and may play a role in preventing or prolonging the recurrence of superficial bladder in some patients.

Based on these preliminary results, this probiotic to reduce the risk of bladder cancer recurrence or progression of superficial bladder cancer when combined with conventional medicine more clinical data was needed. Another clinical trial of 207 patients diagnosed with superficial bladder cancer received transurethral resection followed by intravesical epirubicin twice during a 1-week period [49]. After confirmation of superficial bladder cancer, this group was randomized to further treatment with epirubicin alone or epirubicin and 3 g daily of oral *L. casei* Shirota (Yakult Honsha, Tokyo, Japan) for 1 year. A significantly ($p=0.02$) greater 3-year recurrence-free survival rate was found in the combination group (74.6 %) versus epirubicin alone (59.9 %). However, progression-free and overall survival did not differ between the groups, but this could have been due to the small number of clinical events. Oral probiotic utilization and intravesical instillation of epirubicin may represent one of the more promising and novel combination treatments for superficial bladder cancer after first undergoing transurethral resection.

The probiotic agent used in these past studies can be purchased as a capsule and does not have to be refrigerated [49]. It is usually powdered and contains about 1×10^{10} cells of heat-killed LC Shirota strain per gram (3,000 mg or 3 g per day). Since it has been used in several clinical trials with side effects similar to a placebo and it has been used in Japan for over 30+ years, one should feel more comfortable about the benefit-to-risk ratio favoring benefit. Again, the research appears to demonstrate a benefit for low-grade bladder cancers treated by resection and in some cases intravesical chemotherapy, but has not been tested during or after receiving BCG. Still, the positive human research is interesting enough for potentially using this probiotic and perhaps other lactic acid bacteria in many different bladder cancer scenarios. The average time on the supplement has been 1 year and the average daily dose was 3,000 mg (3 g).

Researchers are not certain, but this probiotic agent appears to improve the body's immune response to bladder tumors based on laboratory research. It could activate natural killer (NK) cells of the immune system and may also induce cancer cell death [50–52]. It is also interesting that the probiotic milk-like product known as "Yakult" (or fermented milk products) contains this same probiotic strain, and this and other milk products (lactic acid bacteria from cultured milk) may be associated with a reduced risk of bladder cancer in several previous epidemiologic studies [53–55]. It is also plausible that this *Lactobacillus* strain simply reduces carcinogenic effects or contact time in the bladder. Perhaps the most fascinating personal observation concerns probiotics commercially and on the Internet, and the perceived profound advocacy and embellishment to support these supplements despite a lack of long-term trials in many disciplines, but one exception is the minimally mentioned (by these same sources) probiotic in the one area of medicine with some adequate clinical data, bladder cancer, and urology.

Chewing Gum

Preliminary evidence from a meta-analysis of 17 randomized trials suggests chewing gum (also known as "sham feeding") has the potential to produce a stimulatory effect on bowel motility and reduce time of ileus in patients after certain abdominal surgical procedures [56]. Interestingly, these benefits also appear to be in the area of urologic surgery, especially radical cystectomy (open or robotic) [57–59]. For example, one prospective randomized comparative study found median time to flatus and bowel movement was significantly reduced with chewing gum versus control (57.1 h vs. 69.6 h and 76.7 h vs. 93.3 h), but no significant difference in time of hospital stay and no adverse effects were noted [57]. This study used sugar-free gum for 30 min three times a day (10 A.M., 3 P.M., and 8 P.M.) on post-op day 1, and this was discontinued after passage of flatus. An observational cohort also found significant reduction in time to flatus (2.4 vs. 2.9 days; $p<0.001$) and bowel movement (3.2 vs. 3.9 days;

$p<0.001$)]. This observational protocol of 102 patients also started chewing on postoperative day 1 (Wrigley's Freedent peppermint flavored), and patients were given 5 sticks per 24 h and instructed to utilize a single piece every 2–4 h [58]. It appeared to have some ability to nonsignificantly reduce the length of hospital stay (4.7 vs. 5.1 days; $p=0.067$). Still, the issues of shortening hospital stay, although pertinent and observed in other studies [56], are not a reasonable consistent expectation, nor the reason for endorsement in my opinion. The preliminary data on bowel recovery as well as the message of patient empowerment immediately after and long after cystectomy to improve outcomes along is reason enough to endorse this behavioral change along with heart-healthy behaviors.

There is a theoretical (not observed in studies) chance of asphyxiation with gum, so the patient should be fully awake and upright when chewing. Overall, the data suggests it should be discussed with the patients after surgery as an option because paralytic ileus is the most common minor postoperative complication after radical cystectomy [57–59], which can result in pain, bloating or abdominal distension, and vomiting.

III. Chronic Prostatitis/Chronic Pelvic Pain Syndrome

There are four types of prostatitis, and some of their characteristics are outlined in Table 9.1 [60].

Type I (acute infection) is the least common but arguably gets a good deal of attention because it can increase PSA levels. However, type III or chronic prostatitis/chronic pelvic pain syndrome (CP/CPPS) is the most common form and the primary subject of this section. CPPS is really a heterogenous syndrome, which is based on individual need for different options, or a well-known phenotype guide known as UPOINT, which has adequate evidence to suggest efficacy [61]. The domains and some commentary for UPOINT include [61]:

- *U*rinary, which involves irritative or obstructive urinary symptoms and high postvoid residual, and alpha-blockers and antimuscarinics are options. It is one of the most commonly diagnosed UPOINT domains.
- *P*sychosocial, which includes depression, stress, or verbalizing helplessness and hopelessness (catastrophizing), and psychologic and cognitive behavioral therapy are options.
- *O*rgan specific (bladder or prostate), which includes specific prostate tenderness, hematospermia, or symptom relief with voiding, and quercetin or pollen extract dietary supplements (e.g., Prosta-Q and Q-Urol or Cernilton) or prescription medications such as pentosan polysulfate are options. This is the one area of CP/CPPS where utilizing dietary supplements is quite common in the field of urology from experts from around the world. This has been the most commonly diagnosed UPOINT domain in some series, followed closely behind by tenderness and then urinary domains.

Table 9.1 The NIH categories for prostatitis and some of the characteristics associated with each classification[a]

	NIH category-other name	Comments	Prostatic fluid
I.	Acute bacterial prostatitis (least common form)	Sudden or acute bacterial infection and PSA can increase	Massage is contraindicated
II.	Chronic bacterial prostatitis	Chronic prostate infection that could increase PSA	Bacteria and WBC
IIIa.	Chronic pelvic pain syndrome: inflammatory	Pelvic pain with prostate inflammation but without infection (generally no impact on PSA)	No bacteria but WBC
IIIb.	Chronic pelvic pain syndrome: noninflammatory	Pelvic pain without prostate inflammation and without infection (generally no impact on PSA)	No bacteria and no WBC
IV.	Asymptomatic inflammatory prostatitis	Incidentally detected and may or may not impact PSA	Bacteria and/or WBC may or may not be present

[a]Note: Category III is the most common form of prostatitis

- *I*nfection, which includes positive cultures of prostatic fluid without a UTI or concomitant urethritis, and antibiotics are an option.
- *N*eurologic/systemic, which includes pain outside the pelvis or systemic pain syndrome, and pregabalin or amitriptyline is an option.
- *T*enderness, which includes pelvic floor spasm or muscle trigger points, and pelvic floor physical therapy or myofascial release is an option. This is also one of the most commonly diagnosed UPOINT domains.

Exercise, Lifestyle Changes, and/or Acupuncture or Percutaneous Tibial Nerve Stimulation and UPOINT?

Still, before drug or supplement treatment should be discussed, it is important to realize a large randomized trial of exercise for CP/CPPS demonstrated impressive results. It would be of interest to immediately add exercise to UPOINT based on these results.

A lifestyle clinical study from Florence, Italy, was double-blind, randomized, and experienced encouraging results because the participants were previously unresponsive to conventional treatments [62]. Participants (average age of 36–38 year, BMI of 22, mean symptom duration of 5.5–6 months) had symptoms of pain in the pelvic region for 3 or more months continuously and scored a minimum of 15 points on NIH-CPSI with at least 6 or more points on the pain subscale. A total of 52 subjects were placed in the exercise group and 51 were assigned to the placebo/stretching group. The outcome measures were the NIH-CPSI, Beck Depression Inventory, State Anxiety Inventory-Y (SAI-Y), and a pain visual analog scale (VAS). These evaluations were determined at baseline, 6 and 18 weeks. The exercise group engaged in vigorous walking three times per week for 40 min each session to achieve 70–80 % of the predicted maximum heart rate for their age. The placebo/stretching group completed a series of stretching exercises, but had to maintain their heart rate under 110 beats per minute for the entire session. Approximately 25 % of the participants dropped out of the study by 18 weeks, which is one of the serious limitations of lifestyle change studies. However, significant differences between the two groups favored the exercise group for total NIH-CPSI ($p=0.006$), pain ($p=0.0009$), quality-of-life subscales ($p=0.02$), and VAS ($p=0.003$). No difference was found for other parameters. Responders considered those that experienced a decrease of 6 or more points in total NIH-CPSI (58 % exercise vs. 43 % placebo), 25–49 % (39 % vs. 35 %), and 50 % (19 % vs. 5 %) or more decrease from baseline in total NIH-CPSI. A 25 % placebo response of this magnitude is expected from other trials. It is of interest that pain is the symptom that is the most influential variable and quality-of-life predictor and should be one of the main targets of any therapy. Exercise is known to induce the release of endogenous opioids and reduces sympathetic activity to the pelvic region [63–65]. It would also be of even more interest in the future to conduct a more intensive exercise aerobic program to determine if pain scores could improve further as has been observed in other chronic pain scenarios [66], and if urinary scores could improve also, as I believe this would be the case.

The other CAM of interest that could be added to UPOINT based on a large meta-analysis is the use of acupuncture or percutaneous tibial nerve stimulation (PTNS), which in my opinion is a conventionally modified form of acupuncture [67]. These techniques have provided the potential to also cause some significant reductions in the NIH-CPSI voiding domain. Large placebo response rates have also been observed, but the overall safety and potential efficacy suggests an immediate role in CP/CPPS.

Dietary Supplements (Cernilton and Quercetin Complex Products)

Pollen extract such as Cernilton appears to have effective anti-inflammatory effects (reduces complement C3/Coeruloplasmin in ejaculate) and have been tested in a variety of clinical trials for CP/CPPS [68]. In the largest and one of the methodologically rigorous clinical trials, the results should be of interest [69]. This large trial included

139 men (70 on intervention and 69 with placebo) of a mean age 39 years and a mean duration of disease and current symptoms of 4.6 years and 8.3 months. A 1-week run-in phase with azithromycin was conducted, and men with elevated residual urine (>50 mL) were excluded. Approximately 45 % of the subjects were on prior medication for CP/CPPS or a related condition. In the intention-to-treat analysis found individual domains of pain ($p=0.009$; mean change −4.50), quality of life ($p=0.03$; mean change −2.23), and total NIH-CPSI ($p=0.01$, mean change −7.66) to be significantly improved after 12 weeks compared to placebo. A 25 % reduction in NIH-CPSI was found in 69 % versus 49 % ($p=0.01$), and a 6-point decrease in NIH-CPSI was found in 62 % versus 43 % ($p=0.03$). Urinary scores/micturition domain did not improve, but side effects were similar to placebo. Cernilton was recommended at two capsules every 8 h, and the active ingredient in each capsule was 60 mg of Cernitin T60 (water soluble) and 3 mg of Cernitin GBX (fat soluble). This is one of the most impressive clinical trials performed to date with a dietary supplement for CP/CPPS.

Currently, there have been seven positive human studies reporting clinical outcomes with pollen extract with CP-CCPS, six with Cernilton (one randomized and five observational/cohort), and one with a product known as "Prostat/Poltit" (1 randomized) [68]. Clinical efficacy ranged from 63 to 87 %, and in the placebo-controlled studies, the placebo groups efficacy rates were 36 to 49 %. The only issue with Cernilton is it has a long history with multiple companies, which can be quite daunting for the average clinician and patient when attempting to order this or another similar product. For example, Cernilton started with A.B. Cernelle, Sweden, and then it was also licensed in the USA by Cernitin America, Utica, OH and discontinued. Graminex LLC (Deshler, Ohio and Saginaw, Michigan) currently sell one option, and the most recent randomized clinical trial was supported by Strathmann AG &Co (Hamburg, Germany) and AB Cernelle (Angelholm, Sweden). There are a variety of dietary supplements suggesting they have the same product outside of Europe, but a comparison with the information from the latest clinical trial is needed [68, 69]. Companies should be rewarded for their commitment to research, but again some background is needed to arrive at the conclusion of a proper product to use for CP/CPPS.

Cernilton from the latest clinical trial was a microbial digestion of a mixture of pollen extracts (Cernitins), which were then extracted [68, 69]. It appears currently that the pollen extract is derived from machine-harvested pollen from species *Secale cereale* (cereal rye or grass), *Phleum pratense* (Timothy grass), and *Zea mays* (corn), and proportion of the mixture of these three species is 30:1.5:1. Pollen extract contains numerous natural compounds from amino acids, carbohydrates, lipids, vitamins, and minerals. Phytosterols and secalosides are also proposed important active ingredients. This complex total extract is comprised of 63 mg of defined pollen extract fractions with two primary components, the hydrophilic T60 fraction and the hydrophobic GBX, both of which apparently have no allergenic properties. Check the label for gluten status (some companies and pollen products like Graminex G63 are gluten free). Again, it is difficult for healthcare professionals outside of Europe and patients to determine the amount of a pollen extract product to utilize. For example, dosages of 2 bid and 1–3 bid have been used in past studies [67]. Since there have been no published overtly negative or neutral effects in studies with Cernilton, regardless of the dosage question this should be an option for patients. There is also some evidence from a meta-analysis of two older placebo-controlled trial that Cernilton (Secale cereale, 2–4 tablets daily) could also have some minimal to moderate efficacy against BPH nocturia, for example (subjective symptoms), but did not appear to improve urinary flow rates, residual volume, or prostate volume compared to placebo [70].

Quercetin is an anti-inflammatory bioflavonoid found in green tea, onions, and red wine. It may also posses the ability to block mast cell cytokine release, which could be the route whereby it may reduce allergic and inflammatory reactions [71]. A rigorously impressive but small ($n=30$) randomized, placebo-controlled trial utilized a dosage of 500 mg twice a day for 4 weeks, and the NIH-CPSI was the primary endpoint [72]. Patients on placebo had a mean improvement from 20.2 to 18.8, and those on quercetin experienced a mean improvement from 21.0 to 13.1 ($p=0.003$). A total of 20 % utilizing placebo and 67 % on quercetin had an improvement of symptoms of 25 % or more. Significant efficacy in reducing pain (10.3–6.2, $p=0.005$) and improving quality-of-life (8–4.9, $p=0.004$) scores with no significant effect on urinary score domain (2.7–1.5) occurred. Symptom duration was a mean of 10.5–11.5 years in this study, and in 17 patients with expressed prostatic secretions on both visits, the WBC count per high-powered field (hpf) was reduced from 16.8 to 5.3 ($p=0.01$), and no significant change occurred in the placebo arm (13.1–8.3). A third group (not placebo controlled, $n=17$) of patients received quercetin with bromelain and papain (digestive enzymes found in pineapple and papaya to enhance absorption), and 82 % experienced a significant improvement in symptoms after 1 month (this product was Prosta-Q) in this open-label study. Since this time these quercetin-derived supplements, primarily Prosta-Q and Q-Urol (Farr Labs, Beverly Hills, CA) have been arguably one of the most commonly utilized CAM products from CP/CPPS based on global distribution with urologists and continues to accumulate positive data in UPOINT patient observational cohort series when used for organ-specific symptoms of UPOINT [61].

IV. Interstitial Cystitis/Painful Bladder Syndrome

Diet and CAM

The largest focus over the past few decades with CAM or dietary supplements is in the area of inflammation reduction and/or to potentially support the GAG (glycosaminoglycan) bladder layer, which becomes potentially compromised and then permeable to noxious solutes, and an inflammatory/allergic response occurs with IC [73]. Pentosan polysulfate (PPS, Elmiron) is FDA approved and an oral prescription for IC, which actually is a synthetic polysaccharide originally created as a substitute for heparin, and has been marketed as helping to replenish the GAG layer. This drug is not without controversy because of large dosages over long periods of time needed for a potential impact, cost, or toxicity, which could include hair loss and bleeding complications in a minority of cases. This is one reason I believe CAM or dietary supplementation in IC has a fairly strong presence in urology. GAG is comprised of chondroitin sulfate (CS) and sodium hyaluronate (SH), which can be increased in the urine of PBS/IC [73]. Thus, a variety of supplements have been tested to either impact the GAG or some aspect of it and/or inflammation as well as to provide ancillary effects. Acid reduction from trigger foods and beverages has also been an enormous area of interest.

Calcium glycerophosphate (Prelief, AkPharma Inc, Pleasantville, NJ) is a widely utilized supplement to reduce meal acidity (two tablets have an approximate total of 690-mg and 130-mg elemental calcium, used before meals of concern, or ¼ teaspoon of powder = 2 tablets), and acidity could trigger IC symptoms, but despite a lack of placebo-controlled clinical trials, patient usage and satisfaction appear very high [74–77]. Surveys of users of these tablets have suggested improved quality of life and reduced pain/discomfort and urgency. The only controversy (apart from a lack of placebo studies) is the issue of urine acidity exacerbating pain because some small studies suggest women experienced no statistical difference in pain sensation for urine at physiologic acidity (pH 5.0) or urine with less acidity (pH 7.5) [78]. Regardless, this acid-neutralizing effect could occur in the gastrointestinal tract, which could translate to some subjective benefit in the pelvic bladder area because bloating and discomfort can be reduced. Whether or not this supplement provides a benefit over other effective calcium antacids such as calcium carbonate has not been tested. However, I am reminded of the profound benefit in symptoms of painful bladder disease from one particular older 3-month small prospective randomized, double-blind, placebo-controlled trial ($n=36$, 35 women, mean age 42 years, range 23–73) of cimetidine

(H2 blocker) [79]. A significant improvement in symptoms ($p<0.001$) and suprapubic pain ($p=0.009$) and even nocturia ($p=0.006$) was also significantly reduced, but histologically the bladder mucosa demonstrated no change in the GAG layer or basement membrane or in muscle collagen deposition. In other words, perhaps the antacid effects of cimetidine and calcium glycerophosphate share a mechanism of action that has been profoundly underappreciated in IC treatment. Regardless, the safety of calcium glycerophosphate appears to be excellent, but the potential issues of ingesting too much calcium (stones, calcification of vascular system, reduced gastric absorption of nutrients, etc.) should always be addressed, so moderation is appreciated.

One ancillary benefit of some of the calcium glycerophosphate surveys with patients is the potential to identify some dietary triggers for IC, which have included citrus fruits, tomatoes, vitamin C, artificial sweeteners, coffee, tea, carbonated and alcoholic beverages, and spicy foods [77]. Many of these trigger foods are an issue for IC, and alternatives should be proffered if they become an issue. For example, vitamin C supplements in the form of pH-neutral or calcium ascorbate (mentioned in Chap. 8) are an option or non-citrus-based fruits are another option along with reduced caffeinated beverages. Meeting with a nutritionist with a history of working with an IC diet is critical. Despite the lack of long-term controlled studies on dietary triggers, the consistent positive impact of these changes for the patient cannot be ignored and could provide substantial relief.

A specific but a comprehensive list of lifestyle options with a focus on stress reduction should be emphasized to IC patients as much as dietary additions or deletions. Recent surveys suggest tremendous benefits for elimination diets (limit foods and beverages that cause flares) or strict dietary change (avoid products list in IC diet guidelines), heat and cold use, meditation and relaxation, stress reduction, acupuncture, exercise, and sleep hygiene [80]. It is interesting in some of these surveys that diet or lifestyle changes appear to work in some cases as well or better than pill interventions. This is exciting and again needs more study and emphasis in the clinical setting.

A retrospective study utilizing the dietary supplement CystoProtek (Media Consumer Healthcare Inc in U.S. and Algonot Internationally), which is currently a combination of chondroitin sulfate, sodium hyaluronate, quercetin, rutin, glucosamine sulfate, and olive kernel extract, has some preliminary positive data. This supplement, utilized for 6 months in 37 patients, produced a reduction of PBS/IC symptoms of 55 % ($p<0.01$) [81]. A larger study of 252 IC/PBS patients who had failed other treatment utilized four tablets per day (mg/capsule: glucosamine sulfate, 120; chondroitin sulfate, 150; hyaluronate sodium, 10; quercetin 150, rutin 20) [82]. Male patients (mean 53 years, $n=25$) had VAS scores reduced by 52 % ($p<0.0001$) after 12 months of treatment, and female patients had a reduction of 49 % after 11 months. More rigorous placebo-controlled trials are needed, but this was interesting and appears to have a GAG mechanism of action. It would also be of interest to simply test a traditional osteoarthritis glucosamine or chondroitin supplement in larger doses (1,500 and/or 1,200 mg/day) to determine how it would rate against this product and other products in this chapter.

L-arginine supplements, including their limitations, were discussed in Chap. 6. The data in IC have been mixed [83], and primarily noneffective [73, 84–86] and even large dosages in some small studies (3 or 10 g for 5 weeks) have not been impressive [85]. Perhaps this is due to the already high levels of nitric oxide in some patients with IC.

A quercetin complex product (Cysta-Q, Farr Labs) at a dosage of one capsule (500 mg each) twice a day after 4 weeks demonstrated a significant reduction in problem index (11.3–5.1; $p=0.000001$), symptom index (11.9–4.5; $p=0.000001$), and mean global assessment score (8.2–3.5; $p=0.000001$) in 20 patients (mean age 53 years, 17 women and 5 men) [87]. This was an open-label trial, and a placebo comparison should be attempted, but side effects similar to placebo and the history of the use of this supplement in urology internationally (USA, Canada, South Africa, etc.) and history in CP/CPPS with a somewhat similar complex suggest a potential role currently for patients with IC. Still, a placebo-controlled comparative is needed.

Other CAM products simply need some form of further rigorous study or placebo-controlled intervention in the future to be discussed and/or recommended. For example, a dry aloe leaf supplement at 900 mg/day and others need further investigation [73], as well as intravesical capsaicin, which can potentially cause desensitization of bladder C-fiber afferents that could otherwise promote painful effects in IC patients [88]. Regardless, it is fascinating and frustrating that only two FDA-approved therapies exist for IC, one oral therapy (pentosan polysulfate sodium) and only one intravesical therapy (dimethyl sulfoxide) [89], and the limitations of these agents abound. This also suggests CAM treatment options and research in the area of IC have a healthy future.

V. Kidney Cancer (Renal Cell)

Obesity is linked to multiple cancers, but kidney cancer (renal cell) has arguably the strongest correlation of almost any cancer type in terms of a higher risk with a greater BMI or waist circumference and other lifestyle factors [90–93]. Hypertension, lack of exercise, smoking, insulin resistance, and even dyslipidemia may also be associated with increased risks of kidney cancer. Exercise is strongly associated with a lower risk from a meta-analysis [94], and increased consumption of fruits and vegetables is correlated moderately to strongly with kidney cancer risk reduction [11, 95]. This is unusual for any cancer currently, since produce intake has not been associated with most cancers when further evaluated with the exception of bladder cancer and cruciferous vegetables. Basically, reducing the risk of cardiovascular disease in general (hypertension, smoking cessation, weight gain, exercise, cholesterol reduction) suggests the potential for a profound benefit against kidney cancer [96–99], which is the theme of this book.

Conclusion

A summary of the CAM options that could negatively and positively impact the risk of multiple urologic conditions is listed in Table 9.2.

Table 9.2 A partial summary list of lifestyle and other CAM interventions for bladder cancer, CP/CPPS, IC/PBS, and kidney cancer

I.	*Bladder cancer. Lifestyle interventions/changes*	*Lifestyle changes commentary*
	Aromatic amine and 4,4′-methylenebis (2-chloroaniline) from occupational exposures-chemical, dye, and rubber industries	A proven risk factor for bladder cancer and one of the most notable occupational risk factors for any cancer
		Other potential and more controversial sources (hair dyes, paints, motor vehicle exhaust, metals, fungicides, and cigarette smoke) are receiving more attention
	Arsenic (inorganic) in drinking water, especially well water, or nonmunicipal sources. Other compounds in water (chromium chlorination by products)	Higher levels and chronic exposure to inorganic (not organic) arsenic can be metabolized to more toxic methylated arsenicals and has been strongly associated with a higher risk of bladder cancer. Having well water tested regularly is a good idea
		Exposure from arsenic in air, food, occupational, and tobacco products may also have some controversial impact on risk. Other compounds in water such as chromium chlorination by products may increase risk
	Fermented (*L. casei* Shirota) or cultured milk (lactic acid bacteria) with probiotics	Several epidemiology studies suggest a lower risk of bladder cancer especially utilizing lactic acid bacteria or the probiotic *L. casei* Shirota (e.g., Yakult drink), which has the most data currently as a dietary supplement to be utilized with some conventional forms of bladder cancer treatment

(continued)

Table 9.2 (continued)

	Fluid intake	Increasing intake is associated with the potential for reducing bladder cancer risk in some large epidemiological studies but not shown to be beneficial after diagnosis and treatment to prevent recurrence (thus far)
	Schistosomiasis infection (*Schistosoma haematobium*)	Proven risk factor for bladder cancer from chronic infection from this parasitic blood fluke. Most cases occur in developing areas of Africa and the Middle East and generally found in more advanced stages, but treatment at these stages is somewhat similar to transitional cell carcinoma (TCC) of the bladder. Eggs deposited in the bladder from this parasite cause irritation and tissue fibrosis that can increase the risk of developing squamous cell carcinoma of the bladder
	Smoking, especially from cigarettes	A proven risk factor is associated with 50 % of the bladder cancers in both men and women, and risk is correlated with the amount and duration of use. Smoking is also correlated with a worse prognosis for current smokers diagnosed with bladder cancer
		Smoking increases the risk of bladder cancer and correlation is as strong or stronger compared to lung cancer. Smoking cessation is needed ASAP. Other forms of smoking (smokeless tobacco, pipe, environmental, etc.) may also increase risk
	Vegetable intake (cruciferous)	Increasing intake associated with a reduction in bladder cancer risk
II.	*Bladder cancer CAM/supplement intervention*	*CAM/dietary supplements commentary*
	Chewing gum	Preliminary evidence suggests chewing gum has the potential for a stimulatory effect on bowel motility and reduces ileus time in patients after radical cystectomy (open or robotic)
	L. casei (LC) Shirota and lactic acid bacteria	3,000 mg (3 g) a day after resection or with certain conventional treatments for 1 year appears to reduce the risk of superficial bladder cancer recurrence from three clinical trials (after resection or intravesical chemotherapy/Epirubicin). Yakult drink may provide a similar benefit also in the area of prevention and treatment. In the most recent trial the preparation contains 1×10^{10} of LC Shirota strain per gram
	Low-dose low-cost multivitamin (e.g., Centrum Silver or children's multivitamin)	Significantly lower modest risk of total cancer risk, and hematuria and nonsignificant reduction in bladder cancer diagnosis (utilized in current, former and never smokers). Safe as a placebo overall
	Megadose vitamins and minerals	Does not further reduce the risk of superficial bladder cancer recurrence when added to BCG or interferon alpha-2b treatment
III.	*Chronic nonbacterial prostatitis/chronic pelvic pain syndrome (CP/CPPS)*	*CAM/dietary supplements commentary*
	Exercise (e.g., vigorous walking three times per week for 40 min each session to achieve 70/80 % of the predicted maximum heart rate for age)	Significant reductions in pain using the NIH-CPSI and improvement in quality of life over 18 weeks. This should arguably be standard treatment (ancillary or monotherapy) for CP/CPPS and in UPOINT clinical guidelines. It improves mental health, increases endorphins, and arguably reduces sympathetic overload. More high-intensity exercise should also be tried and tested for the potential for enhanced pain reduction and quality of life and because no impact on urinary domain of NIH-CPSI has been observed thus far with less intense exercise
	Acupuncture or modified conventional form of electro-acupuncture (posterior tibial nerve stimulation or PTNS)	Significant preliminary reductions in the NIH-CPSI urinary domain for CP/CPPS. Should receive more immediate attention and investigation
	Cernilton (mixed polled extract)	Arguably, the most studied supplement in CP/CPPS with one rigorous positive trial with an intention to treat demonstrated reduction in pain and improved quality of life and six other clinical studies to demonstrate benefit. Finding a reputable Cernilton product is not simple and following the steps in this chapter can be helpful to locate such a product (AB Cernelle, Graminex, Farr Labs...). No impact on urinary domain of NIH-CPSI

(continued)

Table 9.2 (continued)

	Quercetin complex products	A dosage of 500 twice a day in a small randomized trial of Prosta-Q was impressive in terms of pain reduction and quality-of-life improvement. Reduced WBC in prostatic fluid. No impact on urinary domain of NIH-CPSI. Q-Urol supplement has also been used in UPOINT published cohort series
	Saw palmetto	Questionable impact for CP/CPPS at 325 mg/day and controversial based on past methodology of trials and based on lack of BPH activity from STEP and CAMUS clinical trials. Regardless, a controlled or placebo comparison is needed
IV.	*Interstitial cystitis (IC)/painful bladder syndrome (PBS)*	*CAM/dietary supplements commentary*
	Diet (elimination of triggers or restrictive changes) and stress reduction techniques	Published surveys suggest citrus fruits, tomatoes, vitamin C, artificial sweeteners, coffee, tea, carbonated and alcoholic beverages, and spicy foods could be significant triggers. There is a lack of rigorous diet studies, but the consistent input from patient surveys such dietary changes can have profound impacts as well as stress reduction techniques
	Calcium glycerophosphate (acid neutralizer)	Surveys suggest efficacy of this supplement (Prelief) to reduce food or beverage triggers of IC. Lacks rigorous comparative studies against a control such as standard antacids (calcium carbonate), but the patient satisfaction rates in general are excellent with a good safety profile
	Capsaicin (intravesical)	Preliminary research suggests no impact on histamine or prostaglandin E2, but an effect on desensitization of bladder C-fiber afferents that could otherwise initiate painful bladder sensations. Oral supplements have not been studied
	Glucosamine, chondroitin, and hyaluronate complex	Preliminary studies suggest a benefit to reduce IC symptoms (Cystoprotek). It should be tested against a standard osteoarthritis glucosamine mixed product. Intravesical chondroitin is being tested now with some preliminary benefits
	Hyperbaric oxygen	A small preliminary study found some potential benefit. Needs more research
	L-arginine supplementation	Failed to provide a benefit at a variety of dosages in multiple clinical studies. Nitric oxide levels could already be elevated in some patients with IC
	Quercetin complex	Preliminary evidence to suggest a benefit for some IC patients (Cysta-Q). It should be tested in a comparative clinical trial
V.	*Kidney cancer*	*CAM and lifestyle changes commentary*
	Cardiovascular disease risk factors	Virtually every major cardiovascular disease risk factor has been associated with kidney cancer from obesity, smoking, hypertension, physical inactivity, and perhaps poor diet and high cholesterol
	Exercise	One of the strongest relationships of any cancer in terms of risk reduction
	Fruits and veggies	One of the strongest associations with an increase in consumption and a reduced risk of a cancer (from a blood pressure lowering impact)
	Hypertension	Associated with an increased risk of kidney cancer
	Obesity	One of the strongest relationships of any cancer in terms of increased risk
	Smoking	Associated with an increased risk of kidney cancer

Multiple lifestyle changes have the ability to prevent bladder cancer (smoking cessation, reduce arsenic concentrations in water, cruciferous vegetable intake, etc.), and some dietary supplements such as *L. casei* Shirota have the ability to reduce recurrence rates after superficial bladder cancer treatment from three clinical trials. Chronic prostatitis/chronic pelvic pain syndrome (CP/CPPS) can be treated with exercise as well as a variety of dietary supplements (quercetin complex, cernilton, etc.) as is the case with interstitial cystitis/painful bladder syndrome (IC/PBS). For example, elimination and restriction diets based on triggers as well as calcium glycerophosphate, glucosamine, chondroitin, hyaluronate, and quercetin complex may help patients with IC/PBS. And kidney cancer, compared to almost any other cancer, has some of the strongest associations with cardiovascular risk factors, especially obesity and a reduction in risk with exercise and diet. It is time to update these important lifestyle findings in various clinical guidelines for these specific urologic conditions.

References

1. Grossman HB, Stenzl A, Moyad MA, Droller MJ. Bladder cancer: chemoprevention, complementary approaches and budgetary considerations. Scand J Urol Nephrol Suppl. 2008;218:213–33.
2. Vilensky D, Lawrentschuk N, Hersey K, Fleshner NE. A smoking cessation program as a resource for bladder cancer patients. Can Urol Assoc J. 2012;6(5):E167–73.
3. Freedman ND, Silverman DT, Hollenbeck AR, Schatzkin A, Abnet CC. Association between smoking and risk of bladder cancer among men and women. JAMA. 2011;306:737–45.
4. Rink M, Xylinas E, Babjuk M, Hansen J, Pycha A, Comploj E, et al. Impact of smoking on outcomes of patients with a history of recurrent nonmuscle invasive bladder cancer. J Urol. 2012;188:2120–7.
5. Letasiova S, Medveova A, Sovcikova A, Dusinska M, Volkovova K, Mosolu C, et al. Bladder cancer, a review of environmental risk factors. Environ Health. 2012;11 Suppl 1:11.
6. Flore MC, Baker TB. Should clinicians encourage smoking cessation for every patient who smokes? JAMA. 2013;309:1032–3.
7. Stewart SB, Freedland SJ. Influence of obesity on the incidence and treatment of genitourinary malignancies. Urol Oncol. 2011;29:476–86.
8. Chromecki TF, Cha EK, Fajkovic H, Rink M, Ehdaie B, Svatek RS, et al. Obesity is associated with worse oncological outcomes in patients treated with radical cystectomy. BJU Int. 2013;111:249–55.
9. Liu B, Mao Q, Lin Y, Zhou F, Xie L. The association of cruciferous vegetables intake and risk of bladder cancer: a meta-analysis. World J Urol. 2013;31:127–33.
10. Michaud DS, Spiegelman D, Clinton SK, Rimm EB, Willett WC, Glovannucci EL. Fruit and vegetable intake and incidence of bladder cancer in a male prospective cohort. J Natl Cancer Inst. 1999;91:605–13.
11. Lee JE, Mannisto S, Spiegelman D, Hunter DJ, Bernstein L, van den Brandt PA, et al. Intake of fruits, vegetables, and carotenoids and renal cell cancer risk: a pooled analysis of 13 prospective studies. Cancer Epidemiol Biomarkers Prev. 2009;18:1730–9.
12. Zhou J, Smith S, Giovannucci E, Michaud DS. Reexamination of total fluid intake and bladder cancer in the Health Professionals Follow-up Study Cohort. Am J Epidemiol. 2012;175:696–705.
13. Donat SM, Bayuga S, Herr HW, Berwick M. Fluid intake and the risk of tumor recurrence in patients with superficial bladder cancer. J Urol. 2003;170:1777–80.
14. Curhan GC, Willett WC, Rimm EB, Spiegelman D, Stampfer MJ. Prospective study of beverage use and the risk of kidney stones. Am J Epidemiol. 1996;143:240–7.
15. Ferris J, Berbel O, Alonso-Lopez J, Garcia J, Ortega JA. Environmental non-occupational risk factors associated with bladder cancer. Actas Urol Esp. 2013 [Epub ahead of print].
16. Brinkman MT, Karagas MR, Zens MS, Schned AR, Reulen RC, Zeegers MP. Intake of alpha-linolenic acid and other fatty acids in relation to the risk of bladder cancer: results from the New Hampshire case–control study. Br J Nutr. 2011;106:1070–7.
17. Zhang XL, Geng J, Zhang XP, Peng B, Che JP, Yan Y, et al. Statin use and risk of bladder cancer: a meta-analysis. Cancer Causes Control. 2013;24:769–76.
18. Silva RD, Xylinas E, Kluth L, Crivelli JJ, Chrystal J, Chade D, et al. Impact of statin use on oncological outcomes in patients with urothelial carcinoma of the bladder treated with radical cystectomy. J Urol. 2013;190:487–92.
19. Defronzo RA, Mehta RJ, Schnure JJ. Pleiotropic effects of thiazolidinediones: implications for the treatment of patients with type 2 diabetes mellitus. Hosp Pract. 1995;2013(41):132–47.
20. Campbell PT, Newton CC, Patel AV, Jacobs EJ, Gapstur SM. Diabetes and cause-specific mortality in a prospective cohort of one million U.S. adults. Diabetes Care. 2012;35:1835–44.
21. Xu X, Wu J, Mao Y, Zhu Y, Hu Z, Xu X, et al. Diabetes mellitus and risk of bladder cancer: a meta-analysis of cohort studies. PLoS One. 2013;8:e58079.
22. Schuhmacher-Wolz U, Dieter HH, Klein D, Schneider K. Oral exposure to inorganic arsenic: evaluation of its carcinogenic and non-carcinogenic effects. Crit Rev Toxicol. 2009;39:271–98.

23. Zaghloul MS. Bladder cancer and schistosomiasis. J Egypt Natl Canc Inst. 2012;24:151–9.
24. Gaziano JM, Sesso HD, Christen WG, Bubes V, Smith JP, MacFadyen J, et al. Multivitamins in the prevention of cancer in men: the Physicians' Health Study II randomized controlled trial. JAMA. 2012;308:1871–80.
25. Sesso HD, Christen WG, Bubes V, Smith JP, MacFadyen J, Schvartz M, et al. Multivitamins in the prevention of cardiovascular disease in men: the Physicians' Health Study II randomized controlled trial. JAMA. 2012;308:1751–60.
26. Neuhouser ML, Wasserthell-Smoller S, Thomson C, Aragaki A, Anderson GL, Manson JE, et al. Multivitamin use and risk of cancer and cardiovascular disease in the Women's Health Initiative cohorts. Arch Intern Med. 2009;169:294–304.
27. Cole BF, Baron JA, Sandler RS, Polyp Prevention Study Group, et al. Folic acid for the prevention of colorectal adenomas: a randomized clinical trial. JAMA. 2007;297:2351–9.
28. Figueriredo JC, Grau MV, Haile RW, et al. Folic acid and risk of prostate cancer: results from a randomized clinical trial. J Natl Cancer Inst. 2009;101:432–5.
29. Collin SM, Metcalfe C, Refsum H, Lewis SJ, Zuccolo L, Smith GD, et al. Circulating folate, vitamin B12, homocysteine, vitamin B12 transport proteins, and risk of prostate cancer: a case–control study, systematic review, and meta-analysis. Cancer Epidemiol Biomarkers Prev. 2010;19:1632–42.
30. Bailey RL, Mills JL, Yetley EA, Gahche JJ, Pfeiffer CM, Dwyer JT, et al. Unmetabolized serum folic acid and its relation to folic acid intake from diet and supplements in a nationally representative sample of adults aged > or =60 y in the United States. Am J Clin Nutr. 2010;92:383–9.
31. Lippman SM, Klein EA, Goodman PJ, Lucia MS, Thompson IM, Ford LG, et al. Effect of selenium and vitamin E on risk of prostate cancer and other cancers: the Selenium and Vitamin E Cancer Prevention Trial (SELECT). JAMA. 2009;301:39–51.
32. Duffield-Lillico AJ, Slate EH, Reid ME, Turnbull BW, Wilkins PA, Combs Jr GF, Nutritional Prevention of Cancer Study Group, et al. Selenium supplementation and secondary prevention of nonmelanoma skin cancer in a randomized trial. J Natl Cancer Inst. 2003;95:1477–81.
33. Stranges S, Marshall JR, Natarajan R, Donahue RP, Trevisan M, Combs GF, et al. Effects of long-term selenium supplementation on the incidence of type 2 diabetes: a randomized trial. Ann Intern Med. 2007;147:217–23.
34. Lawson KA, Wright ME, Subar A, Mouw T, Hollenbeck A, Schatzkin A, et al. Multivitamin use and risk of prostate cancer in the National Institutes of Health-AARP Diet and Health Study. J Natl Cancer Inst. 2007;99:754–64.
35. Miller 3rd ER, Pastor-Barriuso R, Dalal D, Riemersma RA, Appel LJ, Guallar E. Meta-analysis: high-dosage vitamin E supplementation may increase all-cause mortality. Ann Intern Med. 2005;142:37–46.
36. Clarke R, Halsey J, Lewington S, Lonn E, Armitage J, Manson JE, B-vitamin Treatment Trialists' Collaboration, et al. Effects of lowering homocysteine levels with B vitamins on cardiovascular disease, cancer, and cause-specific mortality. Meta-analysis of 8 randomized trials involving 37,485 individuals. Arch Intern Med. 2010;170:1622–31.
37. Sesso HD, Buring JE, Christen WG, Kurth T, Belanger C, MacFadyen J, et al. Vitamins E and C in the prevention of cardiovascular disease in men: the Physicians' Health Study II randomized controlled trial. JAMA. 2008;300:2123–33.
38. Lamm DL, Riggs DR, Shriver JS, van Gilder PF, Rach JF, De Haven JI. Megadose vitamins in bladder cancer: a double-blind clinical trial. J Urol. 1994;151:21–6.
39. Nepple KG, Lightfoot AJ, Rosevear HM, O'Donnell MA, Lamm DL, Bladder Cancer Genitourinary Oncology Study Group. Bacillus Calmette-Guerin with or without interferon alpha-2b and megadose versus recommended daily allowance vitamins during induction and maintenance intravesical treatment of nonmuscle invasive bladder cancer. J Urol. 2010;184:1915–9.
40. Moyad MA. Dr. Moyad's no bogus science health advice. Ann Arbor, MI: Ann Arbor Media Group; 2010.
41. Morris MC, Tangney CC. A potential design flaw of randomized trials of vitamin supplements. JAMA. 2011;305:1348–9.
42. Tighe P, Ward M, McNulty H, Finnegan O, Dunne A, Strain J, et al. A dose-finding trial of the effect of long-term folic acid intervention: implications for food fortification policy. Am J Clin Nutr. 2011;93:11–8.
43. Hercberg S, Galan P, Preziosi P, Bertrais S, Mennen L, Malvy D, et al. The SU.VI.MAX study: a randomized, placebo-controlled trial of the health effects of antioxidant vitamins and minerals. Arch Intern Med. 2004;164:2335–42.
44. Goossens ME, Buntinx F, Joniau S, Ackaert K, Ameye F, Billet I, et al. Designing the selenium and bladder cancer trial (SELEBLAT), a phase III randomized chemoprevention study with selenium on recurrence of bladder cancer in Belgium. BMC Urol. 2012;12:8.
45. Moyad MA. Selenium and vitamin E supplements for prostate cancer: evidence or embellishment? Urology. 2002;59(4 Suppl 1):9–19.
46. Giovannucci E, Chan AT. Role of vitamin and mineral supplementation and aspirin use in cancer survivors. J Clin Oncol. 2010;28:4081–5.
47. Aso Y, Akazan H, BLP Study Group. Prophylactic effect of a Lactobacillus casei preparation on the recurrence of superficial bladder cancer. Urol Int. 1992;49:125–9.
48. Aso Y, Akaza H, Kotake T, Tsukamoto T, Imai K, Naito S. Prevention effect of a Lactobacillus casei preparation on the recurrence of superficial bladder cancer in a double-blind trial. Eur Urol. 1995;27:104–9.

49. Naito S, Koga H, Yamaguchi A, Fujimoto N, Hasui Y, Kuramoto H, Kyushu University Urological Oncology Group. Prevention of recurrence with epirubicin and Lactobacillus casei after transurethral resection of bladder cancer. J Urol. 2008;179:485–90.
50. Dong H, Rowland I, Thomas LV, Yaqoob P. Immunomodulatory effects of a probiotc drink containing Lactobacillus casei Shirota in healthy older volunteers. Eur J Nutr. 2013; [Epub ahead of print].
51. Dong H, Rowland I, Yaqoob P. Comparative effects of six probiotic strains on immune function in vitro. Br J Nutr. 2012;108:459–70.
52. Dong H, Rowland I, Tuohy KM, Thomas LV, Yaqoob P. Selective effects of Lactobacillus casei Shirota on T cell activation, natural killer cell activity and cytokine production. Clin Exp Immunol. 2010;161:378–88.
53. Ohashi Y, Nakai S, Tsukamoto T, Masumori N, Akaza H, Miyanaga N, et al. Habitual intake of lactic acid bacteria and risk reduction of bladder cancer. Urol Int. 2002;68:273–80.
54. Larsson SC, Andersson SO, Johansson JE, Wolk A. Cultured milk, yogurt, and dairy intake in relation to bladder cancer risk in a prospective study of Swedish women and men. Am J Clin Nutr. 2008;88:1083–7.
55. Keszei AP, Schouten LJ, Goldbohm RA, van den Brandt PA. Dairy intake and the risk of bladder cancer in the Netherlands Cohort Study on Diet and Cancer. Am J Epidemiol. 2010;171:436–46.
56. Li S, Liu Y, Peng Q, Xie L, Wang J, Qin X. Chewing gum reduces postoperative ileus following abdominal surgery: a meta-analysis of 17 randomized controlled trials. J Gastroenterol Hepatol. 2013;28:1122–32.
57. Choi H, Kang SH, Yoon DK, Kang SG, Ko HY, du Moon G, et al. Chewing gum has a stimulatory effect on bowel motility in patients after open or robotic radical cystectomy for bladder cancer: a prospective randomized comparative study. Urology. 2011;77:884–90.
58. Kouba EJ, Wallen EM, Pruthi RS. Gum chewing stimulates bowel motility in patients undergoing radical cystectomy with urinary diversion. Urology. 2007;70:1053–6.
59. Pruthi RS, Nielsen M, Smith A, Nix J, Schultz H, Wallen EM. Fast track program in patients undergoing radical cystectomy: results in 362 consecutive patients. J Am Coll Surg. 2010;210:93–9.
60. Krieger JN, Nyberg Jr L, Nickel JC. NIH consensus definition and classification of prostatitis. JAMA. 1999;282:236–7.
61. Shoskes DA, Nickel JC, Kattan MW. Phenotypically directed multimodal therapy for chronic prostatitis/chronic pelvic pain syndrome: a prospective study using UPOINT. Urology. 2010;75:1249–53.
62. Giubilei G, Mondaini N, Minervini A, Saieva C, Lapini A, Serni S, Bartoletti R, Carini M. Physical activity of men with chronic prostatitis/chronic pelvic pain syndrome not satisfied with conventional treatments-could it represent a valid option? The physical activity and male pelvic pain trial: a double-blind, randomized study. J Urol. 2007;177:159–65.
63. Pool JL. Role of sympathetic nervous system in hypertension and benign prostatic hyperplasia. Br J Clin Pract Suppl. 1994;74:13–7.
64. McVary KT, Rademaker A, Lloyd GL, Gann P. Autonomic nervous system overactivity in men with lower urinary tract symptoms secondary to benign prostatic hyperplasia. J Urol. 2005;174(4 Pt 1):1327–433.
65. Esch T, Stefano GB. The neurobiology of stress management. Neuro Endocrinol Lett. 2010;31:19–39.
66. Murtezani A, Hundozi H, Orovcanec N, Sllamniku S, Osmani T. A comparison of high intensity aerobic exercise and passive modalities for the treatment of workers with chronic low back pain: a randomized, controlled trial. Eur J Phys Rehabil Med. 2011;47:359–66.
67. Cohen JM, Fagin AP, Hariton E, Niska JR, Pierce MW, Kuriyama A, et al. Therapeutic intervention for chronic prostatitis/chronic pelvic pain syndrome (CP/CPPS): a systematic review and meta-analysis. PLoS One. 2012;7:e41941.
68. Wagenlehner FM, Bschleipfer T, Pilatz A, Weidner W. Pollen extract for chronic prostatitis-chronic pelvic pain syndrome. Urol Clin N Am. 2011;38:285–92.
69. Wagenlehner FME, Schneider H, Ludwig M, Schnitker J, Brahler E, Weidner W. A pollen extract (cernilton) in patients with inflammatory chronic-prostatitis-chronic pelvic pain syndrome: a multicentre, randomized, prospective, double-blind, placebo-controlled trial. Eur Urol. 2009;56:544–51.
70. MacDonald R, Ishani A, Rutks I, Wilt TJ. A systematic review of Cernilton for the treatment of benign prostatic hyperplasia. BJU Int. 2000;85:836–41.
71. Weng Z, Zhang B, Asadi S, Sismanopoulos N, Butcher A, Fu X, et al. Quercetin is more effective than cromolyn in blocking human mast cell cytokine release and inhibits contact dermatitis and photosensitivity in human. PLoS One. 2012;7:e33805.
72. Shoskes DA, Zeitlin SI, Shahed A, Rajfer J. Quercetin in men with category III chronic prostatitis: a preliminary prospective, double-blind, placebo-controlled trial. Urology. 1999;54:960–3.
73. Theoharides TC, O'Leary M. Painful bladder syndrome/interstitial cystitis: current concepts and role of nutraceuticals. Sem Prev Altern Med. 2006;14:2–6.
74. Hill JR, Isom-Batz G, Panagopoulos G, Zakariasen K, Kavaler E. Patient perceived outcomes of treatments used for interstitial cystitis. Urology. 2008;71:62–6.
75. Bologna RA, Gomelsky A, Lukban JC, Tu LM, Holzberg AS, Whitmore KE. The efficacy of calcium glycerophosphate in the prevention of food-related flares in interstitial cystitis. Urology. 2001;57 (6 Suppl 1):119–20.
76. Bassaly R, Downes K, Hart S. Dietary consumption triggers in interstitial cystitis pain syndrome patients. Female Pelvic Med Reconstr Surg. 2011;17:36–9.
77. Friedlander JI, Shorter B, Moldwin RM. Diet and its role in interstitial cystitis/bladder pain syndrome (IC/BPS) and comorbid conditions. BJU Int. 2012; 109:1584–91.

78. Nguan C, Franciosi LG, Butterfield NN, Macleod BA, Jens M, Fenster HN. A prospective, double-blind, randomized cross-over study evaluating changes in urinary pH for relieving symptoms of interstitial cystitis. BJU Int. 2005;95:91–4.
79. Thilagarajah R, Wltherow RO, Walker MM. Oral cimetidine gives effective symptom relief in painful bladder disease: a prospective, randomized, double-blind placebo-controlled trial. BJU Int. 2001;87:207–12.
80. O'Hare 3rd PG, Hoffman AR, Allen P, Gordon B, Salin L, Whitmore K. Interstitial cystitis patients' use and rating of complementary and alternative medicine therapies. Int Urogynecol J. 2013;24:977–82.
81. Theoharides TC, Sant GR. A pilot open label study of Cystoprotek in interstitial cystitis. Int J Immunopathol Pharmacol. 2005;18:183–8.
82. Theoharides TC, Kempuraj D, Vakall S, Sant GR. Treatment of refractory interstitial cystitis/painful bladder syndrome with CystoProtek-an oral multi-agent natural supplement. Can J Urol. 2008;15:4410–4.
83. Smith SD, Wheeler MA, Foster Jr HE, Weiss RM. Improvement in interstitial cystitis symptom scores during treatment with oral L-arginine. J Urol. 1997;158(3 Pt 1):703–8.
84. Korting GE, Smith SD, Wheeler MA, Weiss RM, Foster Jr HE. A randomized double-blind trial of oral L-arginine for treatment of interstitial cystitis. J Urol. 1999;161:558–65.
85. Cartledge JJ, Davies AM, Eardley I. A randomized double-blind placebo-controlled crossover trial of the efficacy of L-arginine in the treatment of interstitial cystitis. BJU Int. 2000;85:421–6.
86. Ehren I, Lundberg JO, Adolfsson J, Wiklund NP. Effects of L-arginine treatment on symptoms and bladder nitric oxide levels in patients with interstitial cystitis. Urology. 1998;52:1026–9.
87. Katske F, Shoskes DA, Sender M, Poliakin R, Gagliano K, Rajfer J. Treatment of interstitial cystitis with a quercetin supplement. Tech Urol. 2001;7:44–6.
88. Fageril J, Fraser MO, de Groat WC, Chancellor MB, Flood HD, Smith D, et al. Intravesical capsaicin for the treatment of interstitial cystitis: a pilot study. Can J Urol. 1999;6:737–44.
89. French LM, Bhambore N. Interstitial cystitis/painful bladder syndrome. Am Fam Physician. 2011;83: 1175–81.
90. Lipworth L, Tarone RE, McLaughlin JK. Renal cell cancer among African Americans: an epidemiologic review. BMC Cancer. 2011;11:133.
91. Chow WH, Dong LM, Devesa SS. Epidemiology and risk factors for kidney cancer. Nat Rev Urol. 2010;7:245–57.
92. Moyad MA. Obesity, interrelated mechanisms, and exposures and kidney cancer. Semin Urol Oncol. 2001;19:270–9.
93. Khurana V, Caldito G, Ankem M. Statins might reduce risk of renal cell carcinoma in humans: case–control study of 500,000 veterans. Urology. 2008;71: 118–22.
94. Behrens G, Leitzmann MF. The association between physical activity and renal cancer: systematic review and meta-analysis. Br J Cancer. 2013;108:798–811.
95. Willett WC. Fruits, vegetables, and cancer prevention: turmoil in the produce section. J Natl Cancer Inst. 2010;102:1–2.
96. Macleod LC, Hotaling JM, Wright JL, Davenport MT, Gore JL, Harper J, et al. Risk factors for renal cell carcinoma in the Vitamin and Lifestyle (VITAL) Study. J Urol. 2013; [epub ahead of print].
97. Lai GY, Park Y, Hartge P, Hollenbeck AR, Freedman ND. The association between self-reported diabetes and cancer incidence in the NIH-AARP Diet and Health Study. J Clin Endocrinol Metab. 2013;98:E497–502.
98. Shu X, Lin J, Wood CG, Tannir NM, Wu X. Energy balance, polymorphisms in the mTOR pathway, and renal cell carcinoma risk. J Natl Cancer Inst. 2013;105:424–32.
99. Beebe-Dimmer JL, Colt JS, Ruterbusch JJ, Keele GR, Purdue MP, Wacholder S, et al. Body mass index and renal cell cancer: the influence of race and sex. Epidemiology. 2012;23:821–8.

Review of Lifestyle and CAM for Miscellaneous Urologic Topics (OAB and/or Incontinence, Pediatric Urology, Peyronie's Disease, Premature Ejaculation, UTIs, Miscellaneous): Part Two

10

Introduction

I apologize for the brevity of this chapter, but it is simply a mirror reflection of the dearth of research on lifestyle and CAM in most of these areas. This would also reflect a challenge to those of us working in these areas of urology because there is some much potential here. Randomized trials have and are being designed and implemented in most of these areas, and it is my hope that this chapter will have a similar volume to other chapters in this book when the second or third edition is released. In the meantime, I hope this chapter provides some insight into potential research and benefits of CAM that could be derived in some of these areas.

VI. Overactive Bladder and/or Urinary Incontinence

Minimal research in CAM and overactive bladder (OAB) has been accomplished, but dietary changes including reduction in fluid intake, caffeine, alcohol and acidic foods alone with weight reduction, smoking cessation, and bladder retraining have been of some benefit [1]. Low levels of physical activity and obesity may be an emerging risk factor for OAB and may exacerbate symptoms [2].

Arguably, a modified form of CAM derived from conventional medicine principles applied to acupuncture is percutaneous tibial nerve stimulation (PTNS). Apart from cost issues, it could be argued that PTNS is as effective as pharmacologic therapy with a better side effect profile based on past and recent results from clinical trials [3–5].

Similar issues abound for patients concerned about urinary incontinence from urge to stress and mixed in terms of lifestyle factors, especially obesity and worsening of symptoms, but weight loss could provide significant reduction in symptoms, as exemplified by already completed randomized trials. One randomized weight-loss trial ($n=226$ with intervention and $n=112$ in control, mean age 53 years and BMI of 36 ± 6) resulted in significant greater loss of weekly stress incontinence episodes (65 % vs. 47 %, $p<0.001$) at 12 months and greater percentage of women experiencing more than 70 % improvement in urge incontinence episodes at 18 months [6]. Mean weight loss was 8.0 kg over the entire study.

One of the more novel and exciting areas of incontinence improvement has to be the reduction in the risk of side effects from prostate cancer and other treatments with lifestyle changes. For example, core or abdominal strength training exercise two sessions a week (60 min per session) can result in significant improvement in continence rates and quality of life post-prostatectomy compared to Kegel exercises alone [7]. In a unique prostate cancer radiation series of 440 men given a questionnaire found significantly lower rectal symptom scores ($p<0.001$), better erectile function ($p<0.001$), and urinary function ($p<0.01$) in nonsmoking men who were physically active and had a lower body mass index [8].

M.A. Moyad, *Complementary & Alternative Medicine for Prostate and Urologic Health*,
DOI 10.1007/978-1-4614-8492-9_10, © Springer Science+Business Media New York 2014

VII. Pediatric Urology (Lifestyle, Urinary Tract Infections, Etc.)

Minimal research in pediatric urology and CAM has been accomplished. For example, there is limited evidence for the effectiveness on acupuncture for nocturnal enuresis in children [9, 10]. This is not necessarily a negative finding because it is my belief that pediatric urologic research should first focus on lifestyle changes compared to exotic tablets or herbal products. For example, the high rate of dysfunctional voiding, especially nocturnal enuresis in obese children, and a lower rate of treatment response are concerning [11]. Hypertension, diabetes, and obesity appear to be associated with a higher risk of stone disease [12, 13].

Preventing recurrent urinary tract infections (UTIs) in children with cranberry juice has mixed results [14–16], but I am concerned about the caloric contribution and compliance of these beverages in the age of an obesity epidemic [17]. Overall, the sum of the evidence has resulted in discouraging the use of this beverage to prevent UTI [16]. Dietary supplements of cranberry concentrate appear to have similar data to juice and contribute little to no calories, but a definitive pediatric clinical trial is needed with a high proanthocyanidin (PAC and PAC-A) concentrations, and oxalate contributions from supplements need to be reported [18]. For example, in a successful and more recent pediatric UTI trial, the juice utilized had a total PAC concentration of 37 % [15]. A total of 12 out of 40 participants did not complete the study (six in each group). It would be prudent to report weight or waist changes in future clinical trials.

Probiotic dietary supplements are needed in more urologic clinical trials in pediatric patients. There is the suggestion of certain populations of children, including those with persistent primary vesicoureteral reflux (VUR), benefiting with a *Lactobacillus acidophilus* (10^8 CFU.g 1 g twice a day) and showing similar effects to antibiotics (trimethoprim/sulfamethoxazole) in larger clinical studies ($n = 120$) [19, 20]. This data with probiotics needs to continue to mature, but it is a potentially critical development because antibiotic resistance is an ongoing issue in children with UTI [21], and, interestingly, the benefit of probiotics for antibiotic-associated side effects such as diarrhea is becoming well recognized in conventional medicine [22]. It is also of interest that few dietary studies in pediatric urology have been completed, especially in regard to conditions to UTI. It would seem logical to promote a heart-healthy diet and lifestyle in children to encourage overall health and to reduce the risk of blood sugar changes or weight that could increase the risk of urologic issues.

VIII. Peyronie's Disease

If Peyronie's disease (PD) has an inflammatory component and there are acute, early chronic phases, then the potential for a CAM option to be utilized early with some conventional therapy is practical and logical, especially if "first do no harm" is the approach here. For example, vitamin E supplements have been used with mixed success [23], and some would argue similar to placebo effects or discouraged use from reputable experts [24], but the recent finding of an increased risk of prostate cancer in just a few years of ingesting this supplement from the SELECT is concerning enough [25, 26]. It is for this reason the future of vitamin supplements in PD should be discouraged. Some clinicians have used topical vitamin E cream and perhaps this makes more sense and might be far less concerning, but it does need some clinical controlled testing outside of the office, and the real concern of allergic reactions or contact dermatitis from these topicals is rare in general skin use but should be addressed [27, 28].

Carnitine (acetyl esters) dietary supplements may be able to reduce calcium levels inside endothelial cells, which are found in the penis and elsewhere [29, 30]. This may cause a reduction in fibroblasts and collagen production, which can reduce the risk of plaques or fibrosis. There have been randomized trials of this supplement—for example, acetyl-L-carnitine, 1,000 mg twice a day, compared with 20 mg twice a day of prescription tamoxifen [29]. After 3 months, acetyl-L-carnitine was more effective in reducing pain and curvature and slowing the progression of PD and was better tolerated, but not in reducing plaque size (both significantly accomplished this). This is another example of the need to use the supplement as early as possible (early chronic phase or earlier) in PD with conventional treatment because otherwise the supplement is expected to accomplish an unrealistic outcome.

However, there is a suggestion that propionyl-L-carnitine is more active than acetyl-L-carnitine and L-carnitine [30]. A total of 60 patients with advanced PD were placed in one of two studies—2,000 mg per day for 3 months and verapamil injections (10 mg weekly for 10 weeks) compared to verapamil plus tamoxifen (40 mg per day). The reduction in pain was similar, but a significant reduction in penile curvature, plaque size, need for surgery, and disease progression and increased IIEF occurred in the carnitine group. The group taking tamoxifen instead of the supplement did not experience these benefits. There was also a hint in a second smaller study of resistant PD that the combination of verapamil and carnitine could be beneficial. Yet, despite these positive studies, it has become difficult for some clinicians to promote this instead of vitamin E. This is slightly perplexing since there have been no side effects over that of placebo and perhaps because there has been one study that failed over placebo at 2,000 mg of propionyl-L-carnitine [31]. In all fairness, this should not completely remove the preliminary results with other studies that showed some benefit and good safety.

A total of 300 mg of coenzyme Q10 (CoQ10) per day for 6 months worked significantly better than placebo at reducing plaque size, penile curvature, pain, and improved sexual function and slowed the progression or stabilized this disease in approximately 85 % of the men with early chronic PD within approximately 24 weeks [32]. CoQ10 is a fat-soluble supplement, so it should be taken with food, but keep in mind that it can reduce the effect of the blood thinner warfarin, but at the same time it could enhance the effect of the blood thinner clopidogrel [33]. This is one large study, but it was of interest, and since this supplement has a good safety record, overall, it may be worth a recommendation, and perhaps the same mechanism of action whereby blood pressure has been reduced in some clinical trials of hypertensive patients [33] offers the same mechanism of action on those with PD at the microvascular level. CoQ10 could be used in PD whenever the health care professional desires to use vitamin E dietary supplements with conventional therapy, but these dietary supplements are not low cost, and comparative pricing should still allow for good quality control on this product. Another trial by the same research team using omega-3 fatty acid supplements for PD found no benefit [34].

L-arginine research in PD has not matured yet, but there is a hint of efficacy in a study ($n=74$) utilizing 1,000 mg twice a day of L-arginine along with conventional treatment [35]. L-arginine could increase nitric oxide (NO) and increasing perfusion could allow for an anti-fibrosis effect and could reduce the development of scars and improve healing of wounds [36]. Laboratory studies for some time have suggested that it can prevent inflammation and fibrosis in the liver, kidney, lung, and cardiovascular system. Perhaps the other true benefit for L-arginine might just be an improvement in erectile function in those with PD. Please read the erectile dysfunction chapter of this book because there is plenty of information as to why L-citrulline could be a more ideal and safer dietary supplement compared to L-arginine for NO production. Thus, using 1,500 mg of L-citrulline daily or 2,000 mg of L-arginine daily could be a viable option for PD and is arguable that the one I find has some of the most potential for future research, especially in combination with other therapies [35–37].

Other areas of interest have not been impressive, for example, a topical magnesium sulfate, which could theoretically function as a less potent calcium channel blocker, worked no better compared to a topical placebo [38].

IX. Premature Ejaculation

Topical CAM

Severance secret-cream (also known as "SS-cream" from Cheil Jedang Corporation, Seoul, Korea) is one of the only CAM topical products with notable methodological clinical trials [39, 40]. It is composed of nine ingredients and is applied to the glans penis 1 h before sexual activity and washed or removed after sexual activity. The nine ingredients include:

- Ginseng radix alba
- Angelicae gigantis radix
- Cistanches herba
- Zanthoxyli fructs
- Torlidis semen
- Asiasari radix
- Caryophylli flos
- Cinnamoni cortex
- Bufonis venenum

This cream is not simple to order outside of Korea, but those willing to contact the company have been successful at times or from Internet operations. It had results in a double-blind trial that were impressive ($n=106$, mean age 39 years). The average ejaculatory time went from 1.4 to 10.9 min and was 27 times more effective than the placebo cream in terms of increasing sexual satisfaction [40]. However, 20 % of those using the SS-cream reported mild localized irritation, including burning and pain, and 12 % reported other side effects, such as delayed ejaculation, no ejaculation, or erectile dysfunction. This cream has been criticized for having an unpleasant odor and color, but at least it has clinical evidence in CAM. I rarely recommend complex combinations of herbal or other dietary supplements because they are confusing to buy and replicate and do not necessarily have better evidence compared to a single ingredient or herbal product. SS-cream is an exception because of all of the published clinical evidence. It is my hope that if this cream is as effective as the research suggest, this product will experience more future licensing agreement, but these studies were conducted almost 15 years ago, so I am less optimistic about this possibility.

There are a few of over-the-counter (OTC) creams that can be applied to the penis 5–15 min before intercourse to reduce the sensation that could otherwise lead to a rapid ejaculation [41]. For example, there is a 9.6 % lidocaine spray available in many countries, including the USA, called "Premjact" and others, and it has been available over the counter for almost 25 years; it is easy to order and is one of the best rated. There are also benzocaine (e.g., 5–7.5 %) creams and sprays. A cream or spray that is odorless and alcohol free is desired because it is not as irritating and damaging to the skin. Still, there are no good studies to back it up, but these over-the-counter ingredients are mimics of what has been used by health care professionals for this condition. And, similar to the prescription creams, they can cause temporary desensitization of the penis and the vagina if a condom is not used. For example, there is also a benzocaine cream sold by many companies in the USA. If the cream is utilized for too long (30–45 min), it could result in the loss of difficulty in maintaining an erection because of the penile numbness.

Serotonin Increasing CAM (Drug-Like Mimics)

Dietary supplements that work somewhat like the SSRI drugs need more research, but they have the very preliminary laboratory and indirect clinical research that they may help some men with PE [41]. For example, one of the active ingredients in St. John's wort, "hyperforin," has demonstrated promise [42]. Since delayed ejaculation is actually a side effect of many of the antidepressant drugs, especially the ones that impact serotonin levels or the SSRIs, then this is an adequate area of CAM research for potentially drug mimics. Increased serotonin apparently inhibits the ejaculatory reflex, and there are a small number of dependable CAM serotonin-acting products. The doses of SSRIs needed for PE are generally lower than the ones used for depression.

The problem with using St. John's wort (SJW) is its ability to reduce the efficacy of almost 50 % of the available prescription drugs [43]. SJW (500–1,200 mg/day over 4–12 weeks) has been moderately effective when used as 2–3 divided doses for major depressive disorder (MDD). An SJW extract that is standardized to contain 0.3 % hypericin is the active standardized ingredient, and the most common dosage in clinical trials was 900 mg per day. Clinical trials for PE again will need to utilize a lower dosage, for example, a third to a half of what has been used for depression.

SJW appears to inhibit serotonin uptake and alters levels of multiple brain neurotransmitters including dopamine, norepinephrine, and gamma-aminobutyric acid (GABA). SJW should not be combined with prescription antidepressants including SSRIs, tricyclic antidepressants (TCA), or monoamine oxidase (MAO) inhibitors. It should also be avoided in those individuals on specific drugs such as immunosuppressants, antiretrovirals (anti-HIV drugs), blood thinners like warfarin, oral contraceptives, and chemotherapy drugs. Other side effects of SJW include insomnia, vivid dreams, anxiety, dizziness, and photosensitivity.

5-HTP is an intermediate metabolite in the conversion of L-tryptophan to serotonin. It can be taken with meals, and the dosage range for antidepressant studies should be 50–300 mg (most positive studies used 200–300 mg) [44, 45]. Higher doses are not better because they can actually create nightmares and vivid dreams, and dizziness, nausea, and diarrhea have also been reported. Most importantly, L-5-HTP should not be combined with any other medications that also impact serotonin levels such as antidepressant. This is a controversial supplement [46] because it is a precursor to serotonin, and I do believe it can increase the risk of serotonin syndrome and possibly deplete other neurotransmitters. Still some of these critiques are not necessarily justified and often referred to the L-tryptophan EMS (eosinophilia-myalgia syndrome) that occurred from a unique contaminate from one manufacturer of these supplements. Personally, I was one of the investigators as a student of public health in the state of Florida during this issue 20 years ago, and although devastating it was not due to the supplement itself but, again, a contaminant from one manufacturer. Thus, to refer 5-HTP supplements as potentially causing the same issue is not an educational and objective opinion as to the etiology of this problem long ago.

Regardless, the future of dietary supplements or CAM for PE will rely on a mimic for what is already effective for PE as a prescription drug such as dapoxetine (short-acting SSRI) [47, 48], and serotonin-impacting supplements such as the ones mentioned in this section along with other promising CAM antidepressants such as S-adenosyl methionine (SAM-e) [43] offer some exciting research opportunities. The only issue with SAM-e is that the side effect profile has actually not been notable and may in fact could have less sexual function issues compared to SSRIs, which suggests other prominent mechanisms of action are occurring [49].

Some dietary supplements that improve erectile function or dysfunction (ED) are touted by many Web sites to provide significant benefits to those with isolated PE without ED [41], and this is a misrepresentation and not accurate based on PDE-5 data for those without erectile function issues and should be explained to patients [50]. Similarly, most promising dietary supplements for ED (*Panax ginseng*, L-citrulline, L-arginine) have not demonstrated an ability to assist in the treatment of isolated premature ejaculation (PE) [51] or have not been tested for this condition [41], but this continues to garner some rare positive research when both conditions may be occurring together [52]. Additionally, there are other CAMs that deserve further attention based on preliminary positive clinical research such as acupuncture [53].

X. Urinary Tract Infections

Few studies have researched the potential for cranberry supplements to be a large source of oxalate. One of the classically small but urologic impactful studies to show the importance of CAM research of any size was published back in 2001 [18]. A total of five subjects utilized cranberry supplements at the recommended daily dosage on the label for 7 days, and then urinary oxalate levels increased significantly ($p=0.01$) by an average of over 43 %. If over 10 % consistent increases as noted by these authors can cause calcium and oxalate to bind and crystallize or form a stone, then this is concerning. The average normal intake of oxalate from the diet is about 150 mg per day, but two cranberry tablets from this study could be expected to contain over 350 mg of oxalate per day. Another problem with many cranberry concentrate supplements is that they can contain a good amount or at least some plain vitamin C (known oxalate-increasing compound). Otherwise, it would appear today that for adults inquiring about cranberry juice to prevent recurrent UTIs, a good quality-controlled cranberry supplement is more sensible for adults compared to juice. These pills do not appear to add to the obesity epidemic in terms of caloric contribution (100–150 cal per 8 oz of juice vs. little to no calories with pills) [17] and have worked as well thus far as the juice option for the prevention of UTIs [16]. Also, the impact of cranberry juice for UTIs is being questioned now with added clinical trials, and the compliance rates of drinking cranberry juice daily for months in some trials have been poor. If someone has a high risk for oxalate stone and UTI recurrence, then again some idea of the contribution of the amount of oxalate from the supplement would be of assistance in deciding if the benefit was worth the risk.

Additionally, cranberry supplements have not been shown to increase antibiotic resistance even when inferior or similar in effect to antibiotics [16]. And they have flexible application as long as standardization is closely followed. For example, a 370 ($n = 184$ with cranberry and $n = 186$ for control) subject external beam radiation treatment study (6–7 weeks) for prostate cancer found a 200 mg (30 % PAC) daily cranberry supplement significantly lowered the risk of lower UTI as well as produced significant reductions in UTI symptoms such as dysuria, nocturia, frequency, and urgency [54]. Cranberry supplements in the future should have total PAC levels of 25–30 % or higher to approximate some positive juice products and studies and should primarily consist of higher PAC-A concentrations given as a percentage and/or milligrams per gram (proposed active ingredients) [15, 16, 54], which should always be reported to provide comparisons. Most future studies or products should contain at least 36 mg/day of PACs based on a recent meta-analysis [16].

Other factors impacting UTIs were discussed earlier in the pediatric section, but improved diet and the potential for probiotics from food or supplements to reduce UTIs should continue to receive attention [55]. There is some moderate evidence to suggest some *Lactobacillus* strains could prevent recurrent UTIs [56], and clinicians and patients need to continue to monitor this data because it will be one of the more ample areas of research in the area of CAM and urology. Another hope is lifestyle changes will continue to garner research—for example, the connection between UTI and obesity in males and females should be of ongoing interest [57].

Miscellaneous Urology

This area of the chapter was specifically left open for future references toward novel CAM research and products, which could provide assistance for patients—for example, the use of capsaicin is of interest [58–60], and it is already been used outside of urology. Whether it is improving surgical or procedural recovery times or reducing the toxicity of a standard treatment, it is my hope that this section of the book will accumulate more evidence by the next edition.

Conclusion

A summary of the CAM options that could negatively and positively impact the risk of multiple urologic conditions are listed in Table 10.1.

Multiple lifestyle changes have the ability to prevent OAB and incontinence, including the ability to go beyond Kegel exercises for improvement utilizing more rigorous weight loss and core abdominal exercises. Even side effects of primary prostate cancer treatments appear to be greatly attenuated with these methods and with overall improvement in cardiovascular health. Pediatric urology is beginning to feel the impact of obesity, and methods to curb this epidemic could be derived from urology. Cranberry for UTI prevention in pediatrics appears to have some data, but as with adults the caloric contribution and compliance are concerning and perhaps concentrated, low-calorie supplements are emerging as a better alternative. Peyronie's disease has several CAM options to be utilized with

Table 10.1 A partial summary list of lifestyle and other CAM interventions for OAB and incontinence, Peyronie's disease, premature ejaculation, and UTI

		Commentary
VI.	Overactive bladder (OAB) and/or incontinence	
	"Core" exercises or abdominal-strengthening exercise	May have a more significant impact on continence rates after prostate cancer surgery and in general compared to Kegel exercises alone. May also improve erectile function (not as well tested)
	Percutaneous tibial nerve stimulation (PTNS)	Really a modified form of electrostimulated acupuncture and proven to improve OAB or urge incontinence as well as antimuscarinics and with a better safety profile but cost can be an issue. Still, an underappreciated option for OAB
	Weight loss	May reduce symptoms of OAB Shown in overweight and obese individuals to dramatically reduce stress incontinence and may reduce the urge and mixed incontinence
VII.	Pediatric urology	
	Acupuncture	May have some limited effect for nocturnal enuresis
	Cranberry juice/supplements/probiotics	Higher PAC and PAC-A content appears to demonstrate a better response, but compliance and caloric contributions are a problem. A good clinical trial of cranberry supplements is needed in pediatrics Probiotics such as *Lactobacillus acidophilus* and others have a potential for reducing UTI in pediatric urology (e.g., for VUR) similar to antibiotics but needs more research now because overall research is in early stages
	Obesity	Increases the potential for worse urologic risk and outcomes including kidney stones and incontinence
VIII.	Peyronie's disease	
	CoQ10 supplements	One large controlled trial showed significant impact (plaque size, curvature, erectile function improved and reduced progression) with 300 mg/day for 6 months versus placebo. Needs to be replicated, but it is of interest and CoQ10 is not a low-cost product, so price comparison is needed
	L-arginine and/or L-citrulline	Preliminary research to suggest it can be utilized with conventional treatment to improve outcomes and erectile function at 2,000 mg of L-arginine, for example. L-citrulline at 1,500 mg per day has some efficacy for ED and may be a more effective and safer nitric oxide source in the future
	L-carnitine supplements	Acetyl-L-carnitine appeared to have preliminary data at 1,000 mg twice a day and so does propionyl-L-carnitine, but it has been controversial
	Vitamin E supplements/topical	Vitamin E supplements at 400 IU per day significantly increased the risk of prostate cancer in just a few years of supplementation based on the SELECT trial. So, why use it for Peyronie's disease? Vitamin E topical cream is used by some clinicians and may be safer, but it just needs some clinical research and be careful with allergic rare skin reactions
IX.	Premature ejaculation	
	Acupuncture	Has preliminary positive research that needs further study
	SS-cream	One of the only topical herbal products (nine herbs) to undergo a methodologically rigorous study and have a positive outcome. It is not easy to locate this product outside of Korea (company and Internet source needs to be contacted—it should be licensed in other countries such as the USA)

(continued)

Table 10.1 (continued)

		Commentary
	Anesthetic over-the-counter products (prescription mimics)	9.6 % lidocaine spray is available in many countries including the USA, called "Premjact" (and many other excellent brands), and it has been available over the counter for almost 25 years and is one of the best rated (still needs formal research). There are also benzocaine (e.g., 5–7.5 %), for example, creams and sprays. A cream or spray that is odorless and alcohol free is desired because it is not as irritating and damaging to the skin
	SSRI/dapoxetine CAM or antidepressant dietary supplement mimics	St. John's wort, 5-HTP, and perhaps SAM-e should be tested for their impact on sexual function and PE. All of these impact depression by potentially increasing serotonin, so they would be ideal testing candidates for PE
X.	Urinary tract infections (UTI) Lifestyle and CAM interventions	
	Lifestyle	Consuming dietary products with probiotics as well as maintaining a heart-healthy lifestyle could reduce risk. For example, obesity increases risk of UTI in men and women
	Cranberry juice/supplements	Recent meta-analysis was not favorable for prevention of recurrent UTI and long-term compliance with juice and excessive calories and compliance are always an issue from this source. Cranberry supplements with concentrated PACs (36 mg/day at least for future studies and current products based on meta-analysis), especially PAC-A, have as much efficacy as cranberry juice thus far and have little to no calories and do not appear to create resistance. Does not work as well as antibiotics thus far, but excessive resistance to prophylactic antibiotic use over several months to a year is a big problem. Cranberry supplements should report oxalate content (high in some brands) for better transparency for high-risk stone formers
	Probiotics	*Lactobacillus* strains have some moderate evidence, but this needs to mature. Safety has been good, but consistency of impact has not thus far

conventional treatment, from vitamin E alternatives to NO producers. Over-the-counter creams and anesthetics are an option for some men with premature ejaculation as well as several SSRI-like CAM mimics, which need more research. UTIs apart from cranberry supplements are being inundated by a variety of probiotics claiming success, but few can be recommended right now with good confidence. In the meantime, impacts of lifestyle changes on most of these urologic conditions are arguably profound enough to garner a Nobel Prize if they were truly appreciated. It is time to update these important lifestyle findings in various clinical guidelines for these specific urologic conditions.

Clinicians should constantly challenge students to think about a simplistic project in CAM that could change a treatment paradigm. For example, at the last AUA meeting, I discussed the potential of a lifestyle program for weight loss in patients with BPH and elevated PSA, to determine if this could reduce PSA sufficiently to help facilitate the decision on whether or not to biopsy for some patients. I could see and feel the excitement of this resident during our discussion, and in turn it reminded me of why it made perfect sense decades ago to work in this discipline full time. These are indeed exciting times for CAM and urology.

References

1. McGrother CW, Donaldson MM, Thompson J, Wag A, Tincello DG, Manktelow BN. Etiology of overactive bladder: a diet and lifestyle model for diabetes and obesity in older women. Neurourol Urodyn. 2012;31:487–95.
2. Chancellor MB, Oefelein MG, Vasavada S. Obesity is associated with a more severe overactive bladder disease state that is effectively treated with once-daily administration of trospium chloride extended release. Neurourol Urodyn. 2010;29:551–4.

3. Peters KM, Macdiarmid SA, Wooldridge LS, Leong FC, Shobeiri SA, Rovner ES, et al. Randomized trial of percutaneous tibial nerve stimulation versus extended-release tolterodine: results from the overactive bladder innovative trial. J Urol. 2009;182:1055–61.
4. Vecchioli-Scaldazza C, Morosetti C, Berouz A, Giannubilo W, Ferrara V. Solifenacin succinate versus percutaneous tibial nerve stimulation in women with overactive bladder syndrome: results of a randomized controlled crossover study. Gynecol Obstet Invest. 2013;75:230–4.
5. Burton C, Saija A, Latthe PM. Effectiveness of percutaneous posterior tibial nerve stimulation for overactive bladder: a systematic review and meta-analysis. Neurourol Urodyn. 2012;31:1206–16.
6. Wing RR, West DS, Grady D, Creasman JM, Richter HE, Myers D, Program to Reduce Incontinence by Diet and Exercise Group, et al. Effect of weight loss on urinary incontinence in overweight and obese women: results at 12 and 18 months. J Urol. 2010;184:1005–10.
7. Park SW, Kim TN, Nam JK, Ha HK, Shin DG, Lee W, et al. Recovery of overall exercise ability, quality of life, and continence after 12-week combined exercise intervention in elderly patients who underwent radical prostatectomy: a randomized controlled study. Urology. 2012;80:299–305.
8. Thomas RJ, Holm M, Williams M, Bowman E, Bellamy P, Andreyev J, et al. Lifestyle factors correlate with the risk of late pelvic symptoms after prostatic radiotherapy. Clin Oncol (R Coll Radiol). 2013;25:246–51.
9. Bower WF, Diao M. Acupuncture as a treatment for nocturnal enuresis. Auton Neurosci. 2010;157:63–7.
10. Bower WF, Diao M, Tang JL, Yeung CK. Acupuncture for nocturnal enuresis in children: a systematic review and exploration of rationale. Neurourol Urodyn. 2005;24:267–72.
11. Guven A, Giramonti K, Kogan BA. The effect of obesity on treatment efficacy in children with nocturnal enuresis and voiding dysfunction. J Urol. 2007;178: 1458–62.
12. Schaeffer AJ, Feng Z, Trock BJ, Mathews RI, Neu AM, Gearhart JP, et al. Medical comorbidities associated with pediatric kidney stone disease. Urology. 2011;77:195–9.
13. Kokorowski PJ, Routh JC, Hubert KC, Graham DA, Nelson CP. Association of urolithiasis with systemic conditions among pediatric patients at children's hospitals. J Urol. 2012;188(4 Suppl):1618–22.
14. Salo J, Uhari M, Helminen M, Korppi M, Nieminen T, Pokka T, et al. Cranberry juice for the prevention of recurrences of urinary tract infections in children: a randomized placebo-controlled trial. Clin Infect Dis. 2012;54:340–6.
15. Afshar K, Stothers L, Scott H, MacNelly AE. Cranberry juice for the prevention of pediatric urinary tract infection: a randomized controlled trial. J Urol. 2012;188(4 Suppl):1584–7.
16. Jepson RG, Williams G, Craig JC. Cranberries for preventing urinary tract infections. Cochrane Database Syst Rev. 2012;10, CD001321.
17. Moyad MA. Promoting wellness for prostate cancer. 4th ed. Ann Arbor, MI: Spry; 2013.
18. Terris MK, Issa MM, Tacker JR. Dietary supplementation with cranberry concentrate tablets may increase the risk of nephrolithiasis. Urology. 2001;57:26–9.
19. Yang SS, Chiang IN, Lin CD, Chang SJ. Advances in non-surgical treatments for urinary tract infections in children. World J Urol. 2012;30:69–75.
20. Lee SJ, Shim YH, Cho SJ, Lee JW. Probiotics prophylaxis in children with persistent primary vesicoureteral reflux. Pediatr Nephrol. 2007;22:1315–20.
21. Hempel S, Newberry SJ, Maher AR, Wang Z, Miles JN, Shanman R, et al. Antibiotics for the prevention and treatment of antibiotic-associated diarrhea: a systematic review and meta-analysis. JAMA. 2012;307:1959–69.
22. Conway PH, Cnaan A, Zaoutis T, Henry BV, Grundmeier RW, Keren R. Recurrent urinary tract infections in children: risk factors and association with prophylactic antimicrobials. JAMA. 2007;298:179–86.
23. Paulis G, Brancato T, D'Ascenzo R, De Giorgio G, Nupieri P, Orsolini G, et al. Efficacy of vitamin E in the conservative treatment of Peyronie's disease: legend or reality? A controlled study of 70 cases. Andrology. 2013;1:120–8.
24. Hatzimouratidis K, Eardley I, Giuliano F, Hatzichriststou D, Moncada I, Salonia A, et al. EAU guidelines on penile curvature. Eur Urol. 2012;62: 543–52.
25. Lippman SM, Klein EA, Goodman PJ, Lucia MS, Thompson IM, Ford LG, et al. Effect of selenium and vitamin E on risk of prostate cancer and other cancers: the Selenium and Vitamin E Cancer Prevention Trial (SELECT). JAMA. 2009;301:39–51.
26. Klein EA, Thompson Jr IM, Tangen CM, Crowley JJ, Lucia MS, Goodman PJ, et al. Vitamin E and the risk of prostate cancer: the Selenium and Vitamin E cancer prevention trial (SELECT). JAMA. 2011;306:1549–56.
27. Bazzano C, de Angeles S, Kleist G, Macedo N. Allergic contact dermatitis from topical vitamins A and E. Contact Dermatitis. 1996;35:261–2.
28. Kosari P, Allkhan A, Sockolov M, Feldman SR. Vitamin E and allergic contact dermatitis. Dermatitis. 2010;21:148–53.
29. Biagotti G, Cavallini G. Acetyl-L-carnitine vs. tamoxifen in the oral therapy of Peyronie's disease: a preliminary report. BJU Int. 2001;88:63–7.
30. Cavallini G, Biagiotti G, Koverech A, Vitali G. Oral propionyl-L-carnitine and intraplaque verapamil in the therapy of advanced and resistant Peyronie's disease. BJU Int. 2002;89:895–900.
31. Safarinejad MR, Hosseini SY, Kolahi AA. Comparison of vitamin E and propionyl-L-carnitine, separately or in combination, in patients with early chronic Peyronie's disease: a double-blind, placebo controlled, randomized study. J Urol. 2007;178:1398–403.

32. Safarinejad MR. Safety and efficacy of coenzyme Q10 supplementation in early chronic Peyronie's disease: a double-blind, placebo-controlled randomized study. Int J Impot Res. 2010;22:298–309.
33. Wyman M, Leonard M, Morledge T. Coenzyme Q10: a therapy for hypertension and statin-induced myalgia? Cleve Clin J Med. 2010;77:435–42.
34. Safarinejad MR. Efficacy and safety of omega-3 for treatment of early-stage Peyronie's disease: a prospective, randomized, double-blind placebo-controlled study. J Sex Med. 2009;6:1743–54.
35. Abern MR, Larsen S, Levine LA. Combination of penile traction, intralesional verapamil, and oral therapies for Peyronie's disease. J Sex Med. 2012;9: 288–95.
36. Valente EG, Vernet D, Ferrini MG, Qian A, Rajfer J, Gonzalez-Cadavid NF. L-arginine and phosphodiesterase (PDE) inhibitors counteract fibrosis in the Peyronie's fibrotic plaque and related fibroblast cultures. Nitric Oxide. 2003;9:229–44.
37. Cіociola F, Colpi GM. Peyronie's disease: a "triple oxygenant therapy". Arch Ital Urol Androl. 2013;85: 36–40.
38. Fitch 3rd WP, Easterling WJ, Talbert RL, Bordovsky MJ, Mosier M. Topical verapamil HCl, topical trifluoperazine, and topical magnesium sulfate for the treatment of Peyronie's disease-a placebo-controlled pilot study. J Sex Med. 2007;4:477–84.
39. Choi HK, Jung GW, Moon KH, Xin ZC, Choi YD, Lee WH, et al. Clinical study of SS-cream in patients with lifelong premature ejaculation. Urology. 2000;55:257–61.
40. Choi HK, Xin ZC, Choi YD, Lee WH, Mah SY, Kim DK. Safety and efficacy study with various doses of SS-cream in patients with premature ejaculation in a double-blind, randomized, placebo controlled clinical study. Int J Impot Res. 1999;11:261–4.
41. Moyad MA. Dr. Moyad's guide to male sexual health. Ann Arbor, MI: Spry; 2012.
42. Thomas CA, Tyagi S, Yoshimura N, Chancellor MB, Tyagi P. Effect of hyperforin-enriched extract on pro-ejaculatory effect of 8-hydroxy-2-(di-N-propylamino) tetralin in anesthetized rats. Urology. 2007;70:813–6.
43. Nahas R, Sheikh O. Complementary and alternative medicine for the treatment of major depressive disorder. Can Fam Physician. 2011;57:659–63.
44. Birdsall TC. 5-hydroxytryptophan: a clinically-effective serotonin precursor. Altern Med Rev. 1998; 3:271–80.
45. Iovieno N, Dalton ED, Fava M, Mischoulon D. Second-tier natural antidepressants: review and critique. J Affect Disord. 2011;130:343–57.
46. Turner EH, Loftis JM, Blackwell AD. Serotonin a la carte: supplementation with the serotonin precursor 5-hydroxytrptophan. Pharmacol Ther. 2006;109: 325–38.
47. McMahon CG. Dapoxetine: a new option in the medical management of premature ejaculation. Ther Adv Urol. 2012;4:233–51.
48. McMahon CG. Dapoxetine for premature ejaculation. Expert Opin Pharmacother. 2010;11:1741–52.
49. Dording CM, Mischoulon D, Shyu I, Alpert JE, Papakostas GI. SAMe and sexual functioning. Eur Psychiatry. 2012;27:451–545.
50. Burton TD, Liday C. The comparison of combination SSRI and PDE-5 inhibitor therapy to SSRI monotherapy in men with premature ejaculation. Ann Pharmacother. 2011;45:1000–4.
51. Choi HK, Seong DH, Rha KH. Clinical efficacy of Korean red ginseng for erectile dysfunction. Int J Impot Res. 1995;7:181–6.
52. Choi YD, Park CW, Jang J, Kim SH, Jeon HY, Kim WG, et al. Effects of Korean ginseng berry extract on sexual function in men with erectile dysfunction: a multicenter, placebo-controlled, double-blind clinical study. Int J Impot Res. 2013;25:45–50.
53. Sunay D, Sunay M, Aydogmus Y, Bagbanci S, Arsian J, Karabulut A, et al. Acupuncture versus paroxetine for the treatment of premature ejaculation: a randomized, placebo-controlled clinical trial. Eur Urol. 2011;59:765–71.
54. Bonetta A, Di Pierro FD. Enter-coated, highly standardized cranberry extract reduces risk of UTIs and urinary symptoms during radiotherapy for prostate carcinoma. Cancer Manag Res. 2012;4:281–6.
55. Kontiokari T, Laitinen J, Jarvi L, Pokka T, Sundqvist K, Uhari M. Dietary factors protecting women from urinary tract infection. Am J Clin Nutr. 2003;77: 600–4.
56. Grin PM, Kowalewska PM, Alhazzan W, Fox-Robichaud AE. Lactobacillus for preventing recurrent urinary tract infections in women: meta-analysis. Can J Urol. 2013;20:6607–14.
57. Saliba W, Barnett-Griness O, Rennert G. The association between obesity and urinary tract infection. Eur J Intern Med. 2013;24:127–31.
58. Dasgupta P, Chandiramani V, Parkinson MC, Beckett A, Fowler CJ. Treating the human bladder with capsaicin: is it safe? Eur Urol. 1998;33:28–31.
59. De Ridder D, Chandiramani V, Dasgupta P, Van Poppel H, Baert L, Fowler CJ. Intravesical capsaicin as a treatment for refractory detrusor hyperreflexia: a dual center study with long-term follow-up. J Urol. 1997;158:2087–92.
60. de Seze M, Wiart L, Ferriere J, de Seze MP, Joseph P, Barat M. Intravesical instillation of capsaicin in urology: a review of the literature. Eur Urol. 1999;36: 267–77.

Index

M.A. Moyad, *Complementary & Alternative Medicine for Prostate and Urologic Health*,
DOI 10.1007/978-1-4614-8492-9, © Springer Science+Business Media New York 2014

MIX
Papier aus verantwortungsvollen Quellen
Paper from responsible sources
FSC® C105338

If you have any concerns about our products,
you can contact us on
ProductSafety@springernature.com

In case Publisher is established outside the EU,
the EU authorized representative is:
Springer Nature Customer Service Center GmbH
Europaplatz 3, 69115 Heidelberg, Germany

Printed by Libri Plureos GmbH
in Hamburg, Germany